Alzheimer Disease

Disease

SOURCEBOOK

Fifth Edition

Injury & Trauma Sourcebook

Learning Disabilities Sourcebook, 3rd Edition

Leukemia Sourcebook

Liver Disorders Sourcebook

Medical Tests Sourcebook, 4th Edition

Men's Health Concerns Sourcebook, 3rd Edition

Mental Health Disorders Sourcebook, 4th Edition

Mental Retardation Sourcebook

Movement Disorders Sourcebook, 2nd Edition

Multiple Sclerosis Sourcebook

Muscular Dystrophy Sourcebook

Obesity Sourcebook

Osteoporosis Sourcebook

Pain Sourcebook, 3rd Edition

Pediatric Cancer Sourcebook

Physical & Mental Issues in Aging Sourcebook

Podiatry Sourcebook, 2nd Edition

Pregnancy & Birth Sourcebook, 3rd Edition

Prostate & Urological Disorders Sourcebook

Prostate Cancer Sourcebook

Rehabilitation Sourcebook

Respiratory Disorders Sourcebook, 2nd Edition

Sexually Transmitted Diseases Sourcebook, 4th Edition

Sleep Disorders Sourcebook, 3rd Edition

Smoking Concerns Sourcebook

Sports Injuries Sourcebook, 4th Edition

Stress-Related Disorders Sourcebook, 2nd Edition

Stroke Sourcebook, 2nd Edition

Surgery Sourcebook, 2nd Edition

Thyroid Disorders Sourcebook

Transplantation Sourcebook

Traveler's Health Sourcebook

Urinary Tract & Kidney Diseases & Disorders Sourcebook, 2nd Edition

Vegetarian Sourcebook

Women's Health Concerns Sourcebook, 3rd Edition

Workplace Health & Safety Sourcebook

Worldwide Health Sourcebook

Teen Health Series

Abuse & Violence Information for Teens

Accident & Safety Information for Teens

Alcohol Information for Teens, 2nd Edition

Allergy Information for Teens

Asthma Information for Teens, 2nd Edition

Body Information for Teens

Cancer Information for Teens, 2nd Edition

Complementary & Alternative Medicine Information for Teens

Diabetes Information for Teens, 2nd Edition

Diet Information for Teens, 3rd Edition

Drug Information for Teens, 3rd Edition

Eating Disorders Information for Teens, 2nd Edition

Fitness Information for Teens, 2nd Edition

Learning Disabilities Information for Teens

Mental Health Information for Teens, 3rd Edition

Pregnancy Information for Teens, 2nd Edition

Sexual Health Information for Teens, 3rd Edition

Skin Health Information for Teens, 2nd Edition

Sleep Information for Teens

Sports Injuries Information for Teens, 2nd Edition

Stress Information for Teens

Suicide Information for Teens, 2nd Edition

Tobacco Information for Teens, 2nd Edition

Health Reference Series

Fifth Edition

Alzheimer Disease
SOURCEBOOK

Basic Consumer Health Information about Alzheimer Disease and Other Forms of Dementia, Including Mild Cognitive Impairment, Corticobasal Degeneration, Dementia with Lewy Bodies, Frontotemporal Dementia, Huntington Disease, Parkinson Disease, and Vascular Dementia

Along with Information about Recent Research on the Diagnosis and Prevention of Alzheimer Disease and Genetic Testing, Tips for Maintaining Cognitive Functioning, Strategies for Long-Term Planning, Advice for Caregivers, a Glossary of Related Terms, and Directories of Resources for Additional Help and Information

Edited by
Amy L. Sutton

Omnigraphics

P.O. Box 31-1640, Detroit, MI 48231

Bibliographic Note

Because this page cannot legibly accommodate all the copyright notices, the Bibliographic Note portion of the Preface constitutes an extension of the copyright notice.

Edited by Amy L. Sutton

Health Reference Series

Karen Bellenir, *Managing Editor*
David A. Cooke, MD, FACP, *Medical Consultant*
Elizabeth Collins, *Research and Permissions Coordinator*
Cherry Edwards, *Permissions Assistant*
EdIndex, Services for Publishers, *Indexers*

* * *

Omnigraphics, Inc.

Matthew P. Barbour, *Senior Vice President*
Kevin M. Hayes, *Operations Manager*

* * *

Peter E. Ruffner, *Publisher*

Copyright © 2011 Omnigraphics, Inc.

ISBN 978-0-7808-1150-8

Library of Congress Cataloging-in-Publication Data

Alzheimer disease sourcebook : basic consumer health information about.../ edited by Amy L. Sutton. -- 5th ed.
  p. cm. -- (Health reference series)
  Includes bibliographical references.
  Summary: "Provides basic consumer health information about symptoms, diagnosis, and treatment of Alzheimer disease and other dementias, along with tips for coping with memory loss and related complications and advice for caregivers. Includes index, glossary of related terms and directory of resources"--Provided by publisher.
  ISBN 978-0-7808-1150-8 (hardcover : alk. paper) 1. Alzheimer's disease--Popular works. 2. Dementia--Popular works. I. Sutton, Amy L. II. Title. III. Series.

  RC523.2.A45 2011
  616.8'31--dc23

                                          2011024979

SEP 03 2012

∞

This book is printed on acid-free paper meeting the ANSI Z39.48 Standard. The infinity symbol that appears above indicates that the paper in this book meets that standard.

R
616.831
A478s

Printed in the United States

Table of Contents

Visit www.healthreferenceseries.com to view *A Contents Guide to the Health Reference Series*, a listing of more than 15,000 topics and the volumes in which they are covered.

Part III: Other Dementia Disorders

Part V: Living with AD and Dementias

Part VI: Caregiver Concerns

Part VII: Additional Help and Information

Preface

About This Book

More than five million Americans experience the progressive, incurable, fatal brain disorder known as Alzheimer disease (AD). AD, which accounts for between 50% and 80% of all cases of dementia, destroys brain cells, causes memory loss and confusion, and worsens over time until patients eventually lose the ability to work, walk, and communicate. Each year, Americans spend $172 billion caring for people with AD. In addition, 10.9 million unpaid caregivers—mostly family members and loved ones—offer assistance to AD patients.

Alzheimer Disease Sourcebook, Fifth Edition provides updated information about causes, symptoms, and stages of AD and other forms of dementia, including mild cognitive impairment, corticobasal degeneration, dementia with Lewy bodies, frontotemporal dementia, Huntington disease, Parkinson disease, and dementia caused by infections. It discusses the structure of the brain, how it changes with age, and the cognitive decline and degeneration that occur in dementia. Facts about genetic testing, cognitive and behavioral symptoms, AD clinical trials, and recent research efforts are also included, along with information about legal, financial, and medical planning and coping strategies for caregivers. The book concludes with a glossary of related terms and directories of resources.

How to Use This Book

This book is divided into parts and chapters. Parts focus on broad areas of interest. Chapters are devoted to single topics within a part.

Part I: Facts about the Brain and Cognitive Decline provides information about healthy brain function and examines changes in cognitive
function and memory that occur during the typical aging process. Facts
about the symptoms, causes, risk factors, and prevalence of dementia—
a brain disorder that significantly impairs intellectual functions—are
also included.

*Part II: Alzheimer Disease (AD): The Most Common Type of Demen-
tia* discusses AD, an irreversible and progressive brain disease and
identifies the signs, symptoms, and diagnostic stages of this disorder,
which affects more than five million Americans. Information about the
role that genetics, brain injuries, weight, and substance abuse play
in the development of AD is also presented, along with facts about
younger-onset AD, a form of the disease that affects people under the
age of 65.

Part III: Other Dementia Disorders identifies types, signs, and symptoms of dementia other than AD, including mild cognitive impairment,
corticobasal degeneration, dementia with Lewy bodies, frontotemporal dementia, Huntington disease, Parkinson disease, and vascular
dementia.

*Part IV: Recognizing, Diagnosing, and Treating Symptoms of AD and
Dementias* explains neurocognitive and imaging tools used to assess
and diagnose dementia, such as positron emission tomography, single
photon emission computed tomography, magnetic resonance imaging,
and biomarker testing. Interventions used to manage AD and other
dementias, such as medications for cognitive and behavioral changes,
are identified, and information about participating in AD clinical trials
and studies is included. The part concludes with an explanation of
recent developments in AD and dementia research.

Part V: Living with AD and Dementias describes strategies for maintaining health and wellness after a dementia diagnosis. Patients and
caregivers will find information about nutrition, exercise, and dental
care for dementia patients, tips on telling someone about the diagnosis,
strategies for slowing the rate of cognitive decline, and advice on pain,
sleep problems, and sexuality in people with dementia. Information
about Medicare and financial, legal, and health care planning is also
included.

Part VI: Caregiver Concerns offers advice to those who care for people
with AD or dementia. Strategies for coping with challenging behaviors, communicating, and planning daily activities for someone with

dementia are discussed, along with tips on creating a safe environment at home. Caregivers struggling to control frustration and cope with fatigue will find information about respite, home health, and nursing home care, as well as suggestions on evaluating difficult health decisions near the end of life.

Part VII: Additional Help and Information provides a glossary of terms related to AD and dementia and a directory of organizations that provide health information about AD and dementia. A list of the Alzheimer Disease Resource Centers across the United States is also included.

Bibliographic Note

This volume contains documents and excerpts from publications issued by the following U.S. government agencies: Administration on Aging (AOA); Centers for Medicare and Medicaid Services (CMS); Federal Emergency Management Agency (FEMA); National Cancer Institute (NCI); National Institute of Neurological Disorders and Stroke (NINDS); National Institute on Aging (NIA); National Institute on Alcohol Abuse and Alcoholism (NIAAA); National Institutes of Health (NIH); National Library of Medicine (NLM); U.S. Department of Health and Human Services (HHS); and the U.S. Food and Drug Administration (FDA).

In addition, this volume contains copyrighted documents from the following organizations and individuals: A.D.A.M., Inc.; Alzheimer Society of Canada; Alzheimer's Association; Alzheimer's Caregiver Support Online/State of Florida Department of Elder Affairs/University of Florida Center for Telehealth and Healthcare Communications; Alzheimer's Foundation of America; American Association for Clinical Chemistry; American Geriatrics Society; American Heart Association; Better Hearing Institute; Caring, Inc.; Center for Gerontology at Virginia Polytechnic Institute and State University; Family Caregiver Alliance; Fisher Center for Alzheimer's Research Foundation; Lewy Body Dementia Association; National Down Syndrome Society; National Stroke Association; Northwestern University; Eric Pfeiffer; Richard E. Powers; Project Inform; Psych Central; Remedy Health Media; Society of Nuclear Medicine; and the Suncoast Alzheimer's Gerontology Center at the University of South Florida College of Medicine.

Full citation information is provided on the first page of each chapter or section. Every effort has been made to secure all necessary rights to reprint the copyrighted material. If any omissions have been made, please contact Omnigraphics to make corrections for future editions.

Acknowledgements

Thanks go to the many organizations, agencies, and individuals who have contributed materials for this *Sourcebook* and to medical consultant Dr. David Cooke and prepress service provider WhimsyInk. Special thanks go to managing editor Karen Bellenir and research and permissions coordinator Liz Collins for their help and support.

About the Health Reference Series

The *Health Reference Series* is designed to provide basic medical information for patients, families, caregivers, and the general public. Each volume takes a particular topic and provides comprehensive coverage. This is especially important for people who may be dealing with a newly diagnosed disease or a chronic disorder in themselves or in a family member. People looking for preventive guidance, information about disease warning signs, medical statistics, and risk factors for health problems will also find answers to their questions in the *Health Reference Series*. The *Series*, however, is not intended to serve as a tool for diagnosing illness, in prescribing treatments, or as a substitute for the physician/patient relationship. All people concerned about medical symptoms or the possibility of disease are encouraged to seek professional care from an appropriate health care provider.

A Note about Spelling and Style

Health Reference Series editors use *Stedman's Medical Dictionary* as an authority for questions related to the spelling of medical terms and the *Chicago Manual of Style* for questions related to grammatical structures, punctuation, and other editorial concerns. Consistent adherence is not always possible, however, because the individual volumes within the *Series* include many documents from a wide variety of different producers and copyright holders, and the editor's primary goal is to present material from each source as accurately as is possible following the terms specified by each document's producer. This sometimes means that information in different chapters or sections may follow other guidelines and alternate spelling authorities. For example, occasionally a copyright holder may require that eponymous terms be shown in possessive forms (Crohn's disease *vs.* Crohn disease) or that British spelling norms be retained (leukaemia *vs.* leukemia).

Locating Information within the Health Reference Series

The *Health Reference Series* contains a wealth of information about a wide variety of medical topics. Ensuring easy access to all the fact sheets, research reports, in-depth discussions, and other material contained within the individual books of the *Series* remains one of our highest priorities. As the *Series* continues to grow in size and scope, however, locating the precise information needed by a reader may become more challenging.

A Contents Guide to the Health Reference Series was developed to direct readers to the specific volumes that address their concerns. It presents an extensive list of diseases, treatments, and other topics of general interest compiled from the Tables of Contents and major index headings. To access *A Contents Guide to the Health Reference Series*, visit www.healthreferenceseries.com.

Medical Consultant

Medical consultation services are provided to the *Health Reference Series* editors by David A. Cooke, MD, FACP. Dr. Cooke is a graduate of Brandeis University, and he received his M.D. degree from the University of Michigan. He completed residency training at the University of Wisconsin Hospital and Clinics. He is board-certified in Internal Medicine. Dr. Cooke currently works as part of the University of Michigan Health System and practices in Ann Arbor, MI. In his free time, he enjoys writing, science fiction, and spending time with his family.

Our Advisory Board

We would like to thank the following board members for providing guidance to the development of this *Series*:

- Dr. Lynda Baker, Associate Professor of Library and Information Science, Wayne State University, Detroit, MI

- Nancy Bulgarelli, William Beaumont Hospital Library, Royal Oak, MI

- Karen Imarisio, Bloomfield Township Public Library, Bloomfield Township, MI

- Karen Morgan, Mardigian Library, University of Michigan-Dearborn, Dearborn, MI

- Rosemary Orlando, St. Clair Shores Public Library, St. Clair Shores, MI

Health Reference Series *Update Policy*

The inaugural book in the *Health Reference Series* was the first edition of *Cancer Sourcebook* published in 1989. Since then, the *Series* has been enthusiastically received by librarians and in the medical community. In order to maintain the standard of providing high-quality health information for the layperson the editorial staff at Omnigraphics felt it was necessary to implement a policy of updating volumes when warranted.

Medical researchers have been making tremendous strides, and it is the purpose of the *Health Reference Series* to stay current with the most recent advances. Each decision to update a volume is made on an individual basis. Some of the considerations include how much new information is available and the feedback we receive from people who use the books. If there is a topic you would like to see added to the update list, or an area of medical concern you feel has not been adequately addressed, please write to:

Editor
Health Reference Series
Omnigraphics, Inc.
P.O. Box 31-1640
Detroit, MI 48231
E-mail: editorial@omnigraphics.com

Part One

Facts about the Brain and Cognitive Decline

Chapter 1

The Basics of a Healthy Brain

"Never have I loved my husband of 41 years more than I do today. . . . Though he may not know I'm his wife, he does know that my presence means his favorite foods and drinks are near at hand. . . . I wonder why I can sit daily by his side as I play tapes, relate bits and pieces of news, hold his hand, tell him I love him. Yet I am content when I am with him, though I grieve for the loss of his smile, the sound of my name on his lips."

This excerpt from *Lessons Learned: Shared Experiences in Coping,* by participants of the Duke University Alzheimer Support Groups, gives a glimpse into what a person with Alzheimer disease (AD) and a family caregiver might experience as the disease progresses. The gradual slipping away of mind and memory is frightening and frustrating, both for the person with the disease and for family and friends, and can elicit strong feelings of love, grief, anger, and exhaustion.

AD is an irreversible, progressive brain disease that slowly destroys memory and thinking skills, eventually even the ability to carry out the simplest tasks. In most people with AD, symptoms first appear after age 60. AD is caused by a disease that affects the brain. In the absence of disease, the human brain often can function well into the 10th decade of life.

Excerpted from "Alzheimer's Disease: Unraveling the Mystery," by the National Institute on Aging (NIA, www.nia.nih.gov), part of the National Institutes of Health, September 2008.

Not so long ago, we were not able to do much for people with AD. Today, that situation is changing. Thousands of scientists, voluntary organizations, and health care professionals are studying AD so that they can find ways to manage, treat, and one day prevent this terrible disease.

AD: A Growing National Problem

For many older adults and their families, AD stands in the way of the "Golden Years." It also presents a major problem for our health care system and society as a whole. AD is the most common cause of dementia among older people. Recent estimates of how many people in the United States currently have AD differ, with numbers ranging from 2.4 million to 4.5 million, depending on how AD is measured. But scientists agree that unless the disease can be effectively treated or prevented, the numbers will increase significantly if current population trends continue.

Our aging society makes AD an especially critical issue. A 2005 Census Bureau report on aging in the United States notes that the population age 65 and older is expected to double in size to about 72 million people within the next 25 years. Moreover, the 85 and older age group is now the fastest growing segment of the population. This is all the more important for a neurodegenerative disease like AD because the number of people with the disease doubles for every 5-year age interval beyond age 65.

AD not only affects the people with the disease, of course. The number of AD caregivers—and their needs—can be expected to rise rapidly as the population ages and as the number of people with AD grows. During their years of AD caregiving, spouses, relatives, and friends experience great emotional, physical, and financial challenges. As the disease runs its course and the abilities of people with AD steadily decline, family members face difficult, and often costly, decisions about the long-term care of their loved ones.

The growing number of people with AD and the costs associated with the disease also put a heavy economic burden on society. The national direct and indirect costs of caring for people with AD are estimated to be more than $100 billion a year. A 2004 study provided an equally sobering picture of the impact of AD. It is estimated that if current AD trends continue, total federal Medicare spending to treat beneficiaries with the disease will increase from $62 billion in 2000 to $189 billion in 2015.

For these reasons, AD is an urgent research priority. We need to find ways to manage and treat AD because of its broad-reaching and devastating impact. We now know that the disease process begins many years, perhaps even decades, before symptoms emerge. Discovering ways to identify AD in the earliest stages and halt or slow its progress will benefit individuals, families, and the nation as a whole.

The Healthy Brain

To understand AD, it is important to know a bit about the brain. This part of the text gives an inside view of the normal brain, how it works, and what happens during aging.

The brain is a remarkable organ. Seemingly without effort, it allows us to carry out every element of our daily lives. It manages many body functions, such as breathing, blood circulation, and digestion, without our knowledge or direction. It also directs all the functions we carry out consciously. We can speak, hear, see, move, remember, feel emotions, and make decisions because of the complicated mix of chemical and electrical processes that take place in our brains.

The brain is made of nerve cells and several other cell types. Nerve cells also are called neurons. The neurons of all animals function in basically the same way, even though animals can be very different from each other. Neurons survive and function with the help and support of glial cells, the other main type of cell in the brain. Glial cells hold neurons in place, provide them with nutrients, rid the brain of damaged cells and other cellular debris, and provide insulation to neurons in the brain and spinal cord. In fact, the brain has many more glial cells than neurons—some scientists estimate even 10 times as many.

Another essential feature of the brain is its enormous network of blood vessels. Even though the brain is only about 2 percent of the body's weight, it receives 20 percent of the body's blood supply. Billions of tiny blood vessels, or capillaries, carry oxygen, glucose (the brain's principal source of energy), nutrients, and hormones to brain cells so they can do their work. Capillaries also carry away waste products.

Inside the Human Brain

The brain has many parts, each of which is responsible for particular functions. The following section describes a few key structures and what they do.

The Main Players

Two cerebral hemispheres account for 85 percent of the brain's weight. The billions of neurons in the two hemispheres are connected by thick

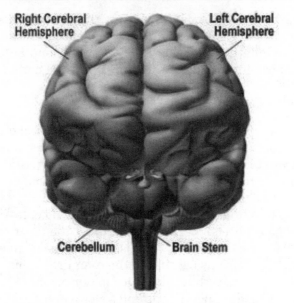

Figure 1.1. A front view of the brain.

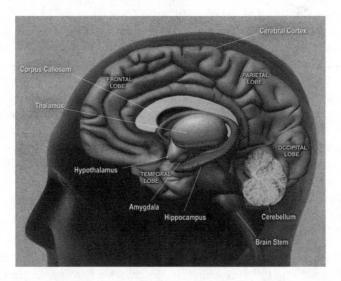

Figure 1.2. A side view of the brain. This illustration shows a three-dimensional side view of one of two cerebral hemispheres of the brain. To help visualize this, imagine looking at the cut side of an avocado sliced long ways in half, with the pit still in the fruit. In this illustration, the pit is several key structures that lie deep within the brain (the hypothalamus, amygdala, and hippocampus) and the brain stem.

bundles of nerve cell fibers called the corpus callosum. Scientists now think that the two hemispheres differ not so much in what they do (the "logical versus artistic" notion), but in how they process information. The left hemisphere appears to focus on details (such as recognizing a particular face in a crowd). The right hemisphere focuses on broad background (such as understanding the relative position of objects in a space). The cerebral hemispheres have an outer layer called the cerebral cortex. This is where the brain processes sensory information received from the outside world, controls voluntary movement, and regulates cognitive functions, such as thinking, learning, speaking, remembering, and making decisions. The hemispheres have four lobes, each of which has different roles:

- The frontal lobe, which is in the front of the brain, controls executive function activities like thinking, organizing, planning, and problem solving, as well as memory, attention, and movement.

- The parietal lobe, which sits behind the frontal lobe, deals with the perception and integration of stimuli from the senses.

- The occipital lobe, which is at the back of the brain, is concerned with vision.

- The temporal lobe, which runs along the side of the brain under the frontal and parietal lobes, deals with the senses of smell, taste, and sound, and the formation and storage of memories.

The cerebellum sits above the brain stem and beneath the occipital lobe. It takes up a little more than 10 percent of the brain. This part of the brain plays roles in balance and coordination. The cerebellum has two hemispheres, which receive information from the eyes, ears, and muscles and joints about the body's movements and position. Once the cerebellum processes that information, it sends instructions to the body through the rest of the brain and spinal cord. The cerebellum's work allows us to move smoothly, maintain our balance, and turn around without even thinking about it. It also is involved with motor learning and remembering how to do things like drive a car or write your name.

The brain stem sits at the base of the brain. It connects the spinal cord with the rest of the brain. Even though it is the smallest of the three main players, its functions are crucial to survival. The brain stem controls the functions that happen automatically to keep us alive—our heart rate, blood pressure, and breathing. It also relays information between the brain and the spinal cord, which then sends out messages to the muscles, skin, and other organs. Sleep and dreaming are also controlled by the brain stem.

Other Crucial Parts

Several other essential parts of the brain lie deep inside the cerebral hemispheres in a network of structures called the limbic system. The limbic system links the brain stem with the higher reasoning elements of the cerebral cortex. It plays a key role in developing and carrying out instinctive behaviors and emotions and also is important in perceiving smells and linking them with memory, emotion, and instinctive behaviors. The limbic system includes the following:

- The amygdala is an almond-shaped structure involved in processing and remembering strong emotions such as fear. It is located in the temporal lobe just in front of the hippocampus.

- The hippocampus is buried in the temporal lobe and is important for learning and short-term memory. This part of the brain is thought to be the site where short-term memories are converted into long-term memories for storage in other brain areas.

- The thalamus, located at the top of the brain stem, receives sensory and limbic information, processes it, and then sends it to the cerebral cortex.

- The hypothalamus, a structure under the thalamus, monitors activities such as body temperature and food intake. It issues instructions to correct any imbalances. The hypothalamus also controls the body's internal clock.

The Brain in Action

Sophisticated brain-imaging techniques allow scientists to monitor brain function in living people and to see how various parts of the brain are used for different kinds of tasks. This is opening up worlds of knowledge about brain function and how it changes with age or disease.

One of these imaging techniques is called positron emission tomography, or PET scanning. Some PET scans measure blood flow and glucose metabolism throughout the brain. During a PET scan, a small amount of a radioactive substance is attached to a compound, such as glucose, and injected into the bloodstream. This tracer substance eventually goes to the brain. When nerve cells in a region of the brain become active, blood flow and glucose metabolism in that region increase. When colored to reflect metabolic activity, increases usually look red and yellow. Shades of blue and black indicate decreased or no activity within a brain region. In essence, a PET scan produces a map of the active brain.

8

Scientists can use PET scans to see what happens in the brain when a person is engaged in a physical or mental activity, at rest, or even while sleeping or dreaming. Certain tracers can track the activity of brain chemicals, for example neurotransmitters such as dopamine and serotonin. Some of these neurotransmitters are changed with age, disease, and drug therapies.

Neurons and Their Jobs

The human brain is made up of billions of neurons. Each has a cell body, an axon, and many dendrites. The cell body contains a nucleus, which controls much of the cell's activities. The cell body also contains other structures, called organelles, that perform specific tasks.

The axon, which is much narrower than the width of a human hair, extends out from the cell body. Axons transmit messages from neuron to neuron. Sometimes, signal transmissions—like those from head to toe—have to travel over very long distances. Axons are covered with an insulating layer called myelin (also called white matter because of its whitish color). Myelin, which is made by a particular kind of glial cell, increases the speed of nerve signal transmissions through the brain.

Dendrites also branch out from the cell body. They receive messages from the axons of other neurons. Each neuron is connected to thousands of other nerve cells through its axon and dendrites.

Groups of neurons in the brain have special jobs. For example, some are involved with thinking, learning, and memory. Others are responsible for receiving information from the sensory organs (such as the eyes and ears) or the skin. Still others communicate with muscles, stimulating them into action.

Several processes all have to work smoothly together for neurons, and the whole organism, to survive and stay healthy. These processes are communication, metabolism, and repair.

Communication

Imagine the many miles of fiber-optic cables that run under our streets. Day and night, millions of televised and telephonic messages flash at incredible speeds, letting people strike deals, give instructions, share a laugh, or learn some news. Miniaturize it, multiply it many-fold, make it much more complex, and you have the brain. Neurons are the great communicators, always in touch with their neighbors.

Neurons communicate with each other through their axons and dendrites. When a dendrite receives an incoming signal (electrical or chemical), an action potential, or nerve impulse, can be generated in the cell body. The action potential travels to the end of the axon and once there, the passage of either electrical current or, more typically, the release of chemical messengers, called neurotransmitters, can be triggered. The neurotransmitters are released from the axon terminal and move across a tiny gap, or synapse, to specific receptor sites on the receiving, or postsynaptic, end of dendrites of nearby neurons. A typical neuron has thousands of synaptic connections, mostly on its many dendrites, with other neurons. Cell bodies also have receptor sites for neurotransmitters.

Once the post-synaptic receptors are activated, they open channels through the cell membrane into the receiving nerve cell's interior or start other processes that determine what the receiving nerve cell will do. Some neurotransmitters inhibit nerve cell function (that is, they make it less likely that the nerve cell will send an electrical signal down its axon). Other neurotransmitters stimulate nerve cells, priming the receiving cell to become active or send an electrical signal down the axon to more neurons in the pathway. A neuron receives signals from many other neurons simultaneously, and the sum of a neuron's neurotransmitter inputs at any one instant will determine whether it sends a signal down its axon to activate or inhibit the action of other neighboring neurons.

During any one moment, millions of these signals are speeding through pathways in the brain, allowing the brain to receive and process information, make adjustments, and send out instructions to various parts of the body.

Metabolism

All cells break down chemicals and nutrients to generate energy and form building blocks that make new cellular molecules such as proteins. This process is called metabolism. To maintain metabolism, the brain needs plenty of blood constantly circulating through its billions of capillaries to supply neurons and other brain cells with oxygen and glucose. Without oxygen and glucose, neurons will quickly die.

Repair

Nerve cells are formed during fetal life and for a short time after birth. Unlike most cells, which have a fairly short lifespan, neurons in the brain live a long time. These cells can live for up to 100 years or longer. To stay healthy, living neurons must constantly maintain and repair themselves. In an adult, when neurons die because of disease or injury, they are not usually replaced. Research, however, shows that in a few brain regions, new neurons can be generated, even in the old brain.

Chapter 2

The Changing Brain in Healthy Aging

In the past several decades, investigators have learned much about what happens in the brain when people have a neurodegenerative disease such as Parkinson disease, Alzheimer disease (AD), or other dementias. Their findings also have revealed much about what happens during healthy aging. Researchers are investigating a number of changes related to healthy aging in hopes of learning more about this process so they can fill gaps in our knowledge about the early stages of AD.

As a person gets older, changes occur in all parts of the body, including the brain:

- Certain parts of the brain shrink, especially the prefrontal cortex (an area at the front of the frontal lobe) and the hippocampus. Both areas are important to learning, memory, planning, and other complex mental activities.

- Changes in neurons and neurotransmitters affect communication between neurons. In certain brain regions, communication between neurons can be reduced because white matter (myelin-covered axons) is degraded or lost.

- Changes in the brain's blood vessels occur. Blood flow can be reduced because arteries narrow and less growth of new capillaries occurs.

Excerpted from "Alzheimer's Disease: Unraveling the Mystery," by the National Institute on Aging (NIA, www.nia.nih.gov), part of the National Institutes of Health, September 2008.

- In some people, structures called plaques and tangles develop outside of and inside neurons, respectively, although in much smaller amounts than in AD.

- Damage by free radicals increases (free radicals are a kind of molecule that reacts easily with other molecules).

- Inflammation increases (inflammation is the complex process that occurs when the body responds to an injury, disease, or abnormal situation).

What effects does aging have on mental function in healthy older people? Some people may notice a modest decline in their ability to learn new things and retrieve information, such as remembering names. They may perform worse on complex tasks of attention, learning, and memory than would a younger person. However, if given enough time to perform the task, the scores of healthy people in their 70s and 80s are often similar to those of young adults. In fact, as they age, adults often improve in other cognitive areas, such as vocabulary and other forms of verbal knowledge.

It also appears that additional brain regions can be activated in older adults during cognitive tasks, such as taking a memory test. Researchers do not fully understand why this happens, but one idea is that the brain engages mechanisms to compensate for difficulties that certain regions may be having. For example, the brain may recruit alternate brain networks in order to perform a task. These findings have led many scientists to believe that major declines in mental abilities are not inevitable as people age. Growing evidence of the adaptive (what scientists call "plastic") capabilities of the older brain provide hope that people may be able to do things to sustain good brain function as they age. A variety of interacting factors, such as lifestyle, overall health, environment, and genetics also may play a role.

Another question that scientists are asking is why some people remain cognitively healthy as they get older while others develop cognitive impairment or dementia. The concept of "cognitive reserve" may provide some insights. Cognitive reserve refers to the brain's ability to operate effectively even when some function is disrupted. It also refers to the amount of damage that the brain can sustain before changes in cognition are evident. People vary in the cognitive reserve they have, and this variability may be because of differences in genetics, education, occupation, lifestyle, leisure activities, or other life experiences. These factors could provide a certain amount of tolerance and ability to adapt to change and damage that occurs during aging. At some point, depending on a person's cognitive reserve and unique mix of genetics, environment, and life experiences, the balance may tip in favor of a disease process that will ultimately lead to dementia. For another person, with a different reserve and a different mix of genetics, environment, and life experiences, the balance may result in no apparent decline in cognitive function with age.

Scientists are increasingly interested in the influence of all these factors on brain health, and studies are revealing some clues about actions people can take that may help preserve healthy brain aging. Fortunately, these actions also benefit a person's overall health. They include the following:

- Controlling risk factors for chronic disease, such as heart disease and diabetes (for example, keeping blood cholesterol and blood pressure at healthy levels and maintaining a healthy weight)

- Enjoying regular exercise and physical activity

- Eating a healthy diet that includes plenty of vegetables and fruits

- Engaging in intellectually stimulating activities and maintaining close social ties with family, friends, and community

ACTIVE Study May Provide Clues to Help Older Adults Stay Mentally Sharp

The phrase "use it or lose it" may make you think of your muscles, but scientists who study brain health in older people have found that it may apply to cognitive skills as well. In 2006, scientists funded by NIA and the National Institute of Nursing Research completed a study of cognitive training in older adults. This study, the Advanced Cognitive Training for Independent and Vital Elderly (ACTIVE) study, was the first randomized controlled trial to demonstrate long-lasting, positive effects of brief cognitive training in older adults.

The ACTIVE study included 2,802 healthy adults age 65 and older who were living independently. Participants were randomly assigned to four groups. Three groups took part in up to 10 computer-based training sessions that targeted a specific cognitive ability—memory, reasoning, and speed of processing (in other words, how fast participants could respond to prompts on a computer screen). The fourth group (the control group) received no cognitive training. Sixty percent of those who completed the initial training also took part in 75-minute "booster" sessions 11 months later. These sessions were designed to maintain improvements gained from the initial training.

The investigators tested the participants at the beginning of the study, after the initial training and booster sessions, and once a year for 5 more years. They found that the improvements from the training roughly counteracted the degree of decline in cognitive performance that would be expected over a 7- to 14-year period among older people without dementia:

- Immediately after the initial training, 87 percent of the processing-speed group, 74 percent of the reasoning group, and 26 percent of the memory group showed improvement in the skills taught.

- After 5 years, people in each group performed better on tests in their respective areas of training than did people in the control group. The reasoning and processing-speed groups who received booster training had the greatest benefit.

The researchers also looked at the training's effects on participants' everyday lives. After 5 years, all three groups who received training reported less difficulty than the control group in tasks such as preparing meals, managing money, and doing housework. However, these results were statistically significant for only the group that had the reasoning training.

As they get older, many people worry about their mental skills getting rusty. The ACTIVE study offers hope that cognitive training may be useful because it showed that relatively brief and targeted cognitive exercises can produce lasting improvements in the skills taught. Next steps for researchers are to determine ways to generalize the training benefits beyond the specific skills taught in ACTIVE and to find out whether cognitive training programs could prevent, delay, or diminish the effects of AD.

Chapter 3

Understanding Memory Loss

We've all forgotten a name, where we put our keys, or if we locked the front door. It's normal to forget things once in a while. However, forgetting how to make change, use the telephone, or find your way home may be signs of a more serious memory problem.

Mary's Story

Mary couldn't find her car keys. She looked on the hook just inside the front door. They weren't there. She searched in her purse. No luck. Finally, she found them on her desk. Yesterday, she forgot her neighbor's name. Her memory was playing tricks on her. She was starting to worry about it.

She decided to see her doctor. After a complete check-up, her doctor said that Mary was fine. Her forgetfulness was just a normal part of getting older. The doctor suggested that Mary take a class, play cards with friends, or help out at the local school to sharpen her memory.

Differences between Mild Forgetfulness and More Serious Memory Problems

What is mild forgetfulness?

It is true that some of us get more forgetful as we age. It may take longer to learn new things, remember certain words, or find our

Excerpted from "Understanding Memory Loss: What to Do When You Have Trouble Remembering," by the National Institute on Aging (NIA, www.nia.nih.gov), part of the National Institutes of Health, September 2010.

glasses. These changes are often signs of mild forgetfulness, not serious memory problems.

See your doctor if you're worried about your forgetfulness. Tell him or her about your concerns. Be sure to make a follow-up appointment to check your memory in the next 6 months to a year. If you think you might forget, ask a family member, friend, or the doctor's office to remind you.

What can I do about mild forgetfulness?

You can do many things to help keep your memory sharp and stay alert. Here are some ways to help your memory:

- Learn a new skill.

- Volunteer in your community, at a school, or at your place of worship.

- Spend time with friends and family.

- Use memory tools such as big calendars, to-do lists, and notes to yourself.

- Put your wallet or purse, keys, and glasses in the same place each day.

- Get lots of rest.

- Exercise and eat well.

- Don't drink a lot of alcohol.

- Get help if you feel depressed for weeks at a time.

What is a serious memory problem?

Serious memory problems make it hard to do everyday things. For example, you may find it hard to drive, shop, or even talk with a friend. Signs of serious memory problems may include the following:

- Asking the same questions over and over again

- Getting lost in places you know well

- Not being able to follow directions

- Becoming more confused about time, people, and places

- Not taking care of yourself—eating poorly, not bathing, or being unsafe

What can I do about serious memory problems?

See your doctor if you are having any of the problems in the preceding text. It's important to find out what might be causing a serious memory problem. Once you know the cause, you can get the right treatment.

Serious Memory Problems: Causes and Treatments

Certain medical conditions can cause serious memory problems. These problems should go away once you get treatment. Some medical conditions that may cause memory problems are the following:

- Bad reaction to certain medicines

- Depression

- Not eating enough healthy foods, or too few vitamins and minerals in your body

- Drinking too much alcohol

- Blood clots or tumors in the brain

- Head injury, such as a concussion from a fall or accident

- Thyroid, kidney, or liver problems

These medical conditions are serious. See your doctor for treatment.

Some emotional problems in older people can cause serious memory problems. Feeling sad, lonely, worried, or bored can cause you to be confused and forgetful.

You may need to see a doctor or counselor for treatment. Once you get help, your memory problems should get better.

Being active, spending more time with family and friends, and learning new skills also can help you feel better and improve your memory.

Mild Cognitive Impairment

As some people grow older, they have more memory problems than other people their age. This condition is called mild cognitive impairment, or MCI. People with MCI can take care of themselves and do their normal activities.

MCI memory problems may include the following:

- Losing things often

17

- Forgetting to go to events and appointments
- Having more trouble coming up with words than other people of the same age

Your doctor can do thinking, memory, and language tests to see if you have MCI. He or she also may suggest that you see a specialist for more tests. Because MCI may be an early sign of Alzheimer disease, it's really important to see your doctor or specialist every 6 to 12 months.

At this time, there is no proven treatment for MCI. Your doctor can check to see if you have any changes in your memory or thinking skills over time.

Alzheimer Disease

Alzheimer disease causes serious memory problems. The signs of Alzheimer disease begin slowly and get worse over time. This is because changes in the brain cause large numbers of brain cells to die.

It may look like simple forgetfulness at first, but over time, people with Alzheimer disease have trouble thinking clearly. They find it hard to do everyday things like shopping, driving, and cooking. As the illness gets worse, people with Alzheimer disease may need someone to take care of all their needs at home or in a nursing home. These needs may include feeding, bathing, and dressing.

Taking certain medicines can help a person in the early or middle stages of Alzheimer disease. These medicines can keep symptoms, such as memory loss, from getting worse for a time. The medicines can have side effects and may not work for everyone. Talk with your doctor about side effects or other concerns you may have. Other medicines can help if you are worried, depressed, or having problems sleeping.

Vascular Dementia

Many people have never heard of vascular dementia. Like Alzheimer disease, it is a medical condition that causes serious memory problems. Unlike Alzheimer disease, signs of vascular dementia may appear suddenly. This is because the memory loss and confusion are caused by small strokes or changes in the blood supply to the brain. If the strokes stop, you may get better or stay the same for a long time. If you have more strokes, you may get worse.

You can take steps to lower your chances of having more strokes. These steps include the following:

- Control your high blood pressure.

- Treat your high cholesterol.

- Take care of your diabetes.

- Stop smoking.

Help for Serious Memory Problems

If you are worried about your memory, see your doctor. If your doctor thinks your memory problems are serious, you may need to have a complete health check-up. The doctor will review your medicines and may test your blood and urine. You also may need to take tests that check your memory, problem solving, counting, and language skills.

In addition, the doctor may suggest a brain scan. Pictures from the scan can show normal and problem areas in the brain. Once the doctor finds out what is causing your memory problems, ask about the best treatment for you.

If your family member or friend has a serious memory problem, you can help the person live as normal a life as possible. You can help the person stay active, go places, and keep up everyday routines. You can remind the person of the time of day, where he or she lives, and what is happening at home and in the world. You also can help the person remember to take medicine or visit the doctor.

Some families use the following things to help with memory problems:

- Big calendars to highlight important dates and events

- Lists of the plans for each day

- Notes about safety in the home

- Written directions for using common household items (most people with Alzheimer disease can still read)

Chapter 4

What Is Dementia?

A woman in her early 50s was admitted to a hospital because of increasingly odd behavior. Her family reported that she had been showing memory problems and strong feelings of jealousy. She also had become disoriented at home and was hiding objects. During a doctor's examination, the woman was unable to remember her husband's name, the year, or how long she had been at the hospital. She could read but did not seem to understand what she read, and she stressed the words in an unusual way. She sometimes became agitated and seemed to have hallucinations and irrational fears.

This woman, known as Auguste D., was the first person reported to have the disease now known as Alzheimer disease (AD) after Alois Alzheimer, the German doctor who first described it. After Auguste D. died in 1906, doctors examined her brain and found that it appeared shrunken and contained several unusual features, including strange clumps of protein called plaques and tangled fibers inside the nerve cells. Memory impairments and other symptoms of dementia, which means "deprived of mind," had been described in older adults since ancient times. However, because Auguste D. began to show symptoms at a relatively early age, doctors did not think her disease could be related to what was then called "senile dementia." The word senile is derived from a Latin term that means, roughly, "old age."

Excerpted from "Dementia: Hope Through Research," by the National Institute of Neurological Disorders and Stroke (NINDS, www.ninds.nih.gov), part of the National Institutes of Health, January 21, 2011.

It is now clear that AD is a major cause of dementia in elderly people as well as in relatively young adults. Furthermore, we know that it is only one of many disorders that can lead to dementia. The U.S. Congress Office of Technology Assessment estimates that as many as 6.8 million people in the United States have dementia, and at least 1.8 million of those are severely affected. Studies in some communities have found that almost half of all people age 85 and older have some form of dementia. Although it is common in very elderly individuals, dementia is not a normal part of the aging process. Many people live into their 90s and even 100s without any symptoms of dementia.

Besides senile dementia, other terms often used to describe dementia include senility and organic brain syndrome. Senility and senile dementia are outdated terms that reflect the formerly widespread belief that dementia was a normal part of aging. Organic brain syndrome is a general term that refers to physical disorders (not psychiatric in origin) that impair mental functions.

Research in the last 30 years has led to a greatly improved understanding of what dementia is, who gets it, and how it develops and affects the brain. This work is beginning to pay off with better diagnostic techniques, improved treatments, and even potential ways of preventing these diseases.

Defining Dementia

Dementia is not a specific disease. It is a descriptive term for a collection of symptoms that can be caused by a number of disorders that affect the brain. People with dementia have significantly impaired intellectual functioning that interferes with normal activities and relationships. They also lose their ability to solve problems and maintain emotional control, and they may experience personality changes and behavioral problems such as agitation, delusions, and hallucinations. While memory loss is a common symptom of dementia, memory loss by itself does not mean that a person has dementia. Doctors diagnose dementia only if two or more brain functions—such as memory, language skills, perception, or cognitive skills including reasoning and judgment—are significantly impaired without loss of consciousness.

There are many disorders that can cause dementia. Some, such as AD, lead to a progressive loss of mental functions. But other types of dementia can be halted or reversed with appropriate treatment.

With AD and many other types of dementia, disease processes cause many nerve cells to stop functioning, lose connections with other neurons, and die. In contrast, normal aging does not result in the loss of large numbers of neurons in the brain.

What Are the Different Kinds of Dementia?

Dementing disorders can be classified many different ways. These classification schemes attempt to group disorders that have particular features in common, such as whether they are progressive or what parts of the brain are affected. Some frequently used classifications include the following:

- **Cortical dementia:** Dementia where the brain damage primarily affects the brain's cortex, or outer layer. Cortical dementias tend to cause problems with memory, language, thinking, and social behavior.

- **Subcortical dementia:** Dementia that affects parts of the brain below the cortex. Subcortical dementia tends to cause changes in emotions and movement in addition to problems with memory.

- **Progressive dementia:** Dementia that gets worse over time, gradually interfering with more and more cognitive abilities.

- **Primary dementia:** Dementia such as AD that does not result from any other disease.

- **Secondary dementia:** Dementia that occurs as a result of a physical disease or injury.

Some types of dementia fit into more than one of these classifications. For example, AD is considered both a progressive and a cortical dementia.

Alzheimer disease is the most common cause of dementia in people aged 65 and older. Experts believe that up to 4 million people in the United States are currently living with the disease: One in 10 people over the age of 65 and nearly half of those over 85 have AD. At least 360,000 Americans are diagnosed with AD each year and about 50,000 are reported to die from it.

In most people, symptoms of AD appear after age 60. However, there are some early-onset forms of the disease, usually linked to a specific gene defect, which may appear as early as age 30. AD usually causes a gradual decline in cognitive abilities, usually during a span of 7 to 10 years. Nearly all brain functions, including memory, movement, language, judgment, behavior, and abstract thinking, are eventually affected. AD is characterized by two abnormalities in the brain—amyloid plaques and neurofibrillary tangles. Amyloid plaques, which are found in the tissue between the nerve cells, are unusual clumps of a protein called beta amyloid along with degenerating bits of neurons and other cells.

Neurofibrillary tangles are bundles of twisted filaments found within neurons. These tangles are largely made up of a protein called tau. In healthy neurons, the tau protein helps the functioning of microtubules, which are part of the cell's structural support and deliver substances throughout the nerve cell. However, in AD, tau is changed in a way that causes it to twist into pairs of helical filaments that collect into tangles. When this happens, the microtubules cannot function correctly and they disintegrate. This collapse of the neuron's transport system may impair communication between nerve cells and cause them to die.

Researchers do not know if amyloid plaques and neurofibrillary tangles are harmful or if they are merely side effects of the disease process that damages neurons and leads to the symptoms of AD. They do know that plaques and tangles usually increase in the brain as AD progresses.

In the early stages of AD, patients may experience memory impairment, lapses of judgment, and subtle changes in personality. As the disorder progresses, memory and language problems worsen and patients begin to have difficulty performing activities of daily living, such as balancing a checkbook or remembering to take medications. They also may have visuospatial problems, such as difficulty navigating an unfamiliar route. They may become disoriented about places and times, may suffer delusions (such as the idea that someone is stealing from them or that their spouse is being unfaithful), and may become short-tempered and hostile. During the late stages of the disease, patients begin to lose the ability to control motor functions. They may have difficulty swallowing and lose bowel and bladder control. They eventually lose the ability to recognize family members and to speak. As AD progresses, it begins to affect the person's emotions and behavior. Most people with AD eventually develop symptoms such as aggression, agitation, depression, sleeplessness, or delusions.

On average, patients with AD live for 8 to 10 years after they are diagnosed. However, some people live as long as 20 years. Patients with AD often die of aspiration pneumonia because they lose the ability to swallow late in the course of the disease.

Vascular dementia is the second most common cause of dementia, after AD. It accounts for up to 20 percent of all dementias and is caused by brain damage from cerebrovascular or cardiovascular problems—

usually strokes. It also may result from genetic diseases, endocarditis (infection of a heart valve), or amyloid angiopathy (a process in which amyloid protein builds up in the brain's blood vessels, sometimes causing hemorrhagic or "bleeding" strokes). In many cases, it may coexist with AD. The incidence of vascular dementia increases with advancing age and is similar in men and women.

Symptoms of vascular dementia often begin suddenly, frequently after a stroke. Patients may have a history of high blood pressure, vascular disease, or previous strokes or heart attacks. Vascular dementia may or may not get worse with time, depending on whether the person has additional strokes. In some cases, symptoms may get better with time. When the disease does get worse, it often progresses in a stepwise manner, with sudden changes in ability. Vascular dementia with brain damage to the mid-brain regions, however, may cause a gradual, progressive cognitive impairment that may look much like AD. Unlike people with AD, people with vascular dementia often maintain their personality and normal levels of emotional responsiveness until the later stages of the disease.

People with vascular dementia frequently wander at night and often have other problems commonly found in people who have had a stroke, including depression and incontinence.

There are several types of vascular dementia, which vary slightly in their causes and symptoms. One type, called multi-infarct dementia (MID), is caused by numerous small strokes in the brain. MID typically includes multiple damaged areas, called infarcts, along with extensive lesions in the white matter, or nerve fibers, of the brain.

Because the infarcts in MID affect isolated areas of the brain, the symptoms are often limited to one side of the body or they may affect just one or a few specific functions, such as language. Neurologists call these "local" or "focal" symptoms, as opposed to the "global" symptoms seen in AD, which affect many functions and are not restricted to one side of the body.

Although not all strokes cause dementia, in some cases a single stroke can damage the brain enough to cause dementia. This condition is called single-infarct dementia. Dementia is more common when the stroke takes place on the left side (hemisphere) of the brain and/or when it involves the hippocampus, a brain structure important for memory.

Another type of vascular dementia is called Binswanger disease. This rare form of dementia is characterized by damage to small blood vessels in the white matter of the brain (white matter is found in the inner layers of the brain and contains many nerve fibers coated with a whitish, fatty substance called myelin). Binswanger disease leads to brain lesions, loss of memory, disordered cognition, and mood changes. Patients with this disease often show signs of abnormal blood pressure, stroke, blood abnormalities, disease of the large blood vessels in the neck, and/or disease of the heart valves. Other prominent features include urinary incontinence, difficulty walking, clumsiness, slowness, lack of facial expression, and speech difficulty. These symptoms, which usually begin after the age of 60, are not always present in all patients and may sometimes appear only temporarily. Treatment of Binswanger disease is symptomatic, and may include the use of medications to control high blood pressure, depression, heart arrhythmias, and low blood pressure. The disorder often includes episodes of partial recovery.

Another type of vascular dementia is linked to a rare hereditary disorder called CADASIL, which stands for cerebral autosomal dominant arteriopathy with subcortical infarct and leukoencephalopathy. CADASIL is linked to abnormalities of a specific gene, Notch3, which is located on chromosome 19. This condition causes multi-infarct dementia as well as stroke, migraine with aura, and mood disorders. The first symptoms usually appear in people who are in their twenties, thirties, or forties and affected individuals often die by age 65. Researchers believe most people with CADASIL go undiagnosed, and the actual prevalence of the disease is not yet known.

Other causes of vascular dementia include vasculitis, an inflammation of the blood vessel system; profound hypotension (low blood pressure); and lesions caused by brain hemorrhage. The autoimmune disease lupus erythematosus and the inflammatory disease temporal arteritis can also damage blood vessels in a way that leads to vascular dementia.

Lewy body dementia (LBD) is one of the most common types of progressive dementia. LBD usually occurs sporadically, in people with no known family history of the disease. However, rare familial cases have occasionally been reported.

In LBD, cells die in the brain's cortex, or outer layer, and in a part of the mid-brain called the substantia nigra. Many of the remaining nerve cells in the substantia nigra contain abnormal structures called Lewy bodies that are the hallmark of the disease. Lewy bodies may also appear in the brain's cortex, or outer layer. Lewy bodies contain a protein called alpha-synuclein that has been linked to Parkinson disease and several other disorders. Researchers, who sometimes refer to these disorders collectively as "synucleinopathies," do not yet know why this protein accumulates inside nerve cells in LBD.

The symptoms of LBD overlap with AD in many ways, and may include memory impairment, poor judgment, and confusion. However, LBD typically also includes visual hallucinations, parkinsonian symptoms such as a shuffling gait and flexed posture, and day-to-day fluctuations in the severity of symptoms. Patients with LBD live an average of 7 years after symptoms begin.

There is no cure for LBD, and treatments are aimed at controlling the parkinsonian and psychiatric symptoms of the disorder. Patients sometimes respond dramatically to treatment with antiparkinsonian drugs and/or cholinesterase inhibitors, such as those used for AD. Some studies indicate that neuroleptic drugs, such as clozapine and olanzapine, also can reduce the psychiatric symptoms of this disease. But neuroleptic drugs may cause severe adverse reactions, so other therapies should be tried first and patients using these drugs should be closely monitored.

Lewy bodies are often found in the brains of people with Parkinson disease and AD. These findings suggest that either LBD is related to these other causes of dementia or that the diseases sometimes coexist in the same person.

Frontotemporal dementia (FTD), sometimes called frontal lobe dementia, describes a group of diseases characterized by degeneration of nerve cells—especially those in the frontal and temporal lobes of the brain. Unlike AD, FTD usually does not include formation of amyloid plaques. In many people with FTD, there is an abnormal form of tau protein in the brain, which accumulates into neurofibrillary tangles. This disrupts normal cell activities and may cause the cells to die.

Experts believe FTD accounts for 2 to 10 percent of all cases of dementia. Symptoms of FTD usually appear between the ages of 40 and 65. In many cases, people with FTD have a family history of dementia, suggesting that there is a strong genetic factor in the disease. The duration of FTD varies, with some patients declining rapidly over 2 to 3 years and others showing only minimal changes for many years. People with FTD live with the disease for an average of 5 to 10 years after diagnosis.

Because structures found in the frontal and temporal lobes of the brain control judgment and social behavior, people with FTD often have problems maintaining normal interactions and following social conventions. They may steal or exhibit impolite and socially inappropriate behavior, and they may neglect their normal responsibilities. Other common symptoms include loss of speech and language, compulsive or repetitive behavior, increased appetite, and motor problems such as stiffness and balance problems. Memory loss also may occur, although it typically appears late in the disease.

In one type of FTD called Pick disease, certain nerve cells become abnormal and swollen before they die. These swollen, or ballooned, neurons are one hallmark of the disease. The brains of people with Pick disease also have abnormal structures called Pick bodies, composed largely of the protein tau, inside the neurons. The cause of Pick disease is unknown, but it runs in some families and thus it is probably due at least in part to a faulty gene or genes. The disease usually begins after age 50 and causes changes in personality and behavior that gradually worsen over time. The symptoms of Pick disease are very similar to those of AD, and may include inappropriate social behavior, loss of mental flexibility, language problems, and difficulty with thinking and concentration. There is currently no way to slow the progressive degeneration found in Pick disease. However, medication may be helpful in reducing aggression and other behavioral problems, and in treating depression.

In some cases, familial FTD is linked to a mutation in the tau gene. This disorder, called frontotemporal dementia with parkinsonism linked to chromosome 17 (FTDP-17), is much like other types of FTD but often includes psychiatric symptoms such as delusions and hallucinations.

Primary progressive aphasia (PPA) is a type of FTD that may begin in people as early as their forties. "Aphasia" is a general term used to refer to deficits in language functions, such as speaking, understanding what others are saying, and naming common objects. In PPA one or more of these functions can become impaired. Symptoms often begin gradually and progress slowly over a period of years. As the disease progresses, memory and attention may also be impaired and patients may show personality and behavior changes. Many, but not all, people with PPA eventually develop symptoms of dementia.

HIV-associated dementia (HAD) results from infection with the human immunodeficiency virus (HIV) that causes AIDS. HAD can cause widespread destruction of the brain's white matter. This leads to a type of dementia that generally includes impaired memory, apathy, social withdrawal, and difficulty concentrating. People with HAD often develop movement problems as well. There is no specific treatment for HAD, but AIDS drugs can delay onset of the disease and may help to reduce symptoms.

Huntington disease (HD) is a hereditary disorder caused by a faulty gene for a protein called huntingtin. The children of people with the disorder have a 50 percent chance of inheriting it. The disease causes degeneration in many regions of the brain and spinal cord. Symptoms of HD usually begin when patients are in their thirties or forties, and the average life expectancy after diagnosis is about 15 years.

Cognitive symptoms of HD typically begin with mild personality changes, such as irritability, anxiety, and depression, and progress to severe dementia. Many patients also show psychotic behavior. HD causes chorea—involuntary jerky, arrhythmic movements of the body—as well as muscle weakness, clumsiness, and gait disturbances.

Dementia pugilistica, also called chronic traumatic encephalopathy or Boxer syndrome, is caused by head trauma, such as that experienced by people who have been punched many times in the head during boxing. The most common symptoms of the condition are dementia and parkinsonism, which can appear many years after the trauma ends. Affected individuals may also develop poor coordination and slurred speech. A single traumatic brain injury may also lead to a disorder called post-traumatic dementia (PTD). PTD is much like dementia pugilistica but usually also includes long-term memory problems. Other symptoms vary depending on which part of the brain was damaged by the injury.

Corticobasal degeneration (CBD) is a progressive disorder characterized by nerve cell loss and atrophy of multiple areas of the brain. Brain cells from people with CBD often have abnormal accumulations of the protein tau. CBD usually progresses gradually over the course of 6 to 8 years. Initial symptoms, which typically begin at or around age 60, may first appear on one side of the body but eventually will affect both sides. Some of the symptoms, such as poor coordination and rigidity, are similar to those found in Parkinson disease. Other symptoms may include memory loss, dementia, visual-spatial problems, apraxia (loss of the ability to make familiar, purposeful movements), hesitant and halting speech, myoclonus (involuntary muscular jerks), and dysphagia (difficulty swallowing). Death is often caused by pneumonia or other secondary problems such as sepsis (severe infection of the blood) or pulmonary embolism (a blood clot in the lungs).

There are no specific treatments available for CBD. Drugs such as clonazepam may help with myoclonus, however, and occupational, physical, and speech therapy can help in managing the disabilities associated with this disease. The symptoms of the disease often do not respond to Parkinson medications or other drugs.

Creutzfeldt-Jakob disease (CJD) is a rare, degenerative, fatal brain disorder that affects about one in every million people per year worldwide. Symptoms usually begin after age 60 and most patients die within 1 year. Many researchers believe CJD results from an abnormal form of a protein called a prion. Most cases of CJD occur sporadically—that is, in people who have no known risk factors for the disease. However, about 5 to 10 percent of cases of CJD in the United States are hereditary, caused by a mutation in the gene for the prion protein. In rare cases, CJD can also be acquired through exposure to diseased brain or nervous system tissue, usually through certain medical procedures. There is no evidence that CJD is contagious through the air or through casual contact with a CJD patient.

Patients with CJD may initially experience problems with muscular coordination; personality changes, including impaired memory, judgment, and thinking; and impaired vision. Other symptoms may include insomnia and depression. As the illness progresses, mental impairment becomes severe. Patients often develop myoclonus and they may go blind. They eventually lose the ability to move and speak, and go into a coma. Pneumonia and other infections often occur in these patients and can lead to death.

CJD belongs to a family of human and animal diseases known as the transmissible spongiform encephalopathies (TSEs). Spongiform refers to the characteristic appearance of infected brains, which become filled with holes until they resemble sponges when viewed under a microscope. CJD is the most common of the known human TSEs. Others include fatal familial insomnia and Gerstmann-Straussler-Scheinker disease.

In recent years, a new type of CJD, called variant CJD (vCJD), has been found in Great Britain and several other European countries. The initial symptoms of vCJD are different from those of classic CJD and the disorder typically occurs in younger patients. Research suggests that vCJD may have resulted from human consumption of beef from cattle with a TSE disease called bovine spongiform encephalopathy (BSE), also known as "mad cow disease."

Other rare hereditary dementias include Gerstmann-Straussler-Scheinker (GSS) disease, fatal familial insomnia, familial British dementia, and familial Danish dementia. Symptoms of GSS typically include ataxia and progressive dementia that begins when people are between 50 and 60 years old. The disease may last for several years before patients eventually die. Fatal familial insomnia causes degeneration of a brain region called the thalamus, which is partially responsible for controlling sleep. It causes a progressive insomnia that eventually leads to a complete inability to sleep. Other symptoms may include poor reflexes, dementia, hallucinations, and eventually coma.

It can be fatal within 7 to 13 months after symptoms begin but may last longer. Familial British dementia and familial Danish dementia have been linked to two different defects in a gene found on chromosome 13. The symptoms of both diseases include progressive dementia, paralysis, and loss of balance.

Secondary Dementias

Dementia may occur in patients who have other disorders that primarily affect movement or other functions. These cases are often referred to as secondary dementias. The relationship between these disorders and the primary dementias is not always clear. For instance, people with advanced Parkinson disease, which is primarily a movement disorder, sometimes develop symptoms of dementia. Many Parkinson patients also have amyloid plaques and neurofibrillary tangles like those found in AD. The two diseases may be linked in a yet-unknown way, or they may simply coexist in some people. People with Parkinson disease and associated dementia sometimes show signs of Lewy body dementia or progressive supranuclear palsy at autopsy, suggesting that these diseases may also overlap with Parkinson disease or that Parkinson disease is sometimes misdiagnosed.

Other disorders that may include symptoms of dementia include multiple sclerosis; presenile dementia with motor neuron disease, also called ALS dementia; olivopontocerebellar atrophy (OPCA); Wilson disease; and normal pressure hydrocephalus (NPH).

Dementias in Children

While it is usually found in adults, dementia can also occur in children. For example, infections and poisoning can lead to dementia in people of any age. In addition, some disorders unique to children can cause dementia.

Niemann-Pick disease is a group of inherited disorders that affect metabolism and are caused by specific genetic mutations. Patients with Niemann-Pick disease cannot properly metabolize cholesterol and other lipids. Consequently, excessive amounts of cholesterol accumulate in the liver and spleen and excessive amounts of other lipids accumulate in the brain. Symptoms may include dementia, confusion, and problems with learning and memory. These diseases usually begin in young school-age children but may also appear during the teen years or early adulthood.

Batten disease is a fatal, hereditary disorder of the nervous system that begins in childhood. Symptoms are linked to a buildup of substances called lipopigments in the body's tissues. The early symptoms include personality and behavior changes, slow learning, clumsiness, or stumbling. Over time, affected children suffer mental impairment, seizures, and progressive loss of sight and motor skills. Eventually, children with Batten disease develop dementia and become blind and bedridden. The disease is often fatal by the late teens or twenties.

Lafora body disease is a rare genetic disease that causes seizures, rapidly progressive dementia, and movement problems. These problems usually begin in late childhood or the early teens. Children with Lafora body disease have microscopic structures called Lafora bodies in the brain, skin, liver, and muscles. Most affected children die within 2 to 10 years after the onset of symptoms.

A number of other childhood-onset disorders can include symptoms of dementia. Among these are mitochondrial myopathies, Rasmussen encephalitis, mucopolysaccharidosis III (Sanfilippo syndrome), neurodegeneration with brain iron accumulation, and leukodystrophies such as Alexander disease, Schilder disease, and metachromatic leukodystrophy.

What Other Conditions Can Cause Dementia?

Doctors have identified many other conditions that can cause dementia or dementia-like symptoms. Many of these conditions are reversible with appropriate treatment.

Reactions to medications: Medications can sometimes lead to reactions or side effects that mimic dementia. These dementia-like effects can occur in reaction to just one drug or they can result from drug interactions. They may have a rapid onset or they may develop slowly over time.

Metabolic problems and endocrine abnormalities: Thyroid problems can lead to apathy, depression, or dementia. Hypoglycemia, a condition in which there is not enough sugar in the bloodstream, can cause confusion or personality changes. Too little or too much sodium or calcium can also trigger mental changes. Some people have an impaired ability to absorb vitamin B12, which creates a condition called pernicious anemia that can cause personality changes, irritability, or depression. Tests can determine if any of these problems are present.

Nutritional deficiencies: Deficiencies of thiamine (vitamin B1) frequently result from chronic alcoholism and can seriously impair mental abilities, in particular memories of recent events. Severe deficiency of vitamin B6 can cause a neurological illness called pellagra that may include dementia. Deficiencies of vitamin B12 also have been linked to dementia in some cases. Dehydration can also cause mental impairment that can resemble dementia.

Infections: Many infections can cause neurological symptoms, including confusion or delirium, due to fever or other side effects of the body's fight to overcome the infection. Meningitis and encephalitis, which are infections of the brain or the membrane that covers it, can cause confusion, sudden severe dementia, withdrawal from social interaction, impaired judgment, or memory loss. Untreated syphilis also can damage the nervous system and cause dementia. In rare cases, Lyme disease can cause memory or thinking difficulties. People in the advanced stages of AIDS [acquired immune deficiency syndrome] also may develop a form of dementia. People with compromised immune systems, such as those with leukemia and AIDS, may also develop an infection called progressive multifocal leukoencephalopathy (PML). PML is caused by a common human polyomavirus, JC virus, and leads to damage or destruction of the myelin sheath that covers nerve cells. PML can lead to confusion, difficulty with thinking or speaking, and other mental problems.

Subdural hematomas: Subdural hematomas, or bleeding between the brain's surface and its outer covering (the dura), can cause dementia-like symptoms and changes in mental function.

Poisoning: Exposure to lead, other heavy metals, or other poisonous substances can lead to symptoms of dementia. These symptoms may or may not resolve after treatment, depending on how badly the brain is damaged. People who have abused substances such as alcohol and recreational drugs sometimes display signs of dementia even after the substance abuse has ended. This condition is known as substance-induced persisting dementia.

Brain tumors: In rare cases, people with brain tumors may develop dementia because of damage to their brains. Symptoms may include changes in personality, psychotic episodes, or problems with speech, language, thinking, and memory.

Anoxia: Anoxia and a related term, hypoxia, are often used interchangeably to describe a state in which there is a diminished supply of oxygen to an organ's tissues. Anoxia may be caused by many different problems, including heart attack, heart surgery, severe asthma, smoke or carbon monoxide inhalation, high-altitude exposure, strangulation, or an overdose of anesthesia. In severe cases of anoxia the patient may be in a stupor or a coma for periods ranging from hours to days, weeks, or months. Recovery depends on the severity of the oxygen deprivation. As recovery proceeds, a variety of psychological and neurological abnormalities, such as dementia or psychosis, may occur. The person also may experience confusion, personality changes, hallucinations, or memory loss.

Heart and lung problems: The brain requires a high level of oxygen in order to carry out its normal functions. Therefore, problems such as chronic lung disease or heart problems that prevent the brain from receiving adequate oxygen can starve brain cells and lead to the symptoms of dementia.

What Conditions Are Not Dementia?

Age-related cognitive decline: As people age, they usually experience slower information processing and mild memory impairment. In addition, their brains frequently decrease in volume and some nerve cells, or neurons, are lost. These changes, called age-related cognitive decline, are normal and are not considered signs of dementia.

Mild cognitive impairment: Some people develop cognitive and memory problems that are not severe enough to be diagnosed as dementia but are more pronounced than the cognitive changes associated with normal aging. This condition is called mild cognitive impairment. Although many patients with this condition later develop dementia, some do not. Many researchers are studying mild cognitive impairment to find ways to treat it or prevent it from progressing to dementia.

Depression: People with depression are frequently passive or unresponsive, and they may appear slow, confused, or forgetful. Other emotional problems can also cause symptoms that sometimes mimic dementia.

Delirium: Delirium is characterized by confusion and rapidly altering mental states. The person may also be disoriented, drowsy, or incoherent, and may exhibit personality changes. Delirium is usually caused by a treatable physical or psychiatric illness, such as poisoning or infections. Patients with delirium often, though not always, make a full recovery after their underlying illness is treated.

Chapter 5

Dementia: Causes and Risk Factors

Causes of Dementia

All forms of dementia result from the death of nerve cells and/or the loss of communication among these cells. The human brain is a very complex and intricate machine and many factors can interfere with its functioning. Researchers have uncovered many of these factors, but they have not yet been able to fit these puzzle pieces together in order to form a complete picture of how dementias develop.

Many types of dementia, including AD, Lewy body dementia, Parkinson dementia, and Pick disease, are characterized by abnormal structures called inclusions in the brain. Because these inclusions, which contain abnormal proteins, are so common in people with dementia, researchers suspect that they play a role in the development of symptoms. However, that role is unknown, and in some cases the inclusions may simply be a side effect of the disease process that leads to the dementia.

Genes clearly play a role in the development of some kinds of dementia. However, in AD and many other disorders, the dementia usually cannot be tied to a single abnormal gene. Instead, these forms of dementia appear to result from a complex interaction of genes, lifestyle factors, and other environmental influences.

Excerpted from "Dementia: Hope Through Research," by the National Institute of Neurological Disorders and Stroke (NINDS, www.ninds.nih.gov), part of the National Institutes of Health, January 21, 2011.

Researchers have identified several genes that influence susceptibility to AD. Mutations in three of the known genes for AD—genes that control the production of proteins such as amyloid precursor protein (APP), presenilin 1, and presenilin 2—are linked to early-onset forms of the disease.

Variations in another gene, called apolipoprotein E (apoE), have been linked to an increased risk of late-onset AD. The apoE gene does not cause the disease by itself, but one version of the gene, called apoE epsilon4 (apoE E4), appears to increase the risk of AD. People with two copies of the apoE E4 gene have about 10 times the risk of developing AD compared to people without apoE E4. This gene variant seems to encourage amyloid deposition in the brain. One study also found that this gene is associated with shorter survival in men with AD. In contrast, another version of the apoE gene, called apoE E2, appears to protect against AD.

Studies have suggested that mutations in another gene, called CYP46, may contribute to an increased risk of developing late-onset sporadic AD. This gene normally produces a protein that helps the brain metabolize cholesterol.

Scientists are trying to determine how beta amyloid influences the development of AD. A number of studies indicate that the buildup of this protein initiates a complex chain of events that culminates in dementia. One study found that beta amyloid buildup in the brain triggers cells called microglia, which act like janitors that mop up potentially harmful substances in the brain, to release a potent neurotoxin called peroxynitrite. This may contribute to nerve cell death in AD. Another study found that beta amyloid causes a protein called p35 to be split into two proteins. One of the resulting proteins triggers changes in the tau protein that lead to formation of neurofibrillary tangles. A third study found that beta amyloid activates cell-death enzymes called caspases that alter the tau protein in a way that causes it to form tangles. Researchers believe these tangles may contribute to the neuron death in AD.

Vascular dementia can be caused by cerebrovascular disease or any other condition that prevents normal blood flow to the brain. Without a normal supply of blood, brain cells cannot obtain the oxygen they need to work correctly, and they often become so deprived that they die.

The causes of other types of dementias vary. Some, such as CJD and GSS, have been tied to abnormal forms of specific proteins. Others, including Huntington disease and FTDP-17, have been linked to defects in a single gene. Post-traumatic dementia is directly related to brain cell death after injury. HIV-associated dementia is clearly tied to infection by the HIV virus, although the exact way the virus causes damage is not yet certain. For other dementias, such as corticobasal degeneration and most types of frontotemporal dementia, the underlying causes have not yet been identified.

What Are the Risk Factors for Dementia?

Researchers have identified several risk factors that affect the likelihood of developing one or more kinds of dementia. Some of these factors are modifiable, while others are not.

Age: The risk of AD, vascular dementia, and several other dementias goes up significantly with advancing age.

Genetics/family history: Researchers have discovered a number of genes that increase the risk of developing AD. Although people with a family history of AD are generally considered to be at heightened risk of developing the disease themselves, many people with a family history never develop the disease, and many without a family history of the disease do get it. In most cases, it is still impossible to predict a specific person's risk of the disorder based on family history alone. Some families with CJD, GSS, or fatal familial insomnia have mutations in the prion protein gene, although these disorders can also occur in people without the gene mutation. Individuals with these mutations are at significantly higher risk of developing these forms of dementia. Abnormal genes are also clearly implicated as risk factors in Huntington disease, FTDP-17, and several other kinds of dementia.

Smoking and alcohol use: Several recent studies have found that smoking significantly increases the risk of mental decline and dementia. People who smoke have a higher risk of atherosclerosis and other types of vascular disease, which may be the underlying causes for the increased dementia risk. Studies also have found that drinking large amounts of alcohol appears to increase the risk of dementia. However, other studies have suggested that people who drink moderately have a lower risk of dementia than either those who drink heavily or those who completely abstain from drinking.

Atherosclerosis: Atherosclerosis is the buildup of plaque—deposits of fatty substances, cholesterol, and other matter—in the inner lining of an artery. Atherosclerosis is a significant risk factor for vascular dementia, because it interferes with the delivery of blood to the brain and can lead to stroke. Studies have also found a possible link between atherosclerosis and AD.

Cholesterol: High levels of low-density lipoprotein (LDL), the so-called bad form of cholesterol, appear to significantly increase a person's risk of developing vascular dementia. Some research has also linked high cholesterol to an increased risk of AD.

Plasma homocysteine: Research has shown that a higher-than-average blood level of homocysteine—a type of amino acid—is a strong risk factor for the development of AD and vascular dementia.

Diabetes: Diabetes is a risk factor for both AD and vascular dementia. It is also a known risk factor for atherosclerosis and stroke, both of which contribute to vascular dementia.

Mild cognitive impairment: While not all people with mild cognitive impairment develop dementia, people with this condition do have a significantly increased risk of dementia compared to the rest of the population. One study found that approximately 40 percent of people over age 65 who were diagnosed with mild cognitive impairment developed dementia within 3 years.

Down syndrome: Studies have found that most people with Down syndrome develop characteristic AD plaques and neurofibrillary tangles by the time they reach middle age. Many, but not all, of these individuals also develop symptoms of dementia.

How Is Dementia Diagnosed?

Doctors employ a number of strategies to diagnose dementia. It is important that they rule out any treatable conditions, such as depression, normal pressure hydrocephalus, or vitamin B12 deficiency, which can cause similar symptoms.

Early, accurate diagnosis of dementia is important for patients and their families because it allows early treatment of symptoms. For people with AD or other progressive dementias, early diagnosis may allow them to plan for the future while they can still help to make decisions. These people also may benefit from drug treatment.

The "gold standard" for diagnosing dementia, autopsy, does not help the patient or caregivers. Therefore, doctors have devised a number of techniques to help identify dementia with reasonable accuracy while the patient is still alive.

Patient History

Doctors often begin their examination of a patient suspected of having dementia by asking questions about the patient's history. For example, they may ask how and when symptoms developed and about the patient's overall medical condition.

They also may try to evaluate the patient's emotional state, although patients with dementia often may be unaware of or in denial about how their disease is affecting them. Family members also may deny the existence of the disease because they do not want to accept the diagnosis and because, at least in the beginning, AD and other forms of dementia can resemble normal aging. Therefore additional steps are necessary to confirm or rule out a diagnosis of dementia.

Physical Examination

A physical examination can help rule out treatable causes of dementia and identify signs of stroke or other disorders that can contribute to dementia. It can also identify signs of other illnesses, such as heart disease or kidney failure, which can overlap with dementia. If a patient is taking medications that may be causing or contributing to his or her symptoms, the doctor may suggest stopping or replacing some medications to see if the symptoms go away.

Neurological Evaluations

Doctors will perform a neurological examination, looking at balance, sensory function, reflexes, and other functions, to identify signs of conditions—for example, movement disorders or stroke—that may affect the patient's diagnosis or are treatable with drugs.

Cognitive and Neuropsychological Tests

Doctors use tests that measure memory, language skills, math skills, and other abilities related to mental functioning to help them diagnose a patient's condition accurately. For example, people with AD often show changes in so-called executive functions (such as problem solving), memory, and the ability to perform once-automatic tasks.

Doctors often use a test called the Mini-Mental State Examination (MMSE) to assess cognitive skills in people with suspected dementia. This test examines orientation, memory, and attention, as well as the ability to name objects, follow verbal and written commands, write a sentence spontaneously, and copy a complex shape. Doctors also use a variety of other tests and rating scales to identify specific types of cognitive problems and abilities.

Brain Scans

Doctors may use brain scans to identify strokes, tumors, or other problems that can cause dementia. Also, cortical atrophy—degeneration of the brain's cortex (outer layer)—is common in many forms of dementia and may be visible on a brain scan. The brain's cortex normally appears very wrinkled, with ridges of tissue (called gyri) separated by "valleys" called sulci. In individuals with cortical atrophy, the progressive loss of neurons causes the ridges to become thinner and the sulci to grow wider. As brain cells die, the ventricles (or fluid-filled cavities in the middle of the brain) expand to fill the available space, becoming much larger than normal. Brain scans also can identify changes in the brain's structure and function that suggest AD.

The most common types of brain scans are computed tomographic (CT) scans and magnetic resonance imaging (MRI). Doctors frequently request a CT scan of the brain when they are examining a patient with suspected dementia. These scans, which use x-rays to detect brain structures, can show evidence of brain atrophy, strokes, and transient ischemic attacks (TIAs), changes to the blood vessels, and other problems such as hydrocephalus and subdural hematomas. MRI scans use magnetic fields and focused radio waves to detect hydrogen atoms in tissues within the body. They can detect the same problems as CT scans but they are better for identifying certain conditions, such as brain atrophy and damage from small TIAs.

Doctors also may use electroencephalograms (EEGs) in people with suspected dementia. In an EEG, electrodes are placed on the scalp over several parts of the brain in order to detect and record patterns of electrical activity and check for abnormalities. This electrical activity can indicate cognitive dysfunction in part or all of the brain. Many patients with moderately severe to severe AD have abnormal EEGs. An EEG may also be used to detect seizures, which occur in about 10 percent of AD patients as well as in many other disorders. EEGs also can help diagnose CJD.

Several other types of brain scans allow researchers to watch the brain as it functions. These scans, called functional brain imaging, are not often used as diagnostic tools, but they are important in research and they may ultimately help identify people with dementia earlier than is currently possible. Functional brain scans include functional MRI (fMRI), single photon-emission computed tomography (SPECT), positron emission tomography (PET), and magnetoencephalography (MEG). fMRI uses radio waves and a strong magnetic field to measure the metabolic changes that take place in active parts of the brain. SPECT shows the distribution of blood in the brain, which generally increases with brain activity. PET scans can detect changes in glucose metabolism, oxygen metabolism, and blood flow, all of which can reveal abnormalities of brain function. MEG shows the electromagnetic fields produced by the brain's neuronal activity.

Laboratory Tests

Doctors may use a variety of laboratory tests to help diagnose dementia and/or rule out other conditions, such as kidney failure, that can contribute to symptoms. A partial list of these tests includes a complete blood count, blood glucose test, urinalysis, drug and alcohol tests (toxicology screen), cerebrospinal fluid analysis (to rule out specific infections that can affect the brain), and analysis of thyroid and thyroid-stimulating hormone levels. A doctor will order only the tests that he or she feels are necessary and/or likely to improve the accuracy of a diagnosis.

Psychiatric Evaluation

A psychiatric evaluation may be obtained to determine if depression or another psychiatric disorder may be causing or contributing to a person's symptoms.

Presymptomatic Testing

Testing people before symptoms begin to determine if they will develop dementia is not possible in most cases. However, in disorders such as Huntington where a known gene defect is clearly linked to the risk of the disease, a genetic test can help identify people who are likely to develop the disease. Since this type of genetic information can be devastating, people should carefully consider whether they want to undergo such testing.

Researchers are examining whether a series of simple cognitive tests, such as matching words with pictures, can predict who will develop dementia. One study suggested that a combination of a verbal learning test and an odor-identification test can help identify AD before symptoms become obvious. Other studies are looking at whether memory tests and brain scans can be useful indicators of future dementia.

Treatment

While treatments to reverse or halt disease progression are not available for most of the dementias, patients can benefit to some extent

41

from treatment with available medications and other measures, such as cognitive training.

Drugs to specifically treat AD and some other progressive dementias are now available and are prescribed for many patients. Although these drugs do not halt the disease or reverse existing brain damage, they can improve symptoms and slow the progression of the disease. This may improve the patient's quality of life, ease the burden on caregivers, and/or delay admission to a nursing home. Many researchers are also examining whether these drugs may be useful for treating other types of dementia.

Many people with dementia, particularly those in the early stages, may benefit from practicing tasks designed to improve performance in specific aspects of cognitive functioning. For example, people can sometimes be taught to use memory aids, such as mnemonics, computerized recall devices, or note taking.

Behavior modification—rewarding appropriate or positive behavior and ignoring inappropriate behavior—also may help control unacceptable or dangerous behaviors.

Alzheimer Disease

Most of the drugs currently approved by the U.S. Food and Drug Administration (FDA) for AD fall into a category called cholinesterase inhibitors. These drugs slow the breakdown of the neurotransmitter acetylcholine, which is reduced in the brains of people with AD. Acetylcholine is important for the formation of memories and it is used in the hippocampus and the cerebral cortex, two brain regions that are affected by AD. There are currently four cholinesterase inhibitors approved for use in the United States: Tacrine (Cognex), donepezil (Aricept), rivastigmine (Exelon), and galantamine (Reminyl). These drugs temporarily improve or stabilize memory and thinking skills in some individuals. Many studies have shown that cholinesterase inhibitors help to slow the decline in mental functions associated with AD, and that they can help reduce behavioral problems and improve the ability to perform everyday tasks. However, none of these drugs can stop or reverse the course of AD.

A fifth drug, memantine (Namenda), is also approved for use in the United States. Unlike other drugs for AD, which affect acetylcholine levels, memantine works by regulating the activity of a neurotransmitter called glutamate that plays a role in learning and memory. Glutamate activity is often disrupted in AD. Because this drug works differently from cholinesterase inhibitors, combining memantine with other AD drugs may be more effective than any single therapy. One controlled clinical trial found that patients receiving donepezil plus memantine had better cognition and other functions than patients receiving donepezil alone.

Doctors may also prescribe other drugs, such as anticonvulsants, sedatives, and antidepressants, to treat seizures, depression, agitation, sleep disorders, and other specific problems that can be associated with dementia. In 2005, research showed that use of "atypical" antipsychotic drugs such as olanzapine and risperidone to treat behavioral problems in elderly people with dementia was associated with an elevated risk of death in these patients. Most of the deaths were caused by heart problems or infections. The FDA has issued a public health advisory to alert patients and their caregivers to this safety issue.

Vascular Dementia

There is no standard drug treatment for vascular dementia, although some of the symptoms, such as depression, can be treated. Most other treatments aim to reduce the risk factors for further brain damage. However, some studies have found that cholinesterase inhibitors, such as galantamine and other AD drugs, can improve cognitive function and behavioral symptoms in patients with early vascular dementia.

The progression of vascular dementia can often be slowed significantly or halted if the underlying vascular risk factors for the disease are treated. To prevent strokes and TIAs, doctors may prescribe medicines to control high blood pressure, high cholesterol, heart disease, and diabetes. Doctors also sometimes prescribe aspirin, warfarin, or other drugs to prevent clots from forming in small blood vessels. When patients have blockages in blood vessels, doctors may recommend surgical procedures, such as carotid endarterectomy, stenting, or angioplasty, to restore the normal blood supply. Medications to relieve restlessness or depression or to help patients sleep better may also be prescribed.

Other Dementias

Some studies have suggested that cholinesterase inhibitors, such as donepezil (Aricept), can reduce behavioral symptoms in some patients with Parkinson dementia.

At present, no medications are approved specifically to treat or prevent FTD and most other types of progressive dementia. However, sedatives, antidepressants, and other medications may be useful in treating specific symptoms and behavioral problems associated with these diseases.

Scientists continue to search for specific treatments to help people with Lewy body dementia. Current treatment is symptomatic, often involving the use of medication to control the parkinsonian and psychiatric symptoms. Although antiparkinsonian medication may help reduce tremor and loss of muscle movement, it may worsen symptoms such as hallucinations and delusions. Also, drugs prescribed for psychiatric symptoms may make the movement problems worse. Several studies have suggested that cholinesterase inhibitors may be able to improve cognitive function and behavioral symptoms in patients with Lewy body disease.

There is no known treatment that can cure or control CJD. Current treatment is aimed at alleviating symptoms and making the patient as comfortable as possible. Opiate drugs can help relieve pain, and the drugs clonazepam and sodium valproate may help relieve myoclonus. During later stages of the disease, treatment focuses on supportive care, such as administering intravenous fluids and changing the person's position frequently to prevent bedsores.

Prevention

Research has revealed a number of factors that may be able to prevent or delay the onset of dementia in some people. For example, studies have shown that people who maintain tight control over their glucose levels tend to score better on tests of cognitive function than those with poorly controlled diabetes.

Several studies also have suggested that people who engage in intellectually stimulating activities, such as social interactions, chess, crossword puzzles, and playing a musical instrument, significantly lower their risk of developing AD and other forms of dementia. Scientists believe mental activities may stimulate the brain in a way that increases the person's "cognitive reserve"—the ability to cope with or compensate for the pathologic changes associated with dementia.

Researchers are studying other steps people can take that may help prevent AD in some cases. So far, none of these factors has been definitively proven to make a difference in the risk of developing the disease. Moreover, most of the studies addressed only AD, and the results may or may not apply to other forms of dementia. Nevertheless, scientists are encouraged by the results of these early studies and many believe it will eventually become possible to prevent some forms of dementia. Possible preventive actions include:

- **Lowering homocysteine:** In one study, elevated blood levels of the amino acid homocysteine were associated with a 2.9 times greater risk of AD and a 4.9 times greater risk of vascular dementia. A preliminary study has shown that high doses of three B vitamins that help lower homocysteine levels—folic acid, B12, and B6—appear to slow the progression of AD. Researchers are conducting a multi-center clinical trial to test this effect in a larger group of patients.

- **Lowering cholesterol levels:** Research has suggested that people with high cholesterol levels have an increased risk of developing AD. Cholesterol is involved in formation of amyloid plaques in the brain. Mutations in a gene called CYP46 and the apoE E4 gene variant, both of which have been linked to an increased risk of AD, are also involved in cholesterol metabolism. Several studies have also found that the use of drugs called statins, which lower cholesterol levels, is associated with a lower likelihood of cognitive impairment.

- **Lowering blood pressure:** Several studies have shown that antihypertensive medicine reduces the odds of cognitive impairment in elderly people with high blood pressure. One large European study found a 55 percent lower risk of dementia in people over 60 who received drug treatment for hypertension. These people had a reduced risk of both AD and vascular dementia.

- **Exercise:** Regular exercise stimulates production of chemicals called growth factors that help neurons survive and adapt to new situations. These gains may help to delay the onset of dementia symptoms. Exercise also may reduce the risk of brain damage from atherosclerosis.

- **Education:** Researchers have found evidence that formal education may help protect people against the effects of AD. In one study, researchers found that people with more years of formal education had relatively less mental decline than people with less schooling, regardless of the number of amyloid plaques and neurofibrillary tangles each person had in his or her brain. The researchers think education may cause the brain to develop robust nerve cell networks that can help compensate for the cell damage caused by AD.

- **Controlling inflammation:** Many studies have suggested that inflammation may contribute to AD. Moreover, autopsies of people who died with AD have shown widespread inflammation in the brain that appeared to be caused by the accumulation of beta amyloid. Another study found that men with high levels of C-reactive protein, a general marker of inflammation, had a significantly increased risk of AD and other kinds of dementia.

- **Nonsteroidal anti-inflammatory drugs (NSAIDs):** Research indicates that long-term use of NSAIDs—ibuprofen, naproxen, and similar drugs—may prevent or delay the onset of AD. Researchers are not sure how these drugs may protect against the disease, but some or all of the effect may be due to reduced inflammation. A 2003 study showed that these drugs also bind to amyloid plaques and may help to dissolve them and prevent formation of new plaques.

The risk of vascular dementia is strongly correlated with risk factors for stroke, including high blood pressure, diabetes, elevated cholesterol levels, and smoking. This type of dementia may be prevented in many cases by changing lifestyle factors, such as excessive weight and high blood pressure, which are associated with an increased risk of cerebrovascular disease. One European study found that treating isolated systolic hypertension (high blood pressure in which only the systolic or top number is high) in people age 60 and older reduced the risk of dementia by 50 percent. These studies strongly suggest that effective use of current treatments can prevent many future cases of vascular dementia.

A study published in 2005 found that people with mild cognitive impairment who took 10 mg/day of the drug donepezil had a significantly reduced risk of developing AD during the first 2 years of treatment, compared to people who received vitamin E or a placebo. By the end of the third year, however, the rate of AD was just as high in the people treated with donepezil as it was in the other two groups.

What Kind of Care Does a Person with Dementia Need?

People with moderate and advanced dementia typically need round-the-clock care and supervision to prevent them from harming themselves or others. They also may need assistance with daily activities such as eating, bathing, and dressing. Meeting these needs takes patience, understanding, and careful thought by the person's caregivers.

A typical home environment can present many dangers and obstacles to a person with dementia, but simple changes can overcome many of these problems. For example, sharp knives, dangerous chemicals, tools, and other hazards should be removed or locked away. Other safety measures include installing bed and bathroom safety rails, removing locks from bedroom and bathroom doors, and lowering the hot water temperature to 120 degrees Fahrenheit (48.9 degrees Celsius) or less to reduce the risk of accidental scalding. People with dementia also should wear some form of identification at all times in case they wander away or become lost. Caregivers can help prevent unsupervised wandering by adding locks or alarms to outside doors.

People with dementia often develop behavior problems because of frustration with specific situations. Understanding and modifying or preventing the situations that trigger these behaviors may help to make life more pleasant for the person with dementia as well as his or her caregivers. For instance, the person may be confused or frustrated by the level of activity or noise in the surrounding environment. Reducing unnecessary activity and noise (such as limiting the number of visitors and turning off the television when it's not in use) may make it easier for the person to understand requests and perform simple tasks. Confusion also may be reduced by simplifying home decorations, removing clutter, keeping familiar objects nearby, and following a predictable routine throughout the day. Calendars and clocks also may help patients orient themselves.

People with dementia should be encouraged to continue their normal leisure activities as long as they are safe and do not cause frustration. Activities such as crafts, games, and music can provide important mental stimulation and improve mood. Some studies have suggested that participating in exercise and intellectually stimulating activities may slow the decline of cognitive function in some people.

Many studies have found that driving is unsafe for people with dementia. They often get lost and they may have problems remembering or following rules of the road. They also may have difficulty processing information quickly and dealing with unexpected circumstances. Even a second of confusion while driving can lead to an accident. Driving with impaired cognitive functions can also endanger others. Some experts have suggested that regular screening for changes in cognition might help to reduce the number of driving accidents among elderly people, and some states now require that doctors report people with AD to their state motor vehicle department. However, in many cases, it is up to the person's family and friends to ensure that the person does not drive.

The emotional and physical burden of caring for someone with dementia can be overwhelming. Support groups can often help caregivers deal with these demands and they can also offer helpful information about the disease and its treatment. It is important that caregivers occasionally have time off from round-the-clock nursing demands. Some communities provide respite facilities or adult day care centers that will care for dementia patients for a period of time, giving the primary caregivers a break. Eventually, many patients with dementia require the services of a full-time nursing home.

What Research Is Being Done?

Current research focuses on many different aspects of dementia. This research promises to improve the lives of people affected by the dementias and may eventually lead to ways of preventing or curing these disorders.

Causes and Prevention

Research on the causes of AD and other dementias includes studies of genetic factors, neurotransmitters, inflammation, factors that influence programmed cell death in the brain, and the roles of tau, beta amyloid, and the associated neurofibrillary tangles and plaques in AD. Some other researchers are trying to determine the possible roles of cholesterol metabolism, oxidative stress (chemical reactions that can damage proteins, DNA, and lipids inside cells), and microglia in the development of AD. Scientists also are investigating the role of aging-related proteins such as the enzyme telomerase.

Since many dementias and other neurodegenerative diseases have been linked to abnormal clumps of proteins in cells, researchers are trying to learn how these clumps develop, how they affect cells, and how the clumping can be prevented.

Some studies are examining whether changes in white matter—nerve fibers lined with myelin—may play a role in the onset of AD. Myelin may erode in AD patients before other changes occur. This may be due to a problem with oligodendrocytes, the cells that produce myelin.

Researchers are searching for additional genes that may contribute to AD, and they have identified a number of gene regions that may be involved. Some researchers suggest that people will eventually be screened for a number of genes that contribute to AD and that they will be able to receive treatments that specifically address their individual genetic risks. However, such individualized screening and treatment is still years away.

Insulin resistance is common in people with AD, but it is not clear whether the insulin resistance contributes to the development of the disease or if it is merely a side effect.

Several studies have found a reduced risk of dementia in people who take cholesterol-lowering drugs called statins. However, it is not yet clear if the apparent effect is due to the drugs or to other factors.

Early studies of estrogen suggested that it might help prevent AD in older women. However, a clinical study of several thousand postmenopausal women aged 65 or older found that combination therapy with estrogen and progestin substantially increased the risk of AD. Estrogen alone also appeared to slightly increase the risk of dementia in this study.

A 2003 study found that people with HIV-associated dementia have different levels of activity for more than 30 different proteins, compared to people who have HIV but no signs of dementia. The study suggests a possible way to screen HIV patients for the first signs of cognitive impairment, and it may lead to ways of intervening to prevent this form of dementia.

Diagnosis

Improving early diagnosis of AD and other types of dementia is important not only for patients and families, but also for researchers who seek to better understand the causes of dementing diseases and find ways to reverse or halt them at early stages. Improved diagnosis can also reduce the risk that people will receive inappropriate treatments.

Some researchers are investigating whether three-dimensional computer models of PET and MRI images can identify brain changes typical of early AD, before any symptoms appear. This research may lead to ways of preventing the symptoms of the disease.

One study found that levels of beta amyloid and tau in spinal fluid can be used to diagnose AD with a sensitivity of 92 percent. If other studies confirm the validity of this test, it may allow doctors to identify people who are beginning to develop the disorder before they start to show symptoms. This would allow treatment at very early stages of the disorder, and may help in testing new treatments to prevent or delay symptoms of the disease. Other researchers have identified factors in the skin and blood of AD patients that are different from those in healthy people. They are trying to determine if these factors can be used to diagnose the disease.

Treatment

Researchers are continually working to develop new drugs for AD and other types of dementia. Many researchers believe a vaccine that reduces the number of amyloid plaques in the brain might ultimately prove to be the most effective treatment for AD. In 2001, researchers began one clinical trial of a vaccine called AN-1792. The study was halted after a number of people developed inflammation of the brain and spinal cord. Despite these problems, one patient appeared to have reduced numbers of amyloid plaques in the brain. Other patients showed little or no cognitive decline during the course of the study, suggesting that the vaccine may slow or halt the disease. Researchers are now trying to find safer and more effective vaccines for AD.

Researchers are also investigating possible methods of gene therapy for AD. In one case, researchers used cells genetically engineered to produce nerve growth factor and transplanted them into monkeys' forebrains. The transplanted cells boosted the amount of nerve growth factors in the brain and seemed to prevent degeneration of acetylcholine-producing neurons in the animals. This suggests that gene therapy might help to reduce or delay symptoms of the disease.

Researchers are now testing a similar therapy in a small number of patients. Other researchers have experimented with gene therapy that adds a gene called neprilysin in a mouse model that produces human beta amyloid. They found that increasing the level of neprilysin greatly reduced the amount of beta amyloid in the mice and halted the amyloid-related brain degeneration. They are now trying to determine whether neprilysin gene therapy can improve cognition in mice.

A clinical trial called the Vitamins to Slow Alzheimer's Disease (VITAL) study is testing whether high doses of three common B vitamins—folic acid, B12, and B6—can reduce homocysteine levels and slow the rate of cognitive decline in AD.

Since many studies have found evidence of brain inflammation in AD, some researchers have proposed that drugs that control inflammation, such as NSAIDs, might prevent the disease or slow its progression. Studies in mice have suggested that these drugs can limit production of amyloid plaques in the brain. Early studies of these drugs in humans have shown promising results. However, a large NIH-funded clinical trial of two NSAIDS (naproxen and celecoxib) to prevent AD was stopped in late 2004 because of an increase in stroke and heart attack in people taking naproxen, and an unrelated study that linked celecoxib to an increased risk of heart attack.

Some studies have suggested that two drugs, pentoxifylline and propentofylline, may be useful in treating vascular dementia. Pentoxifylline improves blood flow, while propentofylline appears to interfere with some of the processes that cause cell death in the brain.

One study is testing the safety and effectiveness of donepezil (Aricept) for treating mild dementia in patients with Parkinson dementia, while another is investigating whether skin patches with the drug selegiline can improve mental function in patients with cognitive problems related to HIV.

Chapter 6

Statistics on Dementia Prevalence and Mortality

Prevalence

Millions of Americans now have Alzheimer's disease or other dementia.

More women than men have Alzheimer's and other dementias, primarily because women live longer, on average, than men, and their longer life expectancy increases the time during which they could develop Alzheimer's or other dementia.

The prevalence of Alzheimer's and other dementias also differs by education; those with fewer years of education appear to have higher rates of Alzheimer's and other dementias. Some researchers believe that having more years of education (compared with those with fewer years) provides a "cognitive reserve" that allows individuals to compensate for symptoms of Alzheimer's or other dementia. However, it is generally believed that these differences reflect socioeconomic factors such as higher rates of disease and less access to medical care in lower socioeconomic groups. Racial and ethnic differences in rates of Alzheimer's disease and other dementias have also been reported, although differences have not been consistently found.

The number of Americans with Alzheimer's and other dementias is increasing every year because of the steady growth in the older

Excerpted from "2009 Alzheimer's Disease Facts and Figures," and reprinted with permission of the Alzheimer's Association. For additional information, call the Alzheimer's Association toll-free helpline, 800-272-3900, or visit their website at www.alz.org. © 2010 Alzheimer's Association. All rights reserved.

population. The number will continue to increase and escalate rapidly in the coming years as the baby boom generation ages.

Figures from different studies on the prevalence and characteristics of people with Alzheimer's and other dementias vary, depending on how each study was conducted. Data from several studies are used in this section to describe the prevalence of these conditions and the proportion of people with the conditions by gender, years of education, race, and cause of dementia. Data sources and methodologies are described, and more detailed information is contained in the End Notes section in the Appendix [of the full report]. Estimates of lifetime risk of Alzheimer's disease and other dementias are also briefly discussed.

Prevalence of Alzheimer's Disease and Other Dementias

Currently, an estimated 5.3 million Americans of all ages have Alzheimer's disease. This figure includes 5.1 million people aged 65 and older and 200,000 individuals under age 65 who have younger-onset Alzheimer's. Based on these estimates, approximately 500,000 Americans under age 65 have Alzheimer's or other dementia. Of these, about 40 percent are estimated to have Alzheimer's disease.

- One in eight persons aged 65 and older (13 percent) have Alzheimer's disease.

- Every 70 seconds, someone in America develops Alzheimer's disease. By mid-century, someone will develop Alzheimer's every 33 seconds.

Prevalence of Alzheimer's Disease and Other Dementias in Women and Men

Women are more likely than men to have Alzheimer's disease and other dementias. Based on estimates from the Aging, Demographics, and Memory Study (ADAMS), 14 percent of all people aged 71 and older have dementia. Women aged 71 and older had higher rates than men: 16 percent for women and 11 percent for men. The 2008 estimate is that 2.4 million women and 1 million men aged 71 and older have dementia.

Further analysis of these data shows that the larger proportion of older women than men who have dementia is primarily explained by the fact that women live longer, on average, than men. Likewise, many studies of the age-specific incidence (new cases) of dementia have found no significant difference by gender.

The same is true for Alzheimer's disease. The larger proportion of older women than men who have Alzheimer's disease is believed to be explained by the fact that women live longer. Again, many studies of the age-specific incidence of Alzheimer's disease show no significant difference for women and men. Thus, it appears that gender is not a risk factor for Alzheimer's disease or other dementia once age is taken into account. Essentially, women are more likely to have Alzheimer's disease and other dementias because they live long enough to develop these conditions and generally live longer than men.

Prevalence of Alzheimer's Disease and Other Dementias by Years of Education

People with fewer years of education appear to be at higher risk for Alzheimer's and other dementias than those with more years of education. Studies of the prevalence of dementia show that having fewer years of education is associated with greater likelihood of having dementia, and incidence studies show that having fewer years of education is associated with a greater risk of developing dementia. One study found, for example, that people with less than 12 years of education had a 15 percent greater risk of developing dementia than people with 12 to 15 years of education and a 35 percent greater risk of developing dementia than people with more than 15 years of education.

Similar findings have been reported for Alzheimer's disease. Studies of the prevalence of Alzheimer's disease show that having fewer years of education is associated with higher likelihood of having Alzheimer's disease, and incidence studies show that having fewer years of education is associated with greater risk of developing Alzheimer's disease.

A number of researchers have noted that years of education may be a surrogate marker for factors that affect access to education, such as socioeconomic status and where one lived as a child. Attaining fewer years of education is generally related to additional factors, such as lower levels of occupational attainment and higher prevalence of physical health conditions in adulthood, that are also associated with the development of dementia.

Prevalence of Alzheimer's Disease and Other Dementias in African-Americans and Whites

African-Americans are frequently reported to be more likely than whites to have Alzheimer's disease and other dementias. However, more detailed analysis of these relationships indicates that the differences may be largely explained by factors other than race. Most analyses that examined racial differences in Alzheimer's and other dementias, and have simultaneously looked at age, gender, years of education, and comorbid conditions, report significant differences on the basis of race do not persist.

Researchers examining racial differences in risk factors for Alzheimer's disease only have reported similar findings. Most analyses that have combined age, gender, years of education, African-American versus white race, and apolipoprotein E (APOE) status have found that the higher prevalence of Alzheimer's disease in African-Americans is primarily explained by these other factors, or that their increased risk is greatly reduced once these factors are taken into account.

Lifetime Risk Estimates for Alzheimer's and Other Dementias

The Framingham original study population was used to estimate short-term (10-year), intermediate (20- and 30-year) and lifetime risks for Alzheimer's disease, as well as overall risk for any dementia. Nearly 2,800 persons 65 years of age and free of dementia were identified in 1975 and provided the basis for an incidence study of dementia, as well as Alzheimer's disease. This group (cohort) was followed for up to 29 years. Key findings included significantly higher lifetime risk for both dementia and Alzheimer's in women compared to men. More than 20 percent of women reaching the age of 65 would ultimately develop dementia (estimated lifetime risk), compared to approximately 17 percent of men. For Alzheimer's, the estimated lifetime risk was nearly one in five for women compared to one in 10 for men. Unpublished data from Framingham indicated that at age 55, the estimated lifetime risk for Alzheimer's was 17 percent in women (approximately one in six women), compared to 9 percent in men (nearly one in 10 men). The unpublished data for any dementia in women who reached 55 was 21 percent, and for men 14 percent. Increases in short- and intermediate-term risks for dementia and Alzheimer's were seen not only at age 65, but also were markedly increased at ages 75 and 85 for both women and men. However, compared with women, the risks were not as high in men. Again, these differences in lifetime risks for women compared with men are largely due to the longer life expectancy for women.

For women, at age 65, the short-term risk for developing dementia over the next 10 years is approximately 1 percent. However, at age 75, for women, the risk of developing dementia over the next 10 years jumps more than sevenfold, and at 85, the risk skyrockets to 20-fold. Similar dramatic increases are seen for Alzheimer's disease. The risk scenario for men follows a similar trajectory.

The Framingham lifetime risk estimates for women are above 20 percent for dementia and clearly higher in women than in men. Although the concept of lifetime risk generally reflects the risk from birth to death, dementia is a condition that usually occurs after age 65. While there is an important minority of people with younger-onset Alzheimer's, the dementia risk prior to age 65 is relatively modest. Estimating the risk in people who have reached the age of at least 65 dementia-free provides a reasonable estimate of lifetime risk in the bulk of the population at risk for dementia.

The definition of Alzheimer's disease and other dementias used in the Framingham study required documentation of moderate to severe disease as well as symptoms lasting a minimum of 6 months. As a result of these requirements, the Framingham study estimates are considered to be conservative. Thus, when one considers the numbers of people with mild to moderate levels of dementia, as well as those with dementia for less than 6 months' duration, the current and future numbers of people at risk for Alzheimer's disease and other dementias far exceed those stated in the Framingham study.

Estimates for the Numbers of People with Alzheimer's Disease, by State

The projected number of people aged 65 and older with Alzheimer's disease varies by region of the country, as well as by state. Comparable projections for prevalence data on dementia by state are not available.

Not only is there substantial variability by state in the projected numbers of people with Alzheimer's, but this variability is also reflected between regions of the country. Some of the difference is clearly due to where the 65-and-older population resides within the United States. However, between 2000 and 2025, it also is clear that across the country, states and regions are expected to experience double-digit percentage increases overall in the numbers of people with Alzheimer's. Compared with the numbers of people with Alzheimer's estimated for 2000, the South, Midwest, and West are expected to experience increases that will result in 30–50 percent (and greater) increases over the 25-year period. Some states in the West (Alaska, Colorado, Idaho, Nevada, Utah, and Wyoming) are projected to experience a doubling (or more) of their populations aged 65 and older with Alzheimer's.

The increased numbers of people with Alzheimer's will have a marked impact on states' infrastructures and healthcare systems, not to mention on families and caregivers. Although the projected increases in the Northeast are not nearly as marked as those in other regions of the United States, it should be noted that this section of the country is the residence of a large proportion of people aged 65 and older with Alzheimer's.

These projections also underscore the fact that the impact of Alzheimer's is not equal across the age groups constituting people aged 65 and older. Although there are dramatic increases in Alzheimer's disease across the elderly age groups, an especially significant impact is expected to occur in the 85 and older age groups.

Causes of Dementia

Alzheimer's disease is the most frequent cause of dementia. As shown in Figure 6.1, Alzheimer's accounts for 70 percent of all cases of dementia in Americans aged 71 and older. Vascular dementia accounts for 17 percent of cases of dementia, and other diseases and conditions, including Parkinson's disease, Lewy body disease, frontotemporal dementia, and normal pressure hydrocephalus, account for the remaining 13 percent.

The proportion of cases of dementia attributable to Alzheimer's disease increases with age. In people aged 90 and older, Alzheimer's disease accounts for 80 percent of all dementias compared with 47 percent for people aged 71–79.

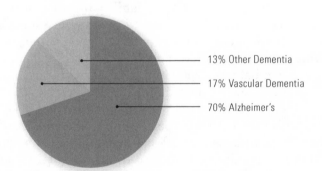

13% Other Dementia

17% Vascular Dementia

70% Alzheimer's

Figure 6.1. *Causes of dementia in people age 71+.*

However, data are beginning to emerge to suggest that attribution of dementia to specific types may not be as clear cut as previously believed. The study by Schneider and colleagues reports that most older community-dwelling residents (mean age at death, approximately 88 years) have changes in the brain suggestive of disease, and that those with dementia often have evidence of multiple types of brain disease.

Of the first 141 autopsies, 80 examined brain tissue from people with intermediate or high likelihood of having Alzheimer's based on clinical evaluation, which included medical history, neuropsychological tests, and physical examination with an emphasis on neurologic function.

Less than half of the 80 autopsies showed evidence of Alzheimer's alone. Nearly a third showed evidence of Alzheimer's and infarcts; 15 percent showed evidence of Alzheimer's and Parkinson's disease/Lewy body disease; 5 percent showed evidence of all three diseases; and 2.5 percent showed evidence of Alzheimer's and brain disease other than infarcts and Parkinson's disease/Lewy body disease. Although 50 percent of participants with no or low likelihood of having Alzheimer's disease based on clinical evaluation also had no evidence of dementia on autopsy, approximately one-third showed evidence of brain infarcts. Thus, there is reason to believe that the causes of dementia may be much more complicated than originally believed.

Looking to the Future

The number of Americans surviving into their 80s and 90s and beyond is expected to grow because of advances in medicine and medical technology, as well as social and environmental conditions. Since the incidence and prevalence of Alzheimer's disease and other dementias increase with age, the number of people with these conditions will also grow rapidly.

- In 2000, there were an estimated 411,000 new (incident) cases of Alzheimer's disease. By 2010, that number is expected to increase to 454,000 new cases per year; by 2029, to 615,000; and by 2050, to 959,000.

- In 2011, the first baby boomers will turn 65. By 2029, all baby boomers will be at least 65 years old.

- The 85 years and older population currently comprises nearly 50 percent of the individuals with Alzheimer's disease, or about 2.7 million people. By the time the first wave of baby boomers reaches age 85 years (2031), there will be an estimated 3.5 million people aged 85 and older with Alzheimer's.

- The number of people aged 65 and older with Alzheimer's disease is estimated to reach 7.7 million in 2030, more than a 50 percent increase from the 5.1 million aged 65 and older who are currently affected.

- By 2050, the number of individuals aged 65 and older with Alzheimer's is projected to number between 11 million and 16 million—unless medical breakthroughs identify ways to prevent or more effectively treat the disease. Barring such developments, by that date, more than 60 percent of people with Alzheimer's disease will be aged 85 or older.

Mortality

Alzheimer's disease was the sixth leading cause of death across all ages in the United States in 2006. It was the fifth-leading cause of death for those aged 65 and older.

In 2006, Alzheimer's disease was reported as the underlying cause of death for 72,914 people. However, underreporting of Alzheimer's disease as an underlying cause of death has been well documented. Death rates from the disease can vary a great deal across states and result from differences in state demographics and reporting practices. On the other hand, death rates among people with Alzheimer's disease dramatically increase with age. From one community-based, 15-year prospective study, the mortality rate for people aged 75–84 with Alzheimer's was nearly 2.5 times greater than for those aged 55–74 with the disease. At age 85 and older, the rate was nearly twice that of those with Alzheimer's aged 75–84. Two-thirds of those dying of dementia did so in nursing homes, compared with 20 percent of cancer patients and 28 percent of people dying from all other conditions.

Deaths from Alzheimer's Disease

While the total number of deaths attributed to other major causes of deaths has been decreasing, those due to Alzheimer's have continued to increase. In 1991, only 14,112 death certificates recorded Alzheimer's disease as the underlying cause. Comparing changes in selected causes of death between 2000 and 2006, deaths attributed to Alzheimer's disease increased 47.1 percent, while those attributed to the number one cause of death, heart disease, decreased 11.5 percent.

Although deaths attributed to Alzheimer's are increasing, under-reporting of this condition on death certificates results in significant underestimates of the public health impact of Alzheimer's. A number of studies have documented substantial underreporting of Alzheimer's disease on death certificates as an underlying or contributory cause of death. Underreporting Alzheimer's disease as the cause of death occurs in the community, as well as in nursing homes.

An increased risk of death may also apply to people newly diagnosed with Alzheimer's. One 2004 study noted that people newly diagnosed with Alzheimer's survived about half as long as those of similar age who did not have the disease. In this study, average survival time was 4 to 6 years after diagnosis, but survival can be as long as 20 years from the first symptoms (although these early symptoms may be fairly subtle and not immediately recognized).

The mechanisms by which dementia leads to death may create ambiguity about the underlying cause of death. Severe dementia frequently causes such complications as immobility, swallowing disorders, or malnutrition. These complications can significantly increase the risk of developing pneumonia, which has been found in several studies to be the most commonly identified cause of death among elderly people with Alzheimer's disease and other dementias. One researcher described the situation as a "blurred distinction between death with dementia and death from dementia."

State-by-State Deaths from Alzheimer's Disease

In terms of relative comparisons, the highest age-adjusted rates for deaths due to Alzheimer's occurred in southern states (Alabama, Louisiana, South Carolina, and Tennessee), with the exceptions of Arizona and Washington State. The age-adjusted rate for Florida would suggest, on the surface, that the risk of mortality from Alzheimer's is more modest in that state compared with others. Florida is home to a large number of people aged 65 years and older, and this is the age group at highest risk for Alzheimer's and death from this disease. However, it may well be that the large number of active, healthy retirees aged 65 years and older living in the state have an impact on producing the more modest levels for age-adjusted relative risks.

Death Rates by Age, Gender, and Ethnicity

Although Alzheimer's disease and death from Alzheimer's can occur in people under age 65, the primary occurrence is in the elderly. However, as can be seen in Table 6.1, death rates for Alzheimer's increase dramatically between the elderly age groups of 65–74, 75–84, and 85+. Increased rates are also apparent between 2004 and 2005 for these older age groups. To put these age-related differences into perspective, for U.S. deaths in 2005, the differences in total mortality rates between 65–74 years and 75–84 years was 2.5-fold, and between 75–84 years and aged 85 and older, 2.6-fold. For diseases of the heart, the differences were 2.9-fold and 3.2-fold, respectively. For all cancers, the differences were 1.7-fold and 1.3-fold respectively. The corresponding differences for Alzheimer's were 8.6-fold and 4.9-fold. The large increase in death rates due to Alzheimer's among America's oldest age groups underscores the impact of having neither a cure for Alzheimer's nor highly effective treatments.

In 2005, the Alzheimer's death rate for females was approximately twice that of males, and this relationship was seen across racial and ethnic groups. White females had the highest death rates for Alzheimer's disease. As can be seen in Table 6.2, there was substantial variability in rates among the racial groups and by gender. However, it should be noted that the lower death rates in non-Hispanic blacks and those of Hispanic origin probably reflect the relatively younger age distributions for those two groups, as compared with non-Hispanic whites, rather than a true lower occurrence of Alzheimer's.

Table 6.1. U.S. Alzheimer Death Rates (per 100,000) by Age, 2000, 2004, and 2005

Age	2000	2004	2005
45–54	0.2	0.2	0.2
55–64	2.0	1.9	2.1
65–74	18.7	19.7	20.5
75–84	139.6	168.7	177.3
85+	667.7	818.8	861.6

Table 6.2. U.S. Alzheimer Death Rates (per 100,000) by Race/Ethnicity and Gender, 2005

	Male	Female
All races*	14.1	33.9
Non-Hispanic Black	7.2	16.9
Hispanic	3.5	7.0
Non-Hispanic White	18.5	44.8

*The lower death rates in non-Hispanic blacks and those of Hispanic origin probably reflect the relatively younger age distributions for those two groups, compared to non-Hispanic whites, rather than a true lower occurrence of Alzheimer's.

Location of Death

A study of national death certificates for 2001 found that 66.9 percent of people aged 65 and older who died of dementia did so in nursing homes. In contrast, 20.6 percent of patients dying from cancer died in nursing homes. Among those dying of other conditions, 28 percent died in nursing homes. Location of death varied significantly across regions of the country. For example, the percentage of dementia deaths in hospitals ranged from 5 percent in Rhode Island to 37 percent in the District of Columbia. Those with dementia died more frequently in the hospital in the Southeastern states.

Part Two

Alzheimer Disease (AD): The Most Common Type of Dementia

Chapter 7

Facts about AD

Alzheimer disease is an irreversible, progressive brain disease that slowly destroys memory and thinking skills, and eventually even the ability to carry out the simplest tasks. In most people with Alzheimer disease, symptoms first appear after age 60.

Alzheimer disease is the most common cause of dementia among older people. Dementia is the loss of cognitive functioning—thinking, remembering, and reasoning—to such an extent that it interferes with a person's daily life and activities. Estimates vary, but experts suggest that as many as 5.1 million Americans may have Alzheimer disease.

Alzheimer disease is named after Dr. Alois Alzheimer. In 1906, Dr. Alzheimer noticed changes in the brain tissue of a woman who had died of an unusual mental illness. Her symptoms included memory loss, language problems, and unpredictable behavior. After she died, he examined her brain and found many abnormal clumps (now called amyloid plaques) and tangled bundles of fibers (now called neurofibrillary tangles). Plaques and tangles in the brain are two of the main features of Alzheimer disease. The third is the loss of connections between nerve cells (neurons) in the brain.

Changes in the Brain in Alzheimer Disease

Although we still don't know what starts the Alzheimer disease process, we do know that damage to the brain begins as many as 10

From "Alzheimer's Disease Fact Sheet," by the National Institute on Aging (NIA, www.nia.nih.gov), part of the National Institutes of Health, February 2010.

to 20 years before any problems are evident. Tangles begin to develop deep in the brain, in an area called the entorhinal cortex, and plaques form in other areas. As more and more plaques and tangles form in particular brain areas, healthy neurons begin to work less efficiently. Then, they lose their ability to function and communicate with each other, and eventually they die. This damaging process spreads to a nearby structure, called the hippocampus, which is essential in forming memories. As the death of neurons increases, affected brain regions begin to shrink. By the final stage of Alzheimer disease, damage is widespread and brain tissue has shrunk significantly.

Very Early Signs and Symptoms

Memory problems are one of the first signs of Alzheimer disease. Some people with memory problems have a condition called amnestic mild cognitive impairment (MCI). People with this condition have more memory problems than normal for people their age, but their symptoms are not as severe as those with Alzheimer disease. More people with MCI, compared with those without MCI, go on to develop Alzheimer disease.

Other changes may also signal the very early stages of Alzheimer disease. For example, brain imaging and biomarker studies of people with MCI and those with a family history of Alzheimer disease are beginning to detect early changes in the brain like those seen in Alzheimer disease. These findings will need to be confirmed by other studies but appear promising. Other recent research has found links between some movement difficulties and MCI. Researchers also have seen links between some problems with the sense of smell and cognitive problems. Such findings offer hope that someday we may have tools that could help detect Alzheimer disease early, track the course of the disease, and monitor response to treatments.

Mild Alzheimer Disease

As Alzheimer disease progresses, memory loss continues and changes in other cognitive abilities appear. Problems can include getting lost, trouble handling money and paying bills, repeating questions, taking longer to complete normal daily tasks, poor judgment, and small mood and personality changes. People often are diagnosed in this stage.

Moderate Alzheimer Disease

In this stage, damage occurs in areas of the brain that control language, reasoning, sensory processing, and conscious thought. Memory loss and confusion increase, and people begin to have problems recognizing family and friends. They may be unable to learn new things, carry out tasks that involve multiple steps (such as getting dressed), or cope with new situations. They may have hallucinations, delusions, and paranoia, and may behave impulsively.

Severe Alzheimer Disease

By the final stage, plaques and tangles have spread throughout the brain and brain tissue has shrunk significantly. People with severe Alzheimer disease cannot communicate and are completely dependent on others for their care. Near the end, the person may be in bed most or all of the time as the body shuts down.

What Causes Alzheimer Disease

Scientists don't yet fully understand what causes Alzheimer disease, but it is clear that it develops because of a complex series of events that take place in the brain over a long period of time. It is likely that the causes include genetic, environmental, and lifestyle factors. Because people differ in their genetic make-up and lifestyle, the importance of these factors for preventing or delaying Alzheimer disease differs from person to person.

The Basics of Alzheimer Disease

Scientists are conducting studies to learn more about plaques, tangles, and other features of Alzheimer disease. They can now visualize plaques by imaging the brains of living individuals. They are also exploring the very earliest steps in the disease process. Findings from these studies will help them understand the causes of Alzheimer disease.

One of the great mysteries of Alzheimer disease is why it largely strikes older adults. Research on how the brain changes normally with age is shedding light on this question. For example, scientists are learning how age-related changes in the brain may harm neurons and contribute to Alzheimer damage. These age-related changes include atrophy (shrinking) of certain parts of the brain, inflammation, and the production of unstable molecules called free radicals.

Genetics

In a very few families, people develop Alzheimer disease in their 30s, 40s, and 50s. Many of these people have a mutation, or permanent change, in one of three genes that they inherited from a parent. We know that these gene mutations cause Alzheimer disease in these "early-onset" familial cases. Not all early-onset cases are caused by such mutations.

Most people with Alzheimer disease have "late-onset" Alzheimer disease, which usually develops after age 60. Many studies have linked a gene called APOE to late-onset Alzheimer disease. This gene has several forms. One of them, APOE e4, increases a person's risk of getting the disease. About 40 percent of all people who develop late-onset Alzheimer disease carry this gene. However, carrying the APOE e4 form of the gene does not necessarily mean that a person will develop Alzheimer disease, and people carrying no APOE e4 forms can also develop the disease.

Most experts believe that additional genes may influence the development of late-onset Alzheimer disease in some way. Scientists around the world are searching for these genes. Researchers have identified variants of the SORL1, CLU, PICALM, and CR1 genes that may play a role in risk of late-onset Alzheimer disease.

Lifestyle Factors

A nutritious diet, physical activity, social engagement, and mentally stimulating pursuits can all help people stay healthy. New research suggests the possibility that these factors also might help to reduce the risk of cognitive decline and Alzheimer disease. Scientists are investigating associations between cognitive decline and vascular and metabolic conditions such as heart disease, stroke, high blood pressure, diabetes, and obesity. Understanding these relationships and testing them in clinical trials will help us understand whether reducing risk factors for these diseases may help with Alzheimer disease as well.

How Alzheimer Disease Is Diagnosed

Alzheimer disease can be definitively diagnosed only after death by linking clinical course with an examination of brain tissue and pathology in an autopsy. But doctors now have several methods and tools to help them determine fairly accurately whether a person who is having memory problems has "possible Alzheimer disease" (dementia may be due to another cause) or "probable Alzheimer disease" (no other cause for dementia can be found). To diagnose Alzheimer disease, doctors do the following:

- Ask questions about the person's overall health, past medical problems, ability to carry out daily activities, and changes in behavior and personality

- Conduct tests of memory, problem solving, attention, counting, and language

- Carry out medical tests, such as tests of blood, urine, or spinal fluid

- Perform brain scans, such as computerized tomography (CT) or magnetic resonance imaging (MRI)

These tests may be repeated to give doctors information about how the person's memory is changing over time.

Early diagnosis is beneficial for several reasons. Having an early diagnosis and starting treatment in the early stages of the disease can help preserve function for months to years, even though the underlying disease process cannot be changed. Having an early diagnosis also helps families plan for the future, make living arrangements, take care of financial and legal matters, and develop support networks.

In addition, an early diagnosis can provide greater opportunities for people to get involved in clinical trials. In a clinical trial, scientists test drugs or treatments to see which are most effective and for whom they work best.

How Alzheimer Disease Is Treated

Alzheimer disease is a complex disease, and no single "magic bullet" is likely to prevent or cure it. That's why current treatments focus on several different aspects, including helping people maintain mental function; managing behavioral symptoms; and slowing, delaying, or preventing the disease.

Helping People with Alzheimer Disease Maintain Mental Function

Four medications are approved by the U.S. Food and Drug Administration to treat Alzheimer disease. Donepezil (Aricept®), rivastigmine (Exelon®), and galantamine (Razadyne®) are used to treat mild to moderate Alzheimer disease (donepezil can be used for severe Alzheimer disease as well). Memantine (Namenda®) is used to treat moderate to severe Alzheimer disease. These drugs work by regulating neurotransmitters (the chemicals that transmit messages between neurons). They may help maintain thinking, memory, and speaking skills, and help with certain behavioral problems. However, these drugs don't change the underlying disease process and may help only for a few months to a few years.

Managing Behavioral Symptoms

Common behavioral symptoms of Alzheimer disease include sleeplessness, agitation, wandering, anxiety, anger, and depression. Scientists are learning why these symptoms occur and are studying new treatments—drug and non-drug—to manage them. Treating behavioral symptoms often makes people with Alzheimer disease more comfortable and makes their care easier for caregivers.

Slowing, Delaying, or Preventing Alzheimer Disease

Alzheimer disease research has developed to a point where scientists can look beyond treating symptoms to think about addressing the underlying disease process. In ongoing clinical trials, scientists are looking at many possible interventions, such as cardiovascular and diabetes treatments, antioxidants, immunization therapy, cognitive training, and physical activity.

Supporting Families and Caregivers

Caring for a person with Alzheimer disease can have high physical, emotional, and financial costs. The demands of day-to-day care, changing family roles, and difficult decisions about placement in a care facility can be hard to handle. Researchers are learning a lot about Alzheimer caregiving, and studies are helping experts develop new ways to support caregivers.

Becoming well-informed about the disease is one important long-term strategy. Programs that teach families about the various stages of Alzheimer disease and about flexible and practical strategies for dealing with difficult caregiving situations provide vital help to those who care for people with Alzheimer disease.

Developing good coping skills and a strong support network of family and friends also are important ways that caregivers can help themselves handle the stresses of caring for a loved one with Alzheimer disease. For example, staying physically active provides physical and emotional benefits.

Some Alzheimer caregivers have found that participating in a support group is a critical lifeline. These support groups allow caregivers to find respite, express concerns, share experiences, get tips, and receive emotional comfort. The Alzheimer's Association, Alzheimer's Disease Centers, and many other organizations sponsor in-person and online support groups across the country. There are a growing number of groups for people in the early stage of Alzheimer disease and their families. Support networks can be especially valuable when caregivers face the difficult decision of whether and when to place a loved one in a nursing home or assisted living facility.

Advancing Our Understanding

Thirty years ago, we knew very little about Alzheimer disease. Since then, scientists have made many important advances. Research supported by NIA and other organizations has expanded knowledge of brain function in healthy older people, identified ways we might lessen normal age-related declines in mental function, and deepened our understanding of the disease. Many scientists and physicians are now working together to untangle the genetic, biological, and environmental factors that, over many years, ultimately result in Alzheimer disease. This effort is bringing us closer to the day when we will be able to manage successfully or even prevent this devastating disease.

Chapter 8

What Happens to the Brain in AD?

The Hallmarks of Alzheimer Disease (AD)

AD disrupts critical metabolic processes that keep neurons healthy. These disruptions cause nerve cells in the brain to stop working, lose connections with other nerve cells, and finally die. The destruction and death of nerve cells causes the memory failure, personality changes, problems in carrying out daily activities, and other features of the disease.

The brains of people with AD have an abundance of two abnormal structures—amyloid plaques and neurofibrillary tangles—that are made of misfolded proteins. This is especially true in certain regions of the brain that are important in memory.

The third main feature of AD is the loss of connections between cells. This leads to diminished cell function and cell death.

Amyloid Plaques

Amyloid plaques are found in the spaces between the brain's nerve cells. They were first described by Dr. Alois Alzheimer in 1906. Plaques consist of largely insoluble deposits of an apparently toxic protein peptide, or fragment, called beta-amyloid.

We now know that some people develop some plaques in their brain tissue as they age. However, the AD brain has many more plaques in

---

Excerpted from "Alzheimer's Disease: Unraveling the Mystery," by the National Institute on Aging (NIA, www.nia.nih.gov), part of the National Institutes of Health, September 2008.

particular brain regions. We still do not know whether amyloid plaques themselves cause AD or whether they are a byproduct of the AD process. We do know that genetic mutations can increase production of beta-amyloid and can cause rare, inherited forms of AD.

Neurofibrillary Tangles

The second hallmark of AD, also described by Dr. Alzheimer, is neurofibrillary tangles. Tangles are abnormal collections of twisted protein threads found inside nerve cells. The chief component of tangles is a protein called tau.

Healthy neurons are internally supported in part by structures called microtubules, which help transport nutrients and other cellular components, such as neurotransmitter-containing vesicles, from the cell body down the axon.

Tau, which usually has a certain number of phosphate molecules attached to it, binds to microtubules and appears to stabilize them. In AD, an abnormally large number of additional phosphate molecules attach to tau. As a result of this hyperphosphorylation, tau disengages from the microtubules and begins to come together with other tau threads. These tau threads form structures called paired helical filaments, which can become enmeshed with one another, forming tangles within the cell. The microtubules can disintegrate in the process, collapsing the neuron's internal transport network. This collapse damages the ability of neurons to communicate with each other.

Loss of Connection between Cells and Cell Death

The third major feature of AD is the gradual loss of connections between neurons. Neurons live to communicate with each other, and this vital function takes place at the synapse. Since the 1980s, new knowledge about plaques and tangles has provided important insights into their possible damage to synapses and on the development of AD.

The AD process not only inhibits communication between neurons but can also damage neurons to the point that they cannot function properly and eventually die. As neurons die throughout the brain, affected regions begin to shrink in a process called brain atrophy. By the final stage of AD, damage is widespread, and brain tissue has shrunk significantly.

The Changing Brain in AD

No one knows exactly what starts the AD process or why some of the normal changes associated with aging become so much more extreme and destructive in people with the disease. We know a lot, however, about what happens in the brain once AD takes hold and about the physical and mental changes that occur over time. The time from diagnosis to death varies—as little as 3 or 4 years if the person is older than 80 when diagnosed to as long as 10 or more years if the person is younger. Several other factors besides age also affect how long a person will live with AD. These factors include the person's sex, the presence of other health problems, and the severity of cognitive problems at diagnosis. Although the course of the disease is not the same in every person with AD, symptoms seem to develop over the same general stages. For a visual representation of how AD spreads, see Figure 8.1.

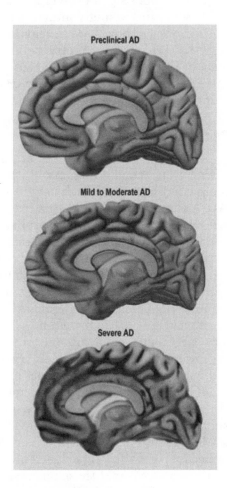

Figure 8.1. AD spreads through the brain.

Preclinical AD

AD begins deep in the brain, in the entorhinal cortex, a brain region that is near the hippocampus and has direct connections to it. Healthy neurons in this region begin to work less efficiently, lose their ability to communicate, and ultimately die. This process gradually spreads to the hippocampus, the brain region that plays a major role in learning and is involved in converting short-term memories to long-term memories. Affected regions begin to atrophy. Ventricles, the fluid-filled spaces inside the brain, begin to enlarge as the process continues.

Scientists believe that these brain changes begin 10 to 20 years before any clinically detectable signs or symptoms of forgetfulness appear. That's why they are increasingly interested in the very early stages of the disease process. They hope to learn more about what happens in the brain that sets a person on the path to developing AD. By knowing more about the early stages, they also hope to be able to develop drugs or other treatments that will slow or stop the disease process before significant impairment occurs.

Very Early Signs and Symptoms

At some point, the damage occurring in the brain begins to show itself in very early clinical signs and symptoms. Much research is being done to identify these early changes, which may be useful in predicting dementia or AD. An important part of this research effort is the development of increasingly sophisticated neuroimaging techniques and the use of biomarkers. Biomarkers are indicators, such as changes in sensory abilities, or substances that appear in body fluids, such as blood, cerebrospinal fluid, or urine. Biomarkers can indicate exposure to a substance, the presence of a disease, or the progression over time of a disease. For example, high blood cholesterol is a biomarker for risk of heart disease. Such tools are critical to helping scientists detect and understand the very early signs and symptoms of AD.

As some people grow older, they develop memory problems greater than those expected for their age. But they do not experience the personality changes or other problems that are characteristic of AD. These people may have a condition called mild cognitive impairment (MCI). MCI has several subtypes. The type most associated with memory loss is called amnestic MCI. People with MCI are a critically important group for research because a much higher percentage of them go on to develop AD than do people without these memory problems. About eight of every 10 people who fit the definition of amnestic MCI go on to develop AD within 7 years. In contrast, 1 to 3 percent of people older than 65 who have normal cognition will develop AD in any one year.

However, researchers are not yet able to say definitively why some people with amnestic MCI do not progress to AD, nor can they say who will or will not go on to develop AD. This raises pressing questions, such as: In cases when MCI progresses to AD, what was happening in the brain that made that transition possible? Can MCI be prevented or its progress to AD delayed?

Scientists also have found that genetic factors may play a role in MCI, as they do in AD. And, they have found that different brain regions appear to be activated during certain mental activities in cognitively healthy people and those with MCI. These changes appear to be related to the early stages of cognitive impairment.

As scientists have sharpened their focus on the early stages of AD, they have begun to see hints of other changes that may signal a developing disease process. For example, in the Religious Orders Study, a large AD research effort that involves older nuns, priests, and religious brothers, investigators have explored whether changes in older adults' ability to move about and use their bodies might be a sign of early AD. The researchers found that participants with MCI had more movement difficulties than the cognitively healthy participants but less than those with AD. Moreover, those with MCI who had lots of trouble moving their legs and feet were more than twice as likely to develop AD as those with good lower body function.

It is not yet clear why people with MCI might have these motor function problems, but the scientists who conducted the study speculate that they may be a sign that damage to blood vessels in the brain or damage from AD is accumulating in areas of the brain responsible for motor function. If further research shows that some people with MCI do have motor function problems in addition to memory problems, the degree of difficulty, especially with walking, may help identify those at risk of progressing to AD.

Other scientists have focused on changes in sensory abilities as possible indicators of early cognitive problems. For example, in one study they found associations between a decline in the ability to detect odors and cognitive problems or dementia.

These findings are tentative, but they are promising because they suggest that, some day, it may be possible to develop ways to improve early detection of MCI or AD. These tools also will help scientists answer questions about causes and very early development of AD, track changes in brain and cognitive function over time, and ultimately track a person's response to treatment for AD.

Mild AD

As AD spreads through the brain, the number of plaques and tangles grows, shrinkage progresses, and more and more of the cerebral cortex is affected. Memory loss continues and changes in other cognitive abilities begin to emerge. The clinical diagnosis of AD is usually made during this stage. Signs of mild AD can include the following:

- Memory loss
- Confusion about the location of familiar places (getting lost begins to occur)
- Taking longer than before to accomplish normal daily tasks
- Trouble handling money and paying bills
- Poor judgment leading to bad decisions
- Loss of spontaneity and sense of initiative
- Mood and personality changes, increased anxiety and/or aggression

In mild AD, a person may seem to be healthy but is actually having more and more trouble making sense of the world around him or her. The realization that something is wrong often comes gradually to the person and his or her family.

Accepting these signs as something other than normal and deciding to go for diagnostic tests can be a big hurdle for people and families. Once this hurdle is overcome, many families are relieved to know what is causing the problems. They also can take comfort in the fact that despite a diagnosis of MCI or early AD, a person can still make meaningful contributions to his or her family and to society for a time.

Moderate AD

By this stage, AD damage has spread to the areas of the cerebral cortex that control language, reasoning, sensory processing, and conscious thought. Affected regions continue to shrink, ventricles enlarge, and signs and symptoms of the disease become more pronounced and widespread. Behavioral problems, such as wandering and agitation, can occur. More intensive supervision and care become necessary, which can be difficult for many spouses and families. The symptoms of this stage can include the following:

- Increasing memory loss and confusion
- Shortened attention span

- Inappropriate outbursts of anger

- Problems recognizing friends and family members

- Difficulty with language and problems with reading, writing, and working with numbers

- Difficulty organizing thoughts and thinking logically

- Inability to learn new things or to cope with new or unexpected situations

- Restlessness, agitation, anxiety, tearfulness, wandering— especially in the late afternoon or at night

- Repetitive statements or movement, occasional muscle twitches

- Hallucinations, delusions, suspiciousness or paranoia, irritability

- Loss of impulse control (shown through undressing at inappropriate times or places or vulgar language)

- An inability to carry out activities that involve multiple steps in sequence, such as dressing, making a pot of coffee, or setting the table

Behavior is the result of complex brain processes, all of which take place in a fraction of a second in the healthy brain. In AD, many of those processes are disturbed, and these disrupted communications between neurons are the basis for many distressing or inappropriate behaviors. For example, a person may angrily refuse to take a bath or get dressed because he does not understand what his caregiver has asked him to do. If he does understand, he may not remember how to do it. The anger can be a mask for his confusion and anxiety. Or, a person with AD may constantly follow her husband or caregiver and fret when the person is out of sight. To a person who cannot remember the past or anticipate the future, the world can be strange and frightening. Sticking close to a trusted and familiar caregiver may be the only thing that makes sense and provides security.

Severe AD

In the last stage of AD, plaques and tangles are widespread throughout the brain, most areas of the brain have shrunk further, and ventricles have enlarged even more. People with AD cannot recognize family and loved ones or communicate in any way. They are completely dependent on others for care. Other symptoms can include the following:

- Weight loss

- Seizures

- Skin infections

- Difficulty swallowing

- Groaning, moaning, or grunting

- Increased sleeping

- Lack of bladder and bowel control

Near the end, the person may be in bed much or all of the time. The most frequent cause of death for people with AD is aspiration pneumonia. This type of pneumonia develops when a person is not able to swallow properly and takes food or liquids into the lungs instead of air.

Chapter 9

Signs and Symptoms of AD

Chapter Contents

Section 9.1

Seven Warning Signs of AD

"The Seven Warning Signs of Alzheimer's Disease," © Eric Pfeiffer, MD. Reprinted with permission from the Suncoast Alzheimer's Gerontology Center at the University of South Florida College of Medicine (http://health.usf .edu/medicine/suncoastalzheimers). This document is undated. Reviewed by David A. Cooke, MD, FACP, February 17, 2011.

The purpose of this list is to alert the public to the early warning signs of one of the most devastating disorders affecting older people—Alzheimer's disease. If someone has several or even most of these symptoms, it does not mean that they definitely have the disease. It does mean that they should be thoroughly examined by a medical specialist trained in evaluating memory disorders, such as a neurologist or a psychiatrist, or by a comprehensive memory disorder clinic, with an entire team of experts knowledgeable about memory problems.

The seven warning signs of Alzheimer's disease are:

1. Asking the same question over and over again.

2. Repeating the same story, word for word, again and again.

3. Forgetting how to cook, or how to make repairs, or how to play cards—activities that were previously done with ease and regularity.

4. Losing one's ability to pay bills or balance one's checkbook.

5. Getting lost in familiar surroundings, or misplacing household objects.

6. Neglecting to bathe, or wearing the same clothes over and over again, while insisting that they have taken a bath or that their clothes are still clean.

7. Relying on someone else, such as a spouse, to make decisions or answer questions they previously would have handled themselves.

Section 9.2

Symptoms of AD

From "Understanding Stages and Symptoms of Alzheimer's Disease," by the National Institute on Aging (NIA, www.nia.nih.gov), part of the National Institutes of Health, February 5, 2009. Adapted from *Caring for People with Alzheimer's Disease: A Manual for Facility Staff* (2nd edition), by Lisa P. Gwyther, 2001. Published by the American Health Care Association (1201 L Street, NW, Washington, DC 20005) and the Alzheimer's Association (919 N. Michigan Ave., Suite 1100, Chicago, IL 60611).

Alzheimer disease (AD) develops slowly and causes changes in the brain long before there are obvious changes in a person's memory, thinking, use of words, or behavior. Stages and changes the person will go through are outlined in the following text.

Common Changes in Mild AD

- Loses spark or zest for life—does not start anything

- Loses recent memory without a change in appearance or casual conversation

- Loses judgment about money

- Has difficulty with new learning and making new memories

- Has trouble finding words—may substitute or make up words that sound like or mean something like the forgotten word

- May stop talking to avoid making mistakes

- Has shorter attention span and less motivation to stay with an activity

- Easily loses way going to familiar places

- Resists change or new things

- Has trouble organizing and thinking logically

- Asks repetitive questions

- Withdraws, loses interest, is irritable, not as sensitive to others' feelings, uncharacteristically angry when frustrated or tired

- Won't make decisions—for example, when asked what she wants to eat, says "I'll have what she is having"

- Takes longer to do routine chores and becomes upset if rushed or if something unexpected happens

- Forgets to pay, pays too much, or forgets how to pay—may hand the checkout person a wallet instead of the correct amount of money

- Forgets to eat, eats only one kind of food, or eats constantly

- Loses or misplaces things by hiding them in odd places or forgets where things go, such as putting clothes in the dishwasher

- Constantly checks, searches, or hoards things of no value

Common Changes in Moderate AD

- Changes in behavior, concern for appearance, hygiene, and sleep become more noticeable

- Mixes up identity of people, such as thinking a son is a brother or that a wife is a stranger

- Poor judgment creates safety issues when left alone—may wander and risk exposure, poisoning, falls, self-neglect, or exploitation

- Has trouble recognizing familiar people and own objects; may take things that belong to others

- Continuously repeats stories, favorite words, statements, or motions like tearing tissues

- Has restless, repetitive movements in late afternoon or evening, such as pacing, trying doorknobs, fingering draperies

- Cannot organize thoughts or follow logical explanations

- Has trouble following written notes or completing tasks

- Makes up stories to fill in gaps in memory—for example might say, "Mama will come for me when she gets off work"

- May be able to read but cannot formulate the correct response to a written request

- May accuse, threaten, curse, fidget, or behave inappropriately, such as kicking, hitting, biting, screaming, or grabbing

- May become sloppy or forget manners

- May see, hear, smell, or taste things that are not there

- May accuse spouse of an affair or family members of stealing

- Naps frequently or awakens at night believing it is time to go to work

- Has more difficulty positioning the body to use the toilet or sit in a chair

- May think mirror image is following him or television story is happening to her

- Needs help finding the toilet, using the shower, remembering to drink, and dressing for the weather or occasion

- Exhibits inappropriate sexual behavior, such as mistaking another individual for a spouse; forgets what is private behavior, and may disrobe or masturbate in public

Common Changes in Severe AD

- Doesn't recognize self or close family

- Speaks in gibberish, is mute, or is difficult to understand

- May refuse to eat, chokes, or forgets to swallow

- May repetitively cry out, pat, or touch everything

- Loses control of bowel and bladder

- Loses weight and skin becomes thin and tears easily

- May look uncomfortable or cry out when transferred or touched

- Forgets how to walk or is too unsteady or weak to stand alone

- May have seizures, frequent infections, falls

- May groan, scream, or mumble loudly

- Sleeps more

- Needs total assistance for all activities of daily living

Chapter 10

Clinical Stages of AD

New York University's Dr. Barry Reisberg outlines the seven major clinical stages of Alzheimer's disease. Dr. Reisberg is the Clinical Director of New York University's Aging and Dementia Research Center. As the principal investigator of studies conducted by the National Institutes of Health, Dr. Reisberg's work has been pivotal in the development of two of the three current pharmaceutical treatment modalities for Alzheimer's. He developed the "Global Deterioration Scale" which is now used in many diagnoses and care settings as the rating scale.

Stage 1: Normal

At any age, persons may potentially be free of objective or subjective symptoms of cognition and functional decline and also free of associated behavioral and mood changes. We call these mentally healthy persons at any age, stage 1, or normal.

Stage 2: Normal Aged Forgetfulness

Half or more of the population of persons over the age of 65 experience subjective complaints of cognitive and/or functional difficulties. The nature of these subjective complaints is characteristic. Elderly

---

"Clinical Stages of Alzheimer's Disease," © 2010 Fisher Center for Alzheimer's Research Foundation. Reprinted with permission. For additional information, visit www.alzinfo.com.

persons with these symptoms believe they can no longer recall names as well as they could 5 or 10 years previously. They also frequently develop the conviction that they can no longer recall where they have placed things as well as previously. Subjectively experienced difficulties in concentration and in finding the correct word when speaking, are also common.

Various terms have been suggested for this condition, but normal aged forgetfulness is probably the most satisfactory terminology. These symptoms which, by definition, are not notable to intimates or other external observers of the person with normal aged forgetfulness, are generally benign. However, there is some recent evidence that persons with these symptoms do decline at greater rates than similarly aged persons and similarly healthy persons who are free of subjective complaints.

Stage 3: Mild Cognitive Impairment

Persons at this stage manifest deficits which are subtle, but which are noted by persons who are closely associated with the stage 3 subject. The subtle deficits may become manifest in diverse ways. For example, the person with mild cognitive impairment (MCI) may noticeably repeat queries. The capacity to perform executive functions also becomes compromised. Commonly, for persons who are still working, job performance may decline. For those who must master new job skills, decrements in these capacities may become evident. For example, the MCI subject may be unable to master new computer skills. MCI subjects who are not employed, but who plan complex social events, such as dinner parties, may manifest declines in their ability to organize such events.

Other MCI subjects may manifest concentration deficits. Many persons with these symptoms begin to experience anxiety, which may be overtly evident.

The prognosis for persons with these subtle symptoms of impairment is variable, even when a select subject group who are free of overt medical or psychological conditions which might account for, or contribute to, the impairments are studied. A substantial proportion of these persons will not decline, even when followed over the course of many years. However, in a majority of persons with stage 3 symptoms, overt decline will occur, and clear symptoms of dementia will become manifest over intervals of approximately 2 to 4 years. In persons who are not called upon to perform complex occupational and/or social tasks, symptoms in this stage may not become evident to family members or friends of the MCI patient. Even when symptoms do become noticeable, MCI subjects are commonly midway or near the end of this stage before concerns result in clinical consultation. Consequently, although progression to the next stage in MCI subjects commonly occurs in 2 to 3 years, the true duration of this stage, when it is a harbinger of subsequently manifest dementia, is probably approximately 7 years.

Management of persons in this stage includes counseling regarding the desirability of continuing in a complex and demanding occupational role. Sometimes, a "strategic withdrawal" in the form of retirement, may alleviate psychological stress and reduce both subjective and overtly manifest anxiety.

Stage 4: Mild Alzheimer's Disease

The diagnosis of Alzheimer's disease can be made with considerable accuracy in this stage. The most common functioning deficit in these patients is a decreased ability to manage instrumental (complex) activities of daily life. Examples of common deficits include decreased ability to manage finances, to prepare meals for guests, and to market for oneself and one's family. The stage 4 patient shown has difficulty writing the correct date and the correct amount on the check. Consequently, her husband has to supervise this activity. The mean duration of this stage is 2 years.

Symptoms of impairment become evident in this stage. For example, seemingly major recent events, such as a recent holiday or a recent visit to a relative, may, or may not, be recalled. Similarly, overt mistakes in recalling the day of the week, month, or season of the year may occur. Patients at this stage can still generally recall their correct current address. They can also generally correctly recall the weather conditions outside and very important current events, such as the name of a prominent head of state. Despite the overt deficits in cognition, persons at this stage can still potentially survive independently in community settings. However, functional capacities become compromised in the performance of instrumental (i.e., complex) activities of daily life. For example, there is a decreased capacity to manage personal finances. For the stage 4 patient who is living independently, this may become evident in the form of difficulties in paying rent and other bills. A spouse may note difficulties in writing the correct date and the correct amount in paying checks. The ability to independently market for food and groceries also becomes compromised in this stage. Persons who previously prepared meals for family members and/or guests begin to manifest decreased performance in these skills. Similarly, the ability to order food from a menu in a restaurant setting begins to be compromised. Frequently, this is manifest in the patient handing the menu to the spouse and saying "you order."

The dominant mood at this stage is frequently what psychiatrists term a flattening of affect and withdrawal. In other words, the patient often seems less emotionally responsive than previously. This absence of emotional responsivity is probably intimately related to the patient's denial of their deficit, which is often also notable at this stage. Although the patient is aware of their deficits, this awareness of decreased intellectual capacity is too painful for most persons and, hence, the psychological defense mechanism known as denial, whereby the patient seeks to hide their deficit, even from themselves where possible, becomes operative. In this context, the flattening of affect occurs because the patient is fearful of revealing their deficits. Consequently, the patient withdraws from participation in activities such as conversations.

In the absence of complicating medical pathology, the diagnosis of AD can be made with considerable certainty from the beginning of this stage. Studies indicate that the duration of this stage of mild AD is a mean of approximately 2 years.

Stage 5: Moderate Alzheimer's Disease

In this stage, deficits are of sufficient magnitude as to prevent catastrophe-free, independent community survival. The characteristic functional change in this stage is incipient deficits in basic activities of daily life. This is manifest in a decrement in the ability to choose proper clothing to wear for the weather conditions and/or for the daily circumstances (occasions). Some patients begin to wear the same clothing day after day unless reminded to change. The spouse or other caregiver begins to counsel regarding the choice of clothing. The mean duration of this stage is 1.5 years.

At this stage, deficits are of sufficient magnitude as to prevent independent, catastrophe-free, community survival. Patients can no longer manage on their own in the community. If they are ostensibly alone in the community then there is generally someone who is assisting in providing adequate and proper food, as well as assuring that the rent and utilities are paid and the patient's finances are taken care of. For those who are not properly watched and/or supervised, predatory strangers may become a problem. Very common reactions for persons at this stage who are not given adequate support are behavioral problems such as anger and suspiciousness.

Cognitively, persons at this stage frequently cannot recall such major events and aspects of their current lives such as the name of the current president, the weather conditions of the day, or their correct current address. Characteristically, some of these important aspects of current life are recalled, but not others. Also, the information is loosely held, so, for example, the patient may recall their correct address on certain occasions, but not others.

Remote memory also suffers to the extent that persons may not recall the names of some of the schools which they attended for many years, and from which they graduated. Orientation may be compromised to the extent that the correct year may not be recalled. Calculation deficits are of such magnitude that an educated person has difficulty counting backward from 20 by 2s.

Functionally, persons at this stage have incipient difficulties with basic activities of daily life. The characteristic deficit of this type is decreased ability to independently choose proper clothing. This stage lasts an average of approximately 1.5 years.

Stage 6: Moderately Severe Alzheimer's Disease

At this stage, the ability to perform basic activities of daily life becomes compromised. Functionally, five successive substages are identifiable. Initially, in stage 6a, patients, in addition to having lost the ability to choose their clothing without assistance, begin to require assistance in putting on their clothing properly. Unless supervised, patients may put their clothing on backward, they may have difficulty putting their arm in the correct sleeve, or they may dress themselves in the wrong sequence.

In the stage of moderately severe Alzheimer's disease, the cognitive deficits are of sufficient magnitude as to interfere with the ability to carry out basic activities of daily life. Generally, the earliest such deficit noted in this stage is decreased ability to put on clothing correctly without assistance. The total duration of the stage of moderately severe AD (stage 6a through 6e) is approximately 2.5 years.

For example, patients may put their street clothes on over their night clothes. At approximately the same point in the evolution of AD, but generally just a little later in the temporal sequence, patients lose the ability to bathe independently without assistance (stage 6b). Characteristically, the earliest and most common deficit in bathing is difficulty adjusting the temperature of the bath water. Initially, once the spouse adjusts the temperature of the bath water, the patient can still potentially otherwise bathe independently. Subsequently, as this stage evolves, additional deficits in bathing independently as well as in dressing independently occur. In this 6b substage, patients generally develop deficits in other modalities of daily hygiene such as properly brushing their teeth independently.

Stages 6c, 6d, 6e

With the further evolution of AD, patients lose the ability to manage independently the mechanics of toileting correctly (stage 6c). Unless supervised, patients may place the toilet tissue in the wrong place. Many patients will forget to flush the toilet properly. As the disease evolves in this stage, patients subsequently become incontinent. Generally, urinary incontinence occurs first (stage 6d), then fecal incontinence occurs (stage 6e). The incontinence can be treated, or even initially prevented entirely in many cases, by frequent toileting. Subsequently, strategies for managing incontinence, including appropriate bedding, absorbent undergarments, etc., become necessary.

In this sixth stage cognitive deficits are generally so severe that persons will display little or no knowledge when queried regarding such major aspects of their current life circumstances as their current address or the weather conditions of the day.

Recall of current events is generally deficient to the extent that the patient cannot name the current national head of state or other, similarly prominent newsworthy figures. Persons at this sixth stage will most often not be able to recall the names of any of the schools which they attended. They may, or may not, recall such basic life events as the names of their parents, their former occupation, and the country in which they were born. They still have some knowledge of their own names; however, patients in this stage begin to confuse their spouse with their deceased parent and otherwise mistake the identity of persons, even close family members, in their own environment. Calculation ability is frequently so severely compromised at this stage that even well-educated patients had difficulty counting backward consecutively from 10 by 1s.

Emotional changes generally become most overt and disturbing in this sixth stage of AD. Although these emotional changes may, in part, have a neurochemical basis, they are also clearly related to the patient's psychological reaction to their circumstances. For example, because of their cognitive deficits, patients can no longer channel their energies into productive activities. Consequently, unless appropriate direction is provided, patients begin to fidget, to pace, to move objects around and place items where they may not belong, or to manifest other forms of purposeless or inappropriate activities. Because of the patient's fear, frustration, and shame regarding their circumstances, as well as other factors, patients frequently develop verbal outbursts, and threatening, or even violent, behavior may occur. Because patients can no longer survive independently, they commonly develop a fear of being left alone. Treatment of these and other behavioral and psychological symptoms which occur at this stage, as well as at other stages of AD, involves counseling regarding appropriate activities and the psychological impact of the illness upon the patient, as well as pharmacological interventions.

The mean duration of this sixth stage of AD is approximately 2.3 years. As this stage comes to an end, the patient, who is doubly incontinent and needs assistance with dressing and bathing, begins to manifest overt breakdown in the ability to articulate speech. Stuttering (verbigeration), neologisms, and/or an increased paucity of speech, become manifest.

Stage 7: Severe Alzheimer's Disease

At this stage, AD patients require continuous assistance with basic activities of daily life for survival. Six consecutive functional substages can be identified over the course of this final seventh stage. Early in this stage, speech has become so circumscribed, as to be limited to approximately a half dozen intelligible words or fewer in the course of an intensive contact and attempt at an interview with numerous queries (stage 7a). As this stage progresses, speech becomes even more limited to, at most, a single intelligible word (stage 7b). Once speech is lost, the ability to ambulate independently (without assistance), is invariably lost (stage 7e). However, ambulatory ability is readily compromised at the end of the sixth stage and in the early portion of the seventh stage by concomitant physical disability, poor care, medication side-effects, or other factors. Conversely, superb care provided in the early seventh stage, and particularly in stage 7b, can postpone the onset of loss of ambulation, potentially for many years. However, under ordinary circumstances, stage 7a has a mean duration of approximately 1 year, and stage 7b has a mean duration of approximately 1.5 years.

In patients who remain alive, stage 7c lasts approximately 1 year, after which patients lose the ability not only to ambulate independently, but also to sit up independently (stage 7d). At this point in the evolution of AD, patients will fall over when seated unless there are arm rests to hold the patient up in the chair.

This 7d substage lasts approximately 1 year. Patients who survive subsequently lose the ability to smile (stage 7e). At this substage only grimacing facial movements are observed in place of smiles. This 7e substage lasts a mean of approximately 1.5 years. It is followed in survivors, by a final 7f substage, in which AD patients additionally lose the ability to hold up their head independently.

With appropriate care and life support, patients can survive in this final substage of AD for a period of years.

With the advent of the seventh stage of AD, certain physical and neurological changes become increasingly evident. One of these changes is physical rigidity. Evident rigidity upon examination of the passive range of motion of major joints, such as the elbow, is present in the great majority of patients, throughout the course of the seventh stage.

In many patients, this rigidity appears to be a precursor to the appearance of overt physical deformities in the form of contractures. Contractures are irreversible deformities which prevent the passive or active range of motion of joints. In the early seventh stage (7a and 7b), approximately 40% of AD patients manifest these deformities. Later in the seventh stage, in immobile patients (from stage 7d to 7f), nearly all AD patients manifest contractures in multiple extremities and joints.

Neurological reflex changes also become evident in the stage 7 AD patient. Particularly notable is the emergence of so-called infantile, primitive or developmental reflexes which are present in the infant but which disappear in the toddler. These reflexes, including the grasp reflex, sucking reflex, and the Babinski plantar extensor reflex, generally begin to re-emerge in the latter part of the sixth stage and are usually present in the stage 7 AD patient. Because of the much greater physical size and strength of the AD patient in comparison with an infant, these reflexes can be very strong and can impact both positively and negatively on the care provided to the AD patient. AD patients commonly die during the course of the seventh stage. The mean point of demise is when patients lose the ability to ambulate and to sit up independently (stages 7c and 7d).

The most frequent proximate cause of death is pneumonia. Aspiration is one common cause of terminal pneumonia. Another common cause of demise in AD is infected decubital ulcerations. AD patients in the seventh stage appear to be more vulnerable to all of the common causes of mortality in the elderly including stroke, heart disease, and cancer. Some patients in this final stage appear to succumb to no identifiable condition other than AD.

Chapter 11

Younger-Onset AD

Alzheimer's is not just a disease of old age.

Younger-onset (or early-onset) Alzheimer's disease affects people who are under age 65.

Many people with younger-onset are in their 40s and 50s. They have families, careers, or are even caregivers themselves when Alzheimer's disease strikes.

Up to 5 percent of people with Alzheimer's have younger-onset. In the United States, that's about 200,000 people. It's important to know you are not alone.

Genetic Link

Most people with younger-onset have the common type of Alzheimer's, which is not directly linked to genes. Doctors do not know why symptoms appear at an unusually young age in these cases.

In a few hundred families worldwide, scientists have found several rare genes that directly cause Alzheimer's. People who inherit these rare genes tend to develop symptoms in their 30s, 40s and 50s.

"Younger-Onset Alzheimer's," is reprinted with permission of the Alzheimer's Association. For additional information, call the Alzheimer's Association toll-free helpline, 800-272-3900, or visit their website at www.alz.org. © 2010 Alzheimer's Association. All rights reserved.

Living with Younger-Onset Alzheimer's

If you have younger-onset Alzheimer's, it's important to know that even after diagnosis, you can live a meaningful and productive life.

You can remain active and take part in activities you enjoy. You can work with family and friends to plan for the future and educate others.

Living with Alzheimer's was not what you had planned. But you have the power to make a new plan with Alzheimer's in the picture.

It's important to know that:

- you are not alone;

- there are many ways to stay active and involved;

- the disease affects each person differently and symptoms will vary;

- the Alzheimer's Association can help you and your family.

Possible Reactions to Diagnosis

After the diagnosis, you may experience a range of emotions:

Relief

Many people have known there was a problem for a long time. It can be validating to know there is a cause for what you are experiencing.

Anger

Your life is taking a different course than the one you and your family had planned.

Denial

The diagnosis seems impossible to believe.

Depression

You may feel sad or hopeless about the life changes you are facing.

Isolation

No one seems to understand what you are going through.

Sense of Loss

It's hard to accept changes in your abilities, or ways you interact with your community or job.

What you can do:

- Join an Alzheimer's Association support group. Some groups are just for people with younger-onset.

- Get involved. Tell your story. Volunteer. Become an advocate.

- Explore new hobbies or interests that are meaningful to you.

- Work with a well-qualified counselor.

- Share your feelings with friends and family, and someone who can help with spiritual needs.

- Visit the message boards and chat rooms on the Alzheimer's Association website at www.alz.org and other Alzheimer-related websites.

Family

Your Spouse or Partner

Many people with Alzheimer's continue to live at home after their diagnosis and it is helpful to work with your family to prepare for changes in the household.

In particular, your spouse or partner may feel a sense of loss or loneliness as a result of the changes the diagnosis brings.

What you can do to help your spouse or partner:

- Continue to take part in all the activities that you can. Adapt activities to fit what you are comfortable with and enjoy doing.

- Find new activities that you can do together. Sometimes be-friending another couple in the same situation offers new possibilities for support.

- Talk with your spouse or partner about how he or she can assist you—and what you can still do on your own.

- Work with your spouse or partner to put together a file with information you may need later about caregiver services and their costs, including housekeeping and respite (caregiver relief) care.

- Discuss with a professional counselor any role changes in the relationship as well as sexuality issues.

- Continue to find ways for you and your spouse or partner to fulfill the need for intimacy.

- Encourage your spouse or partner to attend a support group for caregivers and stay connected with family and friends.

Your Children

Children often experience a wide range of emotions.

Younger children may be afraid that they will get the disease or that they did something to cause it.

Teenagers may become resentful when they have to take on more responsibilities for helping around the home. Or, they may feel embarrassed that their parent is "different."

College-bound children may be reluctant to leave home to attend school.

What you can do to help your children:

- Talk openly about the changes you are experiencing because of the disease.

- Find out what their emotional needs are. Find ways to support them, like meeting with a counselor who specializes in children who have a loved one with Alzheimer's.

- Notify school social workers and teachers about your situation. Give them information about the disease.

- Invite children to attend support group meetings. Include them in counseling sessions.

- Don't pull away. Try to find activities together you can still enjoy together. If you can't drive, plan a hike or bike ride. Check out public transportation in your area.

- Make it okay to laugh. Sometimes humor lightens the mood and makes coping easier.

- Record your thoughts, feelings, and wisdom in writing, audio, or video. Your children will appreciate this when they grow older.

Important life stages you might want to discuss include:

- graduation;

- dating;

- marriage;

- births;

- deaths.

Friends

Friends, co-workers, and neighbors may not understand what is happening to you. Some may keep their distance or resist keeping in touch.

Often they may not know what to do or say. They may be waiting for you to reach out to them.

What you can do to help your friends:

- Share your experiences of living with Alzheimer's disease.

- Invite them to Alzheimer's Association education programs and events.

- Continue social activities as much as possible. Seek out local programs specifically for people with dementia.

- Let your friends know what you are still comfortable doing.

- Let them know when you need help and support—and tell them what they can do.

Job

You may find work-related tasks more difficult to perform as the disease advances. Talk to your doctor to plan when and what you'll tell your employer about the disease, and at what point you should no longer work. If available, use employee assistance programs offered at work.

The Alzheimer's Association has information about the disease that you can share with your employer. Visit www.alz.org or contact your local chapter.

What you can do about your job:

- Continue to work as long as you, your employer, and your doctor feel you are able.

- If you feel overwhelmed at work, take time off. Talk to your doctor and employer about leave of absence options.

- If you are still able to work, ask your employer for work accommodations available to you under the Americans with Disabilities Act.

- Use a daily planning calendar, memos, and other memory aids to help you organize the details of your job.

- Ask your employer if you can switch to a position that better matches your abilities and strengths—or consider reducing your work hours.

- Look into early retirement options.

- Educate yourself, as well as your spouse, partner, or close friend or relative, about the benefits available to you and how to claim them.

Planning for the Future

When you are in the early stages of Alzheimer's, it's important to take steps immediately to plan for the future.

Finances

If your earnings are the family's main source of income, you may be concerned about financially supporting your family now and in the future. Insurance and other benefits may be more difficult to obtain. Future health care costs should be considered.

Steps to plan for your financial future:

- Meet with a qualified financial consultant or an attorney to discuss current and future investments, insurance, and retirement options. See if long-term care insurance is still an option.

- Find out about government assistance programs such as Social Security, Medicare, and Medicaid.

- Review your employer-provided or personal disability insurance policies.

- Organize financial documents and other important information in one place. Go over them with your spouse or partner.

Legal documents include:
- birth certificate;
- insurance policies;
- retirement accounts;
- Social Security information;
- wills;
- research college scholarship and grant money for your children.

Access to Social Security

The Social Security Administration (SSA) has added early-onset Alzheimer's (or younger-onset) to the list of conditions under its Compassionate Allowance Initiative, giving those with the disease expedited access to Social Security Disability Insurance (SSDI) and Supplemental Security Income (SSI). Use our helpful checklist to make sure you have information and resources you need to apply for Social Security Disability and Supplemental Income benefits. Find the checklist and get more information at alz.org/SSDI.

Legal Issues

- Work with a well-qualified attorney to make legal plans.

- Legally appoint a person you trust to make financial and health care decisions on your behalf when you cannot. Tell the person your wishes for the future, including where you want to live and what types of treatments you want or don't want.

Care and Family

- Find adult day care programs and residential care settings that know how to assist people with younger-onset Alzheimer's.

- Gather all of the thoughts, memories, and family history you want to pass on to your loved ones. Work together on family projects to celebrate the past and present.

Well-Being and Safety

Two of the most important ways you can take good care of yourself are to stay healthy and safe.

What you can do about your health:

- Get regular check-ups.

- Exercise regularly, with your doctor's approval.

- Rest when you are tired.

- Adopt a healthy diet.

- Take any prescribed medications according to directions.

- Cut down on alcohol—it can make your symptoms worse.

- Ask for help when you need it.

- Reduce stress in your daily life, and learn new ways to relax.
- Stay socially engaged.

Safety

Symptoms of Alzheimer's, like loss of memory and decision-making ability, can bring about new safety needs.

What you can do about your safety:

- Keep important phone numbers nearby.
- Post reminders to lock doors and turn off electrical appliances.
- Arrange for an in-home helper to assist you when your spouse, partner, or caregiver needs to be away from home.
- Arrange for other ways to get around when it is no longer safe for you to drive.
- Enroll in MedicAlert®+Alzheimer's Association Safe Return® for services to assist you should you ever become lost.
- Purchase the Alzheimer's Association Comfort Zone™, a new web-based GPS location management service that can help families achieve some peace of mind. Comfort Zone™ uses the internet and a small device to ensure that you and your family are always connected.

Chapter 12

The Genetics of AD

Chapter Contents

Section 12.1

Genes Play an Important Role in the Development of AD

Excerpted from "Alzheimer's Disease Genetics Fact Sheet," by the National Institute on Aging (NIA, www.nia.nih.gov), part of the National Institutes of Health, March 4, 2011.

Scientists don't yet fully understand what causes Alzheimer disease (AD). However, the more they learn about AD, the more they realize that genes play an important role in the development of this devastating disease. Research conducted and funded by the National Institute on Aging (NIA) and others is advancing the field of AD genetics.

The Genetics of Disease

Some diseases are caused by a genetic mutation, or permanent change, in one specific gene. If a person inherits a genetic mutation that is linked to a certain disease from a parent, then he or she will usually get the disease. Cystic fibrosis, muscular dystrophy, and Huntington disease are examples of single-gene disorders.

In other diseases, a genetic variant, or a change in a gene, may occur, but it doesn't necessarily cause the person to develop the disease. More than one gene variant may be necessary to cause the disease, or the variant may increase a person's risk of developing the disease. When this happens, the changed gene is called a genetic risk factor.

The Genetics of AD

AD is an irreversible, progressive brain disease characterized by the development of amyloid plaques and neurofibrillary tangles, the loss of connections between nerve cells in the brain, and the death of these nerve cells. AD has two types—early-onset and late-onset. Both types have genetic links.

Early-Onset AD

Early-onset AD is a rare form of AD, affecting only about 5 percent of all people who have AD. It develops in people ages 30 to 60.

Some cases of early-onset AD, called familial AD (FAD), are inherited. FAD is caused by a number of different gene mutations on chromosomes 21, 14, and 1, and each of these mutations causes abnormal proteins to be formed. Mutations on chromosome 21 cause the formation of abnormal amyloid precursor protein (APP). A mutation on chromosome 14 causes abnormal presenilin 1 to be made, and a mutation on chromosome 1 leads to abnormal presenilin 2.

Even if only one of these mutated genes is inherited from a parent, the person will almost always develop early-onset AD. This inheritance pattern is referred to as "autosomal dominant" inheritance. In other words, offspring in the same generation have a 50/50 chance of developing FAD if one of their parents had it.

Scientists know that each of these mutations causes an increased amount of the beta-amyloid protein to be formed. Beta-amyloid, a major component of AD plaques, is formed from APP.

These early-onset findings were critical because they showed that genetics were involved in AD, and they helped identify key players in the AD process. The studies also helped explain some of the variation in the age at which AD develops.

Late-Onset AD

Most cases of Alzheimer disease are of the late-onset form, developing after age 60. Scientists studying the genetics of AD have found that the mutations seen in early-onset AD are not involved in this form of the disease.

Although a specific gene has not been identified as the cause of late-onset AD, one predisposing genetic risk factor does appear to increase a person's risk of developing the disease. This increased risk is related to the apolipoprotein E (APOE) gene found on chromosome 19. APOE contains the instructions needed to make a protein that helps carry cholesterol in the bloodstream. APOE comes in several different forms, or alleles. Three forms—APOE e2, APOE e3, and APOE e4—occur most frequently.

- APOE e2 is relatively rare and may provide some protection against the disease. If AD does occur in a person with this allele, it develops later in life than it would in someone with the APOE e4 gene.

- APOE e3 is the most common allele. Researchers think it plays a neutral role in AD—neither decreasing nor increasing risk.

- APOE e4 occurs in about 40 percent of all people who develop late-onset AD and is present in about 25 to 30 percent of the population. People with AD are more likely to have an APOE e4 allele than people who do not develop AD. However, many people with AD do not have an APOE e4 allele.

Dozens of studies have confirmed that the APOE e4 allele increases the risk of developing AD, but how that happens is not yet understood. These studies also have helped explain some of the variation in the age at which AD develops, as people who inherit one or two APOE e4 alleles tend to develop AD at an earlier age than those who do not have any. APOE e4 is called a risk-factor gene because it increases a person's risk of developing AD. However, inheriting an APOE e4 allele does not mean that a person will definitely develop AD. Some people with one or two APOE e4 alleles never get the disease, and others who develop AD do not have any APOE e4 alleles.

Scientists believe that four to seven other AD risk-factor genes exist and are using a new approach called a genome-wide association study (GWAS) to help speed the discovery process. Another possible risk-factor gene, SORL1, was discovered in 2007. This gene is involved in transporting APP within cells, and its association with AD has been identified and confirmed in three separate studies. Researchers found that when SORL1 is present at low levels or in a variant form, beta-amyloid levels increase and may harm neurons.

DNA, Chromosomes, and Genes

The nucleus of almost every human cell contains a "blueprint" that carries the instructions a cell needs to do its job. The blueprint is made up of DNA, which is present in long strands that would stretch to nearly 6 feet in length if attached end to end. The DNA is packed tightly together with proteins into compact structures called chromosomes in the nucleus of each cell. Each cell has 46 chromosomes in 23 pairs. The DNA in nearly all cells of an individual is identical.

Each chromosome contains many thousands of segments, called genes. People inherit two copies of each gene from their parents, except for genes on the X and Y chromosomes, which, among other functions, determine a person's sex. The gene tells the cell how to make specific proteins, which determine the different kinds of cells that make up an organism and direct almost every aspect of the cell's construction, operation, and repair. Even slight alterations in a gene can produce an abnormal protein, which may lead to cell malfunction and, eventually, to disease. Other changes in genes may not cause disease but can increase a person's risk of developing a particular disease.

APOE Testing

A blood test is available that can identify which APOE alleles a person has, but it is not yet possible to predict who will or will not develop AD. Because APOE e4 is only a risk factor for AD, this blood test cannot say for sure whether a person will develop AD or not. Some researchers believe that screening measures may never be able to predict AD with 100 percent accuracy. However, a small battery of tests for other risk-factor genes might eventually be useful.

At present, APOE testing is used in a research setting to identify study participants who may have an increased risk of developing AD. This knowledge helps scientists look for early brain changes in participants and compare the effectiveness of treatments for people with different APOE profiles. Most researchers believe that the APOE test is useful for studying AD risk in large groups of people but not for determining any one person's specific risk. Someday, perhaps, screening in otherwise healthy people may be useful if an accurate and reliable test is developed and effective ways to treat or prevent AD become available.

Section 12.2

Gene Linked to AD Plays Key Role in Cell Survival

From "Gene Linked to Alzheimer's Disease Plays Key
Role in Cell Survival," by the National Institutes of Health
(NIH, www.nih.gov), June 10, 2010.

Scientists have discovered that a gene linked to Alzheimer disease may play a beneficial role in cell survival by enabling neurons to clear away toxic proteins. A study funded by the National Institute on Aging (NIA), part of the National Institutes of Health, shows the presenilin 1 (PS1) gene is essential to the function of lysosomes, the cell component that digests and recycles unwanted proteins. However, mutations in the PS1 gene—a known risk factor for a rare, early onset form of Alzheimer disease—disrupt this crucial process.

Ralph Nixon, MD, PhD, of the Nathan Kline Institute, Orangeburg, NY, and New York University Langone Medical Center, directed the study involving researchers from the United States, Europe, Japan, and Canada. Also supported in part by the Alzheimer's Association, the study appears in the June 10, 2010, online issue of *Cell*.

Researchers have theorized for more than a decade that PS1 mutations linked to early-onset Alzheimer disease, a rare form of the disease that usually affects people between ages 30 and 60, may trigger abnormally high levels of beta-amyloid protein to clump together in the brain.

Amyloid deposits and tau protein tangles are hallmarks of both early-onset and the sporadic, more common form of the disease found in people aged 60 and older. These new findings, however, suggest PS1 mutations may play a more general role in the development of early-onset Alzheimer disease.

"This study expands our understanding of the role presenilin 1 mutations may play in Alzheimer's pathology," said NIA Director Richard J. Hodes, MD. "While more research is needed, lysosome disruption may be worth exploring as a potential target for new therapeutics to treat, prevent, or delay this progressive and debilitating disease."

Working in cells from Alzheimer disease mouse models and in skin cells from Alzheimer patients with the mutated gene, the researchers found the following:

- The PS1 gene activates lysosome enzymes that digest waste proteins during a process called autophagy. This is the cell's main method of recycling unwanted proteins and other cellular debris. While these waste proteins occur naturally, they are over-produced in neurological disorders like Alzheimer and Parkinson disease, and can be toxic to brain cells.

- Mutations in the PS1 gene disrupt autophagy. This impairs the ability of neurons to remove waste proteins and other debris. Neurons then may fill with sacs containing potentially toxic amyloid fragments and other unwanted proteins.

- Other genetic mutations may be risk factors for similar disruptions to autophagy found in the more common, sporadic form of the disease in people age 60 and older, and in other neurological disorders like Parkinson disease.

"It has become increasingly clear that many factors may drive the development and progression of this very complex disease," said Nixon, the principal investigator. "I believe we will need to explore an array of therapeutic targets, including ones to normalize or moderate disrupted autophagy."

Section 12.3

Variations of Apolipoprotein E Linked to Increased Risk of AD

From "APOE," by *Genetics Home Reference* (ghr.nlm.nih.gov),
part of the National Library of Medicine and National
Institutes of Health, February 27, 2011.

What is the official name of the APOE gene?

The official name of this gene is apolipoprotein E.

APOE is the gene's official symbol. The APOE gene is also known by other names, which are listed in the following text.

What is the normal function of the APOE gene?

The APOE gene provides instructions for making a protein called apolipoprotein E. This protein combines with fats (lipids) in the body to form molecules called lipoproteins. Lipoproteins are responsible for packaging cholesterol and other fats and carrying them through the bloodstream. Apolipoprotein E is a major component of a specific type of lipoprotein called very low-density lipoproteins (VLDLs). VLDLs remove excess cholesterol from the blood and carry it to the liver for processing. Maintaining normal levels of cholesterol is essential for the prevention of disorders that affect the heart and blood vessels (cardiovascular diseases), including heart attack and stroke.

There are at least three slightly different versions (alleles) of the APOE gene. The major alleles are called e2, e3, and e4. The most common allele is e3, which is found in more than half of the general population.

How are changes in the APOE gene related to health conditions?

Alzheimer disease (increased risk from variations of the APOE gene): The e4 version of the APOE gene increases an individual's risk for developing late-onset Alzheimer disease. People who inherit one copy of the APOE e4 allele have an increased chance of developing the disease; those who inherit two copies of the allele are at even greater risk. The APOE e4 allele may also be associated with an earlier onset of memory loss and other symptoms.

It is not known how the APOE e4 allele is related to the risk of Alzheimer disease. However, researchers have found that this allele is associated with an increased number of protein clumps, called amyloid plaques, in the brain tissue of affected people. A buildup of toxic amyloid beta peptide and amyloid plaques may lead to the death of neurons and the progressive signs and symptoms of this disorder.

It is important to note that people with the APOE e4 allele inherit an increased risk of developing Alzheimer disease, not the disease itself. Not all people with Alzheimer disease have the APOE e4 allele, and not all people who have this allele will develop the disease.

Other disorders (associated with the APOE gene): Variants of apolipoprotein E have been studied extensively as risk factors for many different conditions. For example, APOE alleles have been shown to influence the risk of cardiovascular diseases. People who carry at least one copy of the APOE e4 allele have an increased chance of developing atherosclerosis, which is an accumulation of fatty deposits and scar-like tissue in the lining of the arteries. This progressive narrowing of the arteries increases the risk of heart attack and stroke.

The APOE e2 allele has been shown to greatly increase the risk of a rare condition called hyperlipoproteinemia type III. Most people with this disorder have two copies of the APOE e2 allele, leading researchers to conclude that the e2 allele plays a critical role in the development of the condition. Hyperlipoproteinemia type III is characterized by increased blood levels of cholesterol, certain fats called triglycerides, and molecules called beta-very low-density lipoproteins (beta-VLDLs), which carry cholesterol and lipoproteins in the bloodstream. A buildup of cholesterol and other fatty materials can lead to the formation of small, yellow skin growths called xanthomas and the development of atherosclerosis.

APOE gene variants have also been studied as a potential risk factor for age-related macular degeneration, an eye disease that is a leading cause of vision loss among older people worldwide. Some studies have suggested that having at least one copy of the APOE e4 allele may help protect against this disease or delay the onset of vision loss, while having at least one copy of the APOE e2 allele may increase the risk of this disease or cause symptoms to appear earlier. However, other studies have not found these associations. More research is needed to clarify what role, if any, APOE gene variants play in the development of age-related macular degeneration.

Chapter 13

Health Conditions Linked to AD

Chapter Contents

Section 13.1

Down Syndrome and AD

"Alzheimer's and Down Syndrome," © 2010 National Down Syndrome Society. Reprinted with permission. To view this document and other information, including a resource and further reading list, visit www.ndsss.org.

Alzheimer's Disease, a degenerative neurological disorder characterized by progressive memory loss, personality changes, and loss of functional motor capabilities, is far more common in individuals with Down syndrome than the general population. However, not all individuals with Down syndrome will develop Alzheimer's disease, and even those showing Alzheimer's-type symptoms may not have Alzheimer's disease since other conditions can mimic the symptoms.

How common is Alzheimer's disease in individuals with Down syndrome?

Estimates vary, but a reasonable conclusion is that 25 percent or more of individuals with Down syndrome over age 35 show clinical signs and symptoms of Alzheimer's-type dementia. The percentage increases with age. In the general population, Alzheimer's disease does not usually develop before age 50, and the highest incidence (in people over age 65) is between five and 10 percent. The incidence of Alzheimer's disease in the Down syndrome population is estimated to be three to five times greater than in the general population, and oftentimes, symptoms begin much earlier.

What are the symptoms of Alzheimer's disease?

Early symptoms include loss of memory and logical thinking, personality change, decline in daily living skills, new onset of seizures, changes in coordination and gait, and loss of continence in bladder and bowel habits.

How is a final diagnosis made?

Alzheimer's disease is difficult to diagnose. It is important to be certain Alzheimer's-type symptoms do not arise from other conditions, namely thyroid disorders, clinical depression, brain tumor, recurrent brain strokes, metabolic imbalances, and various neurological conditions.

The diagnosis of Alzheimer's disease is made on the basis of clinical history, showing a slow, steady decrease in cognitive function and a variety of laboratory tests which provide contributory evidence, including electroencephalogram, brain stem auditory evoked response, computerized transaxial tomography, and magnetic resonance imaging, among other tests and measurements.

Is there a baseline test that can be repeated at intervals to determine specific decrease in cognitive function?

Psychologists often use questionnaires answered by family members, companions, or caretakers that assist in the early detection of dementia. It is recommended that individuals with Down syndrome be tested at age 30 to provide a baseline reading, and periodically thereafter. If the tests show deterioration, further tests must be made to rule out conditions that present similar or overlapping symptoms.

What information has research yielded about a link between Alzheimer's disease and Down syndrome?

Current research investigating how certain genes on Chromosome 21 may predispose individuals with Down syndrome to Alzheimer's disease. A number of centers are testing therapies in Down syndrome that appear to benefit patients with Alzheimer's disease in the general population.

Section 13.2

Obesity May Raise Risk of AD and Dementia

People who carry a gene that predisposes them to obesity also appear to have smaller brains, researchers report. And having a smaller brain, research shows, may increase the risk for Alzheimer's in old age.

The findings, published online in the [April 19, 2010] *Proceedings of the National Academy of Sciences,* underscore scientists' growing understanding of the links between obesity and Alzheimer's disease.

The gene, called FTO [fat mass and obesity associated], adds about an inch to the waistline and about 2 to 7 pounds in weight, on average, but makes your brain look like it is 16 years older, said Dr. Paul Thompson, a brain researcher at the University of California, Los Angeles, and one of the study's authors. The gene may lead to weight gain by suppressing the body's responses to feeling full.

The FTO gene is surprisingly common, being present in 46 percent of Western and Central Europeans as well as those of European ancestry. It's also present in more than half of West Africans and in more than one in six Chinese.

For the study, the scientists generated three-dimensional maps of the brain in 206 healthy older men and women. The study was part of the ongoing Alzheimer's Disease Neuroimaging Initiative that is looking at factors that help to protect the brain as we age.

Those who had the FTO gene had smaller brains—from 8 to 12 percent smaller in key brain areas important for memory, perception, and thinking. Differences in cholesterol or blood pressure levels did not affect the association between weight and smaller brains.

A growing body of evidence indicates that shrinkage of the brain may be an early sign of Alzheimer's disease, occurring years before obvious memory loss and other symptoms appear. While the brain tends to lose volume with age, excess shrinkage may predispose to Alzheimer's. One theory is that having fewer brain cells reduces the brain's so-called cognitive reserve, making it harder for the brain to compensate when cells are lost as Alzheimer's disease progresses. With more than a billion adults overweight and 300 million obese around the world, it is important to understand the links between body weight and Alzheimer's disease. Obesity is not just bad for the brain: It also raises the risk of diabetes, high blood pressure, and heart disease, all of which have also been linked to an increased risk for Alzheimer's disease.

Other studies have pointed to the links between obesity—and belly fat in particular—and Alzheimer's. A Swedish study from earlier this year [2010], for example, found that women who store fat on their waist in their 40s and 50s are more than twice as likely to develop Alzheimer's in old age than their trimmer peers. And a large study from California last year [2009] found that men and women with thick middles at midlife were nearly three times more likely to suffer from Alzheimer's decades later than their slender peers.

Research has shown that Amish people who carry the FTO obesity gene and who remain physically active may not be heavier than their peers. Other studies have shown that exercise can help to keep weight down and may protect against Alzheimer's in old age.

Advancing age remains the most important risk factor for Alzheimer's: The older you are, the more likely you are to develop the disease. Smoking, high blood pressure, years of schooling, and genetic factors may also contribute to risk, other research has shown.

By ALZinfo.org, the Alzheimer's Information Site. Reviewed by William J. Netzer, PhD, Fisher Center for Alzheimer's Research Foundation at The Rockefeller University.

Source

April J. Ho, Jason L. Stein, Sue Hua, et al: "A Commonly Carried Allele of the Obesity-Related FTO Gene Is Associated with Reduced Brain Volume in the Healthy Elderly." *Proceedings of the National Academy of Sciences,* April 19, 2010, online publication doi: 10.1073/pnas.091878107

Section 13.3

Type 2 Diabetes and AD Risk

Nearly 21 million Americans in the United States have diabetes, a disease that makes the body less able to convert sugar to energy. More than 6 million of these people don't even know they have it. Most people with diabetes have Type 2, which is linked to lack of exercise and being overweight.

When diabetes is not controlled, too much sugar remains in the blood. Over time, this can damage organs, including the brain.

Scientists are finding more evidence that could link Type 2 diabetes with Alzheimer's disease, the most common form of dementia and the seventh leading cause of death in the United States. Several research studies following large groups over many years suggest that adults with Type 2 diabetes have a higher risk of later developing Alzheimer's.

Alzheimer's disease is a progressive and fatal brain disorder that gradually destroys a person's memory and ability to learn, reason, make judgments, communicate and carry out daily activities. As Alzheimer's progresses, individuals may have changes in personality and behavior, such as anxiety, suspiciousness or agitation, as well as delusions.

More than 5 million people have Alzheimer's in the United States, and that number will start to soar as baby boomers enter their 60s when the risk for Alzheimer's begins to rise. And people with diabetes may be at even greater risk for Alzheimer's.

High Blood Sugar Often Is an Early Warning Sign

An estimated 54 million U.S. adults have prediabetes, or blood sugar levels that are higher than normal but not yet in the diabetic range. Most of these people will develop Type 2 diabetes within 10 years.

High blood sugar may also be a sign of insulin resistance. In this disorder, the body becomes unresponsive to insulin, a hormone that helps blood sugar move into cells and fuel vital processes. At first, the body makes more insulin to get the energy it needs. Eventually, the body is making all the insulin it can. If cells grow more insulin resistant, blood sugar will rise higher, and diabetes will develop.

Excess blood sugar and insulin can both damage the body. Doctors do not routinely measure insulin levels because the tests are complicated and expensive. Other signs of insulin resistance are:

- a big waist (at least 40 inches in men and 35 inches in women);

- blood pressure above 130/85;

- low levels of HDL (high-density lipoprotein), or "good" cholesterol.

Who Gets Diabetes?

While anyone can get diabetes, it tends to run in families and to affect certain ethnic groups more than others. Hispanic Americans are at greater risk for developing diabetes than other racial or ethnic groups:

- Hispanic Americans are at very high risk for developing Type 2 diabetes.

- The risk for developing diabetes over their lifetimes is higher for Hispanics than for any other ethnic group.

- Hispanics are almost twice as likely to develop diabetes as non-Hispanic whites.

- Diabetes rates more than double in Hispanics who are obese.

- Of those born in 2000, diabetes will affect half of all Hispanic females; four in 10 Hispanics and African Americans; and one in three Americans overall.

Who Gets Alzheimer's?

- The greatest risk factor is increasing age—one out of eight people aged 65 and older have Alzheimer's and nearly one out of every two over age 85 has it.

- It is estimated that nearly 500,000 people under the age of 65 have early-onset Alzheimer's disease or other dementias.

- Family history can play a part in developing Alzheimer's. Research shows that those with a parent, brother or sister, or child with Alzheimer's are more likely to develop Alzheimer's. When diseases tend to run in families, either heredity (genetics) or environmental factors or both may play a role.

What Is the Alzheimer's–Diabetes Link?

Doctors don't know yet what causes Alzheimer's disease or exactly how Alzheimer's and diabetes are connected. But they do know that high blood sugar or insulin can harm the brain in several ways:

- Diabetes raises the risk of heart disease and stroke, which hurt the heart and blood vessels. Damaged blood vessels in the brain may contribute to Alzheimer's disease.

- The brain depends on many different chemicals, which may be unbalanced by too much insulin. Some of these changes may help trigger Alzheimer's disease.

- High blood sugar causes inflammation. This may damage brain cells and help Alzheimer's to develop.

How to Reduce the Risk of Diabetes

Preventing diabetes may not stop Alzheimer's from developing. But simple lifestyle changes can help avoid diabetes and cut the risk:

- Losing at least 5 percent of body weight—just 10 pounds in someone weighing 200 pounds

- Exercising at least 30 minutes 5 days each week

- Eating a healthy, low-fat diet

As immigrants adapt to and integrate with life in the United States, they adopt habits of the mainstream culture, including eating a diet with less fiber and more prepared fast food. Hispanics are less likely than non-Hispanic whites to regularly see a physician or community professional to help monitor and control their health. This may delay an early diagnosis of diabetes—and Alzheimer's disease—and prevent them from getting treatment when it is most effective.

It's important to work with your doctor to detect the first signs of diabetes or other health concerns. Test your weight, blood pressure, cholesterol, and blood sugar regularly. Even if you get diabetes, treating it may help prevent other complications, such as Alzheimer's disease.

Chapter 14

Traumatic Brain Injury, AD, and Dementia

What is a traumatic brain injury (TBI)?

TBI, a form of acquired brain injury, occurs when a sudden trauma causes damage to the brain. The damage can be focal—confined to one area of the brain—or diffuse—involving more than one area of the brain. TBI can result from a closed head injury or a penetrating head injury. A closed injury occurs when the head suddenly and violently hits an object but the object does not break through the skull. A penetrating injury occurs when an object pierces the skull and enters brain tissue.

What are the signs and symptoms of TBI?

Symptoms of a TBI can be mild, moderate, or severe, depending on the extent of the damage to the brain. Some symptoms are evident immediately, whereas others do not surface until several days or weeks after the injury. A person with a mild TBI may remain conscious or may experience a loss of consciousness for a few seconds or minutes. The person may also feel dazed or not like himself for several days or weeks after the initial injury. Other symptoms of mild TBI include headache, confusion, lightheadedness, dizziness, blurred vision or tired eyes, ringing in the ears, bad taste in the mouth, fatigue or lethargy,

Excerpted from "Traumatic Brain Injury: Hope Through Research," by the National Institute on Neurological Disorders and Stroke (NINDS, www.ninds.nih .gov), part of the National Institutes of Health, January 4, 2011.

a change in sleep patterns, behavioral or mood changes, and trouble with memory, concentration, attention, or thinking.

A person with a moderate or severe TBI may show these same symptoms, but may also have a headache that gets worse or does not go away, repeated vomiting or nausea, convulsions or seizures, inability to awaken from sleep, dilation of one or both pupils of the eyes, slurred speech, weakness or numbness in the extremities, loss of coordination, and/or increased confusion, restlessness, or agitation. Small children with moderate to severe TBI may show some of these signs as well as signs specific to young children, such as persistent crying, inability to be consoled, and/or refusal to nurse or eat. Anyone with signs of moderate or severe TBI should receive medical attention as soon as possible.

What are the causes of and risk factors for TBI?

Half of all TBIs are due to transportation accidents involving automobiles, motorcycles, bicycles, and pedestrians. These accidents are the major cause of TBI in people under age 75. For those 75 and older, falls cause the majority of TBIs. Approximately 20 percent of TBIs are due to violence, such as firearm assaults and child abuse, and about 3 percent are due to sports injuries. Fully half of TBI incidents involve alcohol use.

The cause of the TBI plays a role in determining the patient's outcome. For example, approximately 91 percent of firearm TBIs (two-thirds of which may be suicidal in intent) result in death, while only 11 percent of TBIs from falls result in death.

Transportation accidents involving automobiles, motorcycles, bicycles, and pedestrians account for half of all TBIs and are the major cause of TBIs in people under age 75.

What are the different types of TBI?

Concussion is the most minor and the most common type of TBI. Technically, a concussion is a short loss of consciousness in response to a head injury, but in common language the term has come to mean any minor injury to the head or brain.

Other injuries are more severe. As the first line of defense, the skull is particularly vulnerable to injury. Skull fractures occur when the bone of the skull cracks or breaks. A depressed skull fracture occurs when pieces of the broken skull press into the tissue of the brain. A penetrating skull fracture occurs when something pierces the skull, such as a bullet, leaving a distinct and localized injury to brain tissue.

Skull fractures can cause bruising of brain tissue called a contusion. A contusion is a distinct area of swollen brain tissue mixed with blood released from broken blood vessels. A contusion can also occur in response to shaking of the brain back and forth within the confines of the skull, an injury called contrecoup. This injury often occurs in car accidents after high-speed stops and in shaken baby syndrome, a severe form of head injury that occurs when a baby is shaken forcibly enough to cause the brain to bounce against the skull.

In addition, contrecoup can cause diffuse axonal injury, also called shearing, which involves damage to individual nerve cells (neurons) and loss of connections among neurons. This can lead to a breakdown of overall communication among neurons in the brain.

Damage to a major blood vessel in the head can cause a hematoma, or heavy bleeding into or around the brain. Three types of hematomas can cause brain damage. An epidural hematoma involves bleeding into the area between the skull and the dura. With a subdural hematoma, bleeding is confined to the area between the dura and the arachnoid membrane. Bleeding within the brain itself is called intracerebral hematoma.

Another insult to the brain that can cause injury is anoxia. Anoxia is a condition in which there is an absence of oxygen supply to an organ's tissues, even if there is adequate blood flow to the tissue. Hypoxia refers to a decrease in oxygen supply rather than a complete absence of oxygen. Without oxygen, the cells of the brain die within several minutes. This type of injury is often seen in near-drowning victims, in heart attack patients, or in people who suffer significant blood loss from other injuries that decrease blood flow to the brain.

Are there long-term problems associated with a TBI?

In addition to the immediate post-injury complications, other long-term problems can develop after a TBI. These include Parkinson disease and other motor problems, Alzheimer disease, dementia pugilistica, and post-traumatic dementia.

Alzheimer disease (AD): AD is a progressive, neurodegenerative disease characterized by dementia, memory loss, and deteriorating cognitive abilities. Recent research suggests an association between head injury in early adulthood and the development of AD later in life; the more severe the head injury, the greater the risk of developing AD. Some evidence indicates that a head injury may interact with other factors to trigger the disease and may hasten the onset of the disease in individuals already at risk. For example, people who have a particular form of the protein apolipoprotein E (apoE4) and suffer a head injury fall into this increased risk category. (ApoE4 is a naturally occurring protein that helps transport cholesterol through the bloodstream.)

Parkinson disease and other motor problems: Movement disorders as a result of TBI are rare but can occur. Parkinson disease may develop years after TBI as a result of damage to the basal ganglia. Symptoms of Parkinson disease include tremor or trembling, rigidity or stiffness, slow movement (bradykinesia), inability to move (akinesia), shuffling walk, and stooped posture. Despite many scientific advances in recent years, Parkinson disease remains a chronic and progressive disorder, meaning that it is incurable and will progress in severity until the end of life. Other movement disorders that may develop after TBI include tremor, ataxia (uncoordinated muscle movements), and myoclonus (shock-like contractions of muscles).

Dementia pugilistica: Also called chronic traumatic encephalopathy, dementia pugilistica primarily affects career boxers. The most common symptoms of the condition are dementia and parkinsonism caused by repetitive blows to the head over a long period of time. Symptoms begin anywhere between 6 and 40 years after the start of a boxing career, with an average onset of about 16 years.

Post-traumatic dementia: The symptoms of post-traumatic dementia are very similar to those of dementia pugilistica, except that post-traumatic dementia is also characterized by long-term memory problems and is caused by a single, severe TBI that results in a coma.

Chapter 15

Other Factors That Influence AD Risk

Chapter Contents

Section 15.1

Alcohol Abuse Linked to AD and Dementia

From "Alcohol Use and the Risk of Developing Alzheimer's Disease," by Suzanne L. Tyas, PhD, published in *Alcohol Research & Health,* by the National Institute on Alcohol Abuse and Alcoholism (NIAAA, www.niaaa .nih.gov), part of the National Institutes of Health, 2001. Reviewed and revised by David A. Cooke, MD, FACP, February 17, 2011.

Alzheimer disease (AD) is a degenerative brain disorder character-ized by a progressive loss of memory and other detrimental cognitive changes as well as lowered life expectancy (Morris 1999). It is the leading cause of dementia in the United States. Aside from the sub-stantial personal costs, AD is a major economic burden on health care and social services (Ernst and Hay 1994; Leon et al. 1998). Estimates of the number of people with AD in the United States in 1997 ranged from 1 million to more than 4 million, and these figures are expected to quadruple within 50 years unless effective interventions are devel-oped (Brookmeyer et al. 1998). The risk of AD increases exponentially with age (Kawas and Katzman 1999); consequently, as the population ages, the importance of AD as a public health concern grows, as does the need for research on the cause of AD and on strategies for its pre-vention and treatment.

Studying factors that influence the risk of developing AD may lead to the identification of those at high risk for developing it, strategies for prevention or intervention, and clues to the cause of the disease. Both genetic and environmental factors have been implicated in the development of AD (Kawas and Katzman 1999), but the cause of AD remains unknown, and no cure or universally effective treatment has yet been developed.

Alcohol consumption is one possible risk factor for AD. Alcoholism is associated with extensive cognitive problems (Evert and Oscar-Berman 1995), including alcoholic dementia (Smith and Atkinson 1997). Be-cause alcohol's effects on cognition, brain disorders, and brain chem-istry share some features with AD's effects on these three areas, it is plausible that alcohol use might also increase the risk of developing AD (Tyas 1996). Investigating whether and to what degree alcohol use is related to AD is made more difficult by the challenges of diagnosing and distinguishing alcoholic dementia and AD. Such studies are important, however, because alcohol use is a common but preventable exposure, an association between alcohol and AD is biologically plausible, and knowledge of the effect of alcohol on AD may provide clues to the cause of AD.

This article briefly reviews biological evidence suggesting that alcohol use may be associated with AD. It also focuses on the evidence from epidemiologic studies that link people's consumption of alcohol to whether they develop AD, considers the influence of tobacco use on the relationship between alcohol use and AD, and examines the epidemiologic evidence of the connection between alcohol consumption and types of cognitive impairment other than AD.

Effects of Alcohol Use on Brain Disorders and Cognition

Heavy alcohol consumption has both immediate and long-term detrimental effects on the brain and neuropsychological functioning (Delin and Lee 1992; Evert and Oscar-Berman 1995). Heavy drinking accelerates shrinkage, or atrophy, of the brain, which in turn is a critical determinant of neurodegenerative changes and cognitive decline in aging (Meyer et al. 1998).

Changes observed with alcohol-related brain disorders, however, may be no more than superficially similar to those seen with aging or AD. In contrast to aging and AD, alcohol's effects on the brain may be reversible (Carlen and Wilkinson 1987). Atrophy decreases after abstinence from alcohol (Kril and Halliday 1999). A study that further investigated cerebral atrophy in alcoholics and age-matched control subjects found no significant differences in the number of nerve cells in the brain (i.e., neurons) between the two groups and that most of the loss occurred in the white matter, which consists largely of nerve fibers that connect neurons (Jensen and Pakkenberg 1993). The researchers concluded that, because neurons did not appear to be lost, disrupted functions could be restored after abstinence as neuronal connections were reestablished. This conclusion is supported by research that also showed no neuronal loss in alcoholics compared with nonalcoholics but did show significant loss of brain cells that provide support for neurons (i.e., glial cells) which, in contrast to neurons, can be regenerated (Korbo 1999). That alcoholics can show improved cognitive performance after abstinence provides additional evidence of a reversible effect (Reed et al. 1992). Other studies, however, have reported neuronal loss with chronic alcohol abuse (Kril and Halliday 1999), including loss of neurons (i.e., cholinergic neurons) that contain or are stimulated by a certain chemical messenger in the brain (i.e., the neurotransmitter acetylcholine) (Arendt 1993). Cholinergic neurons are specifically affected in AD.

Improvement in cognitive function, or at least the lack of a progressive cognitive deficit, is one of the major factors used to determine whether a patient has alcoholic dementia rather than AD (Smith and Atkinson 1997). Recent work suggesting that characteristic neuropsychological profiles exist for alcoholic dementia and AD may prove useful in distinguishing the two disorders (Saxton et al. 2000). The diagnosis of alcoholic dementia, however, is itself somewhat controversial. Alcoholic dementia may have multiple causes. Pathological findings consistent with AD, nutritional deficiencies, trauma, and, in particular, stroke, also have been found in demented alcoholics (Fisman et al. 1996). The difficulty in distinguishing alcoholic dementia from AD has been attributed to a shared substrate of brain damage in the two disorders (Arendt 1993). A diagnosis of alcoholic dementia may be appropriate for some demented patients who have a history of alcohol abuse, but the effects of more moderate levels of drinking on cognitive function (for anyone) are not known. Thus, despite evidence of an association between alcohol use and neuropathologic and cognitive deficits, including alcoholic dementia, it is not yet clear whether alcohol use at either heavy or more moderate levels of consumption is associated with AD.

Biological Mechanisms

Both alcohol and AD substantially affect the cholinergic system, and thus it is plausible that alcohol use could be linked to AD through their common effects on this system. Early studies of AD from the 1980s focused on the cholinergic system because it was known to play an important role in memory. Its role in AD was confirmed, and deficits in the cholinergic system, such as lower levels of acetylcholine and fewer receptors (proteins that bind to neurotransmitters), are now well established in AD. Although other neurotransmitter systems have since been implicated in AD, current treatment strategies still include repletion of cholinergic deficits (Forette and Boller 1999).

The cholinergic system also is affected by alcohol use. Chronic alcohol use causes degeneration of cholinergic neurons (Arendt 1993). Alcohol has been shown to decrease acetylcholine levels, reducing its synthesis and release. These deficits may aggravate the reductions already present in AD. Improvement of cognitive function in alcoholics after abstention from alcohol suggests that the cognitive deficits may reflect neurochemical alterations rather than neuronal loss (Kril and Halliday 1999). Alcohol-related memory loss can be partially reversed by compounds that stimulate the cholinergic system (e.g., nicotine) (Arendt 1993), illustrating the importance of the cholinergic system in alcohol's effects on memory. Alcohol-induced cholinergic receptor losses in alcoholics with AD may contribute to the clinical symptoms of dementia. Alcohol does not appear to accelerate the AD process but instead induces its effects on the cholinergic system, independent of the cholinergic deficits caused by AD (Freund and Ballinger 1992). In addition, alcohol has extensive effects on neurotransmitter systems other than the cholinergic system and may also affect AD through these pathways (Diamond and Gordon 1997).

Alcohol may interact with both the brain and the aging process. In rodents, for example, age-related impairments in learning and memory are aggravated by alcohol consumption (Freund 1982). Alcohol-related brain damage appears to differ in young and old alcoholics (Kril and Halliday 1999). Although it has been suggested that alcohol abuse may accelerate aging-related changes in the brain at any age and that older adults may be more vulnerable to alcohol's effects and thus show more age-related cognitive changes, these hypotheses of premature aging have been questioned (Evert and Oscar-Berman 1995). Arendt (1993) has suggested that the degenerative changes associated with aging, chronic alcohol abuse, and AD are on a continuum and that they may be quantitatively different but not qualitatively so.

Although a link between alcohol use and AD is plausible, whether such a relationship does exist or what the characteristics of such an association would be has not yet been established. For example, alcohol might affect whether one developed AD, when one developed it, or the progression of AD once one had developed it. Observing no association between increased numbers of senile plaques (a characteristic marker of AD found in the brain) and alcohol-related receptor loss, Freund and Ballinger (1992) concluded that alcohol consumption did not appear to accelerate the AD process. Although it has been neither proven nor disproven that alcohol increases the risk of developing AD nor lowers the age at onset, this study suggests that alcohol does not appear to affect progression of the disease. This hypothesis is supported by a study that reported that past heavy alcohol consumption was not associated with progression of AD over a 1-year interval (Rosen et al. 1993). Other researchers, however, have found past or current alcohol abuse to be a significant predictor of rate of decline in AD (e.g., Teri et al. 1990).

Epidemiologic Studies of Alcohol Use and Alzheimer Disease

Many studies have examined the effects of alcohol and alcoholism on cognitive function and the brain. However, relatively few epidemiologic studies have focused on whether people who drink alcohol have a greater or lesser chance of developing AD.

Epidemiologic studies of alcohol use and AD in the 1980s and early 1990s generally were based on a case-control design, which identifies people with AD (i.e., cases) and a corresponding group of people without AD (i.e., control subjects) and then investigates whether alcohol consumption differs between these two groups. Relatively quick and inexpensive, the case-control design is a standard epidemiologic approach used to identify potential risk factors and to determine whether more extensive studies are warranted.

A summary of 11 of these case-control studies showed that nine of the studies found no significant relationship between alcohol use and AD, one found that alcohol use increased the risk, and one found that alcohol use decreased the risk of AD (Tyas 1996). Most of these studies examined drinking status of study participants (whether they consumed alcohol at a specific, usually high level) rather than using more detailed measures of amount consumed. These case-control studies, however, may not have found a significant association because they had too few subjects (often less than 100 cases) and thus lacked statistical power. This possibility was addressed in two reports from a meta-analysis (Graves et al. 1991; van Duijn and Hofman 1992) that pooled the data from four individual case-control studies. However, the researchers did not find significant results for low, moderate, or high alcohol consumption even with this larger sample. Graves and colleagues (1991) conducted another meta-analysis that included a fifth study, which had used a different definition of alcohol use, but they still did not find a significant association between alcohol use and AD. Meta-analyses have increased power to detect significant associations but are still limited by the flaws of their constituent individual studies.

Subsequent case-control (Wang et al. 1997) and cross-sectional studies (Callahan et al. 1996) also have failed to provide evidence of an association between alcohol use and AD. One case-control study that did find a significant effect reported a reduced risk of AD in men with "high" alcohol use (i.e., more than two drinks per day), taking into account smoking status, education, and the status of a genetic marker for AD (apolipoprotein E allele, a variant of a gene) (Cupples et al. 2000).

Although the weight of evidence from the studies summarized in the preceding text suggests that alcohol use is not related to AD, any conclusions must take into account the methodological limitations of these types of studies. The early studies often failed to account for confounding factors; drinkers differ from nondrinkers in many characteristics such as tobacco use and educational level and it may be those characteristics that are related to the risk of AD rather than alcohol use per se.

The case-control design also has inherent limitations. One notable weakness is that it is essentially cross-sectional. Longitudinal studies collect data on alcohol use at baseline and follow study participants over time to determine if they develop AD. Because high levels of alcohol use are associated with greater mortality, drinkers may be more likely than nondrinkers to die before developing AD, so a protective association between alcohol use and AD may simply reflect selective mortality. Clearly, longitudinal studies provide a better design from which to address issues such as selective mortality.

In addition, case-control studies collect information on alcohol use after diagnosis of AD. But because the cognitive deficits characteristic of AD mean that self-reported information cannot be obtained from study participants, proxy respondents (e.g., family members) are required. A proxy's report is unlikely to correspond perfectly with the information that the study respondent would have provided. This problem is exacerbated if this source of error is not consistent across cases and controls (i.e., studies that use proxy reports for cases should also use proxy reports for controls). A methodological flaw in some of the case-control studies of AD (e.g., Cupples et al. 2000) has been the use of proxy-reported information for cases but self-reported data for controls.

Because of the methodological limitations of case-control studies, evidence from cohort studies—a stronger, longitudinal design—is usually given more weight, even though they also may have limitations (e.g., determination of AD based on clinical records rather than personal examination as per standard diagnostic criteria [Räihä et al. 1998]). Cohort studies generally have found no significant effect of alcohol use on the risk of developing AD (Brayne et al. 1998; Broe et al. 1998; Hebert et al. 1992; Katzman et al. 1989; Räihä et al. 1998; Tyas et al. 2001; Yoshitake et al. 1995), although some evidence of a protective effect of moderate wine consumption (defined as three to four glasses per day) has been reported—that is, moderate wine consumption has been associated with a decreased risk for AD (Leibovici et al. 1999; Orgogozo et al. 1997). A meta-analysis of 15 prospective studies (Anstey et al, 2009) found a lower risk of AD in "drinkers" than "nondrinkers," and no increase in risk for AD among "heavy drinkers."

It is reasonable to expect that the effect of alcohol use on the risk of developing AD might differ depending on the level of alcohol consumption studied, but this does not seem to explain the study results. The cohort studies that found no association between alcohol use and AD used a variety of measures of alcohol consumption, from drinking status (Yoshitake et al. 1995), to amount of alcohol consumed (Broe et al. 1998), to alcohol abuse (Brayne et al. 1998). Both studies reporting protective effects (Leibovici et al. 1999; Orgogozo et al. 1997) were based in France and focused on wine consumption. It is possible that a protective effect is specific to this situation—that wine rather than other types of alcohol, in the drinking pattern and context of French culture, could be protective. In the study by Leibovici and colleagues (1999), however, the decreased risk of AD with alcohol use was reversed to become a significantly increased risk when the participants' place of residence was considered (i.e., in the community or in an institution). Specifically, moderate wine consumption was associated with a lower risk of AD when place of residence was not considered, but with an increased risk when it was included in the analyses. In addition, the significant protective effect of moderate wine consumption reported in the French longitudinal study (Orgogozo et al. 1997) was based on very few cases of AD. Although overall most epidemiologic studies, regardless of the design, do not support an association between alcohol use and AD, further longitudinal studies are needed that overcome the methodological limitations of previous studies. The apparent lack of association between alcohol use and AD in epidemiological studies contrasts with alcohol's proven effects on cognition, neuropathology, and neurochemistry, and its association with dementias other than AD. If it is determined that alcohol does influence the risk of AD, then understanding the mechanism by which it exerts this effect may provide clues to causal pathways, interventions, and prevention.

Alcohol, Tobacco, and Alzheimer Disease

The effect of alcohol use on AD may be modified by other concurrent factors, such as tobacco use. Tobacco and alcohol use are related: "smokers drink and drinkers smoke" (National Institute on Alcohol Abuse and Alcoholism [NIAAA] 1998). The heaviest drinkers are the most likely to smoke, and 70 percent to almost 100 percent of alcoholics in treatment programs report smoking (Bobo and Husten 2000; NIAAA

1998). Conversely, a smoker is 10 times more likely than a nonsmoker to become an alcoholic (NIAAA 1998).

The prevalence of concurrent alcohol and tobacco dependence suggests that alcohol and tobacco may share mechanisms that lead to dependence (Anthony and Echeagaray-Wagner 2000). These mechanisms may have a genetic basis (Madden et al. 2000). Tobacco and alcohol use may be related at least partially because both nicotine and alcohol affect brain nicotinic cholinergic receptors (Collins 1990; Little 2000). Stimulation of these receptors is thought to contribute to the therapeutic effects of galantamine (Reminyl), a new treatment for AD (Maelicke et al. 2001; Newhouse et al. 2001).

Research shows that alcohol and tobacco use interact to influence the risk of certain diseases, such as cancer (U.S. Department of Health and Human Services 1989). Nicotine counteracts some of alcohol's negative effects on cognition, including increased reaction time, impaired time judgment, and slowing of brain wave activity (Arendt 1993). Epidemiologic studies have begun to investigate the effect of an interaction between smoking and drinking on AD. Adjusting for smoking status had little effect on the association between alcohol use and AD in the case-control study by Cupples and colleagues (2000).

However, an analysis of three case-control data sets (Tyas et al. 2000) has provided some support for the hypothesis that smoking influences the effect of alcohol use on AD. In one of the data sets, the risk of AD was significantly increased in drinkers. Study participants who smoked as well as drank, however, had a lower risk than those who only drank. The pattern in the other two data sets varied depending on whether the participants had a history of hypertension. A pattern similar to that of the first data set, but only marginally significant, was found for hypertensive subjects in a second data set, with the risk of AD for people who were both smokers and drinkers lower than the risk for those who were just smokers or just drinkers. It is not clear whether the effect of hypertension reflects a physiological interaction of hypertension with smoking, drinking, and AD. Few analyses on the interaction of tobacco and alcohol use have been published, but one study (Brenner et al. 1993) did find that the association between smoking and AD varied by the hypertensive status of study participants.

The observation that alcohol and tobacco use appear to influence each other's association with AD is consistent with evidence of a biological interaction between smoking and drinking. This observation also may be attributed, however, to the increased overall mortality of people who both smoke and drink, a possibility that can only be ruled out by longitudinal research. The apparent importance of hypertension suggests that a vascular mechanism may be involved in the interaction of alcohol and tobacco use on the risk of developing AD.

Epidemiologic Studies of Alcohol Use and Cognitive Impairment

Although epidemiologic studies do not generally support an association between alcohol consumption and AD, the lack of such a relationship could reflect methodological limitations, such as the difficulty in discriminating AD cases with a history of heavy alcohol consumption from cases of alcoholic dementia. It thus may also be useful to consider evidence from epidemiologic studies examining the association between alcohol use and cognitive outcomes other than AD. The ways in which alcohol use influences the risk of developing cognitive impairment might be similar to those by which it may affect AD, and some types of cognitive impairment themselves may increase the risk of developing AD.

Overall, the results of epidemiologic studies of alcohol use and cognitive impairment are consistent with results from studies of alcohol use and AD. Most studies, regardless of design, found no significant association between alcohol use and cognitive impairment (Cervilla et al. 2000b; Christian et al. 1995; Dent et al. 1997; DiCarlo et al. 2000; Dufouil et al. 2000; Edelstein et al. 1998; Elwood et al. 1999; Hebert et al. 1993). Those studies which did report a significant effect of alcohol use generally found that the results varied by gender (Dufouil et al. 1997), by apolipoprotein E allele status (Carmelli et al. 1999; Dufouil et al. 2000), or by vascular risk factors (e.g., cardiovascular disease and diabetes) (Launer et al. 1996). Evidence of these subgroup effects is not yet compelling; for example, in people with the apolipoprotein E allele, alcohol use increased the risk of cognitive impairment in one study (Dufouil et al. 2000) but decreased it in another (Carmelli et al. 1999). In another study, apolipoprotein status had no effect (Cervilla et al. 2000a). However, investigation of the effects of alcohol use on AD within these gender, genetic, or vascular risk subgroups may prove informative.

Does Alcohol Use Cause Alzheimer Disease?

Although an increased risk of AD with alcohol use is plausible based on biological evidence, the epidemiologic evidence does not support an association. In the few studies that report a significant association, alcohol consumption is more often found to reduce the risk of AD than to increase it. However, methodological factors could create an apparent protective effect of alcohol use on AD. Such factors include selective mortality of drinkers and diagnosing AD patients with heavy alcohol use as having alcoholic dementia rather than AD. In addition, in some studies reporting a protective effect of alcohol (e.g., Cupples et al. 2000), proxy respondents provided information for the cases whereas self-reported information was used for controls. If proxy reports of drinking underestimate actual exposure (McLaughlin et al. 1990), the alcohol use of cases (i.e., study participants with AD) would be artificially lowered compared with control subjects. The apparent association between alcohol use and a reduced risk of AD might therefore merely reflect bias in proxy reports rather than any true effect. Other recent reports of a protective effect (Orgogozo et al. 1997; Leibovici et al. 1999) may have been affected by sample size and the selection of confounding factors, such as community or institutional residence, included in the analyses.

Most studies, including the meta-analysis of case-control studies (Graves et al. 1991; van Duijn and Hofman 1992) and individual cohort studies of AD (Brayne et al. 1998; Broe et al. 1998; Hebert et al. 1992; Katzman et al. 1989; Räihä et al. 1998; Tyas et al. 2001; Yoshitake et al. 1995) have not found a significant association. Epidemiologic studies of alcohol use and cognitive impairment overall have come to similar conclusions, although some evidence exists for a heterogeneous effect of alcohol use on cognitive impairment across gender, genetic, or vascular subgroups.

The effect of alcohol use on the risk of AD has been explored much less extensively than the effect of other potential risk factors, such as tobacco use. The possibility of a protective effect of moderate drinking on AD, raised in a few studies, may not be compelling, but methodological issues need to be resolved before such an association can be definitively dismissed. Moderate drinking has been reported to have some beneficial vascular effects (NIAAA 2000), which could possibly reduce the risk of AD. The nonsignificant association between alcohol use and risk of AD reported by most studies does not necessarily mean that alcohol has no effect. It may instead reflect a balance between the beneficial vascular effects of alcohol and its detrimental effects on the brain, and the relative weight of these two factors may differ within specific subgroups.

Limitations of Current Studies

Because AD has few established risk factors, most studies have examined alcohol use as only one possibly relevant exposure among many, necessitating superficial treatment. Future studies need to collect more detailed information about lifetime alcohol exposure because imprecision in estimating lifetime exposure may obscure associations, as may inconsistent definitions of drinking status or level of consumption. Evidence that alcohol's effects on AD might vary within subgroups also supports more extensive data collection on variables that characterize these subgroups.

One methodological challenge of both case-control and cohort studies is the separation of AD from alcoholic dementia. AD cannot be definitively diagnosed clinically but instead requires confirmation based on examination of the brain after death. Even when AD is accurately diagnosed before death, study participants still represent a heterogeneous group, differing in age at onset, duration, and genetic basis of AD. Case-control studies may introduce bias by using heavy alcohol consumption as an exclusionary criterion for AD cases but not for controls (e.g., Graves et al. 1991). As alcoholic dementia has not been uniformly diagnosed across epidemiologic studies, the discrimination of alcoholic dementia from AD also is problematic.

Priorities for Future Research

Further longitudinal studies that overcome the methodological limitations described above are needed to address basic issues such as selective survival bias. Better measures of lifetime alcohol exposure will help delineate critical exposure periods. Fundamental questions on the biological association between alcohol and AD remain unanswered, such as whether alcohol is associated with pathological and pharmacological changes characteristic of AD. Research is needed to clarify the effects of alcohol on cognitive abilities and the mechanisms by which alcohol may act to influence the risk of developing AD.

Additional priority areas include research into the possibility of concurrent detrimental and beneficial effects of alcohol on AD across all levels of alcohol consumption. Investigating the effect of alcohol use within gender, genetic, vascular, or other subgroups might reveal associations with AD more clearly.

Conclusions

Although it is biologically plausible that drinking increases the risk of AD, epidemiologic studies have not supported this hypothesis. Currently, no strong evidence suggests that alcohol use influences the risk of developing AD, but further research is needed before the effect of alcohol use on AD is fully understood.

References

Anstey, K.J.; Mack, H.A.; Cherbuin, N. Alcohol consumption as a risk factor for dementia and cognitive decline: Meta-analysis of prospective studies. American *Journal of Geriatric Psychiatry* 17(7): 542–55.

Anthony, J.C., and Echeagaray-Wagner, F. Epidemiologic analysis of alcohol and tobacco use: Patterns of co-occurring consumption and dependence in the United States. *Alcohol Research & Health* 24(4):201–208, 2000.

Arendt, T. The cholinergic deafferentation of the cerebral cortex induced by chronic consumption of alcohol: Reversal by cholinergic drugs and transplantation. In: Hunt, W.A., and Nixon, S.J., eds. *Alcohol-Induced Brain Damage.* Rockville, MD: U.S. Department of Health and Human Services, 1993. pp. 431–460.

Bobo, J.K., and Husten, C. Sociocultural influences on smoking and drinking. *Alcohol Research & Health* 24(4):225–232, 2000.

Brayne, C.; Gill, C.; Huppert, F.A.; Barkley, C.; Gehlhaar, E.; Girling, D.M.; O'Connor, D.W.; and Paykel, E.S. Vascular risks and incident dementia: Results from a cohort study of the very old. *Dementia and Geriatric Cognitive Disorders* 9: 175–180, 1998.

Brenner, D.E.; Kukull, WA; Van Belle, G.; Bowen, J.D.; McCormick, W.C.; Teri, L.; and Larson, E.B. Relationship between cigarette smoking and Alzheimer's disease in a population-based case-control study. *Neurology* 43:293–300, 1993.

Broe, G.A.; Creasey, H.; Jorm, A.F.; Bennett, H.P.; Casey, B.; Waite, L.M.; Grayson, D.A.; and Cullen, J. Health habits and risk of cognitive impairment and dementia in old age: A prospective study on the effects of exercise, smoking, and alcohol consumption. Australia and New Zealand *Journal of Public Health* 22:621–623, 1998.

Brookmeyer, R.; Gray, S.; and Kawas, C. Projections of Alzheimer's disease in the United States and the public health impact of delaying disease onset. *American Journal of Public Health* 88:1337–1342, 1998.

Callahan, C.M.; Hall, K.S.; Hui, S.L.; Musick, B.S.; Unverzagt, F.W.; and Hendrie, H.C. Relationship of age, education, and occupation with dementia among a community-based sample of African Americans. *Archives of Neurology* 53:134–140, 1996.

Carlen, P.L., and Wilkinson, D.A. Reversibility of alcohol-related brain damage: Clinical and experimental observations. *Acta Medica Scandinavica* (Suppl.) 717:19–26, 1987.

Carmelli, D.; Swan, G.E.; Reed, T.; Schellenberg, G.D.; and Christian, J.C. The effect of apolipoprotein E in the relationships of smoking and drinking to cognitive function. *Neuroepidemiology* 18:125–133, 1999.

Cervilla, J.A.; Prince, M.; Joels, S.; Lovestone, S.; and Mann, A. Long-term predictors of cognitive outcome in a cohort of older people with hypertension. *British Journal of Psychiatry* 177(1 Pt 1):66–71, 2000a.

Cervilla, J.A.; Prince, M.; and Mann, A. Smoking, drinking, and incident cognitive impairment: A cohort community based study included in the Gospel Oak project. *Journal of Neurology, Neurosurgery and Psychiatry* 68:622–626, 2000b.

Christian, J.C.; Reed, T.; Carmelli, D.; Page, W.F.; Norton, J.A., Jr.; and Breitner, J.C.S. Self-reported alcohol intake and cognition in aging twins. *Journal of Studies on Alcohol* 56:414–416, 1995.

Collins, A.C. Interactions of ethanol and nicotine at the receptor level. In: Galanter, M., ed. Recent Developments in Alcoholism. Volume 8: *Combined Alcohol and Other Drug Dependence.* New York: Plenum Press, 1990. pp. 221–231.

Cupples, L.A.; Weinberg, J.; Beiser, A.; Auerbach, S.H.; Volicer, L.; Cipolloni, P.B.; Wells, J.; Growdon, J.H.; D'Agostino, R.B.; Wolf, P.A.; and Farrer, L.A. Effects of smoking, alcohol and APOE genotype on Alzheimer disease: The MIRAGE study. *Alzheimer's Reports* 3(2):105–114, 2000.

Delin, C.R., and Lee, T.H. Drinking and the brain: Current evidence. *Alcohol and Alcoholism* 27(2):117–126, 1992.

Dent, O.F.; Sulway, M.R.; Broe, G.A.; Creasey, H.; Kos, S.C.; Jorm, A.F.; Tennant, C.; and Fairley, M.J. Alcohol consumption and cognitive performance in a random sample of Australian soldiers who served in the second world war. *British Medical Journal* 314:1655–1657, 1997.

Diamond, I., and Gordon, A.S. Cellular and molecular neuroscience of alcoholism. *Physiological Reviews* 77(1):1–20, 1997.

Dicarlo, A.; Baldereschi, M.; Amaducci, L.; et al. Cognitive impairment without dementia in older people: Prevalence, vascular risk factors, impact on disability. The Italian Longitudinal Study on Aging. *Journal of the American Geriatrics Society* 48:775–782, 2000.

Dufouil, C.; Ducimetière, P.; and Alpérovitch, A. Sex differences in the association between alcohol consumption and cognitive performance. *American Journal of Epidemiology* 146:405–412, 1997.

Dufouil, C.; Tzourio, C.; Brayne, C.; Berr, C.; Amouyel, P.; and Alpéro-vitch, A. Influence of apolipoprotein E genotype on the risk of cognitive deterioration in moderate drinkers and smokers. *Epidemiology* 11:280–284, 2000.

Edelstein, S.L.; Kritz-Silverstein, D.; and Barrett-Connor, E.L. Prospective association of smoking and alcohol use with cognitive function in an elderly cohort. *Journal of Women's Health* 7(10): 1271–1281, 1998.

Elwood, P.C.; Gallacher, J.E.J.; Hopkinson, C.A.; Pickering, J.; Rabbitt, P.; Stollery, B.; Brayne, C.; Huppert, F.A.; and Bayer, A. Smoking, drinking, and other life style factors and cognitive function in men in the Caerphilly cohort. *Journal of Epidemiology and Community Health* 53:9–14, 1999.

Ernst, R.L., and Hay, J.W. The U.S. economic and social costs of Alzheimer's disease revisited. *American Journal of Public Health* 84:1261–1264, 1994.

Evert, D.L., and Oscar-Berman, M. Alcohol-related cognitive impairments: An overview of how alcoholism may affect the workings of the brain. *Alcohol Health & Research World* 19(2):89–96, 1995.

Fisman, M.; Ramsay, D.; and Weiser, M. Dementia in the elderly male alcoholic—A retrospective clinicopathologic study. *International Journal of Geriatric Psychiatry* 11:209–218, 1996.

Forette, F., and Boller, F. Trends in Alzheimer's disease treatment and prevention. In: Iqbal, K.; Swaab, D.F.; Winblad, B.; and Wisniewski, H.M., eds. *Alzheimer's Disease and Related Disorders: Etiology, Pathogenesis, and Therapeutics.* Chichester: John Wiley & Sons, 1999. pp. 623–631.

Freund, G. The interaction of chronic alcohol consumption and aging on brain structure and function. *Alcoholism: Clinical and Experimental Research* 6(1):13–21, 1982.

Freund, G., and Ballinger, W.E., Jr. Alzheimer's disease and alcoholism: Possible interactions. *Alcohol* 9:233–240, 1992.

Graves, A.B.; Van Duijn, C.; Chandra, V.; Fratiglioni, L.; Heyman, A.; Jorm, A.F.; et al. Alcohol and tobacco consumption as risk factors for Alzheimer's disease: A collaborative re-analysis of case-control studies. *International Journal of Epidemiology* 20(2) Suppl. 2:S48–S57, 1991.

Hebert, L.E.; Scherr, P.A.; Beckett, L.A.; et al. Relation of smoking and alcohol consumption to incident Alzheimer's Disease. *American Journal of Epidemiology* 135(4):347–355, 1992.

Hebert, L.E.; Scherr, P.A.; Beckett, L.A.; et al. Relation of smoking and low-to-moderate alcohol consumption to change in cognitive function: A longitudinal study in a defined community of older persons. *American Journal of Epidemiology* 137:881–891, 1993.

Jensen, G.B., and Pakkenberg, B. Do alcoholics drink their neurons away? *The Lancet* 342:1201–1204, 1993.

Katzman, R.; Aronson, M.; Fuld, P.; et al. Development of dementing illnesses in an 80-year-old volunteer cohort. *Annals of Neurology* 25:317–324, 1989.

Kawas, C.H., and Katzman, R. Epidemiology of dementia and Alzheimer disease. In: Terry, R.D.; Katzman, R.; Bick, K.L.; and Sisodia, S.S., eds. *Alzheimer Disease.* Philadelphia: Lippincott Williams & Wilkins, 1999. pp. 95–116.

Korbo, L. Glial cell loss in the hippocampus of alcoholics. *Alcoholism: Clinical and Experimental Research* 23(1):164–168, 1999.

Kril, J.J., and Halliday, G.M. Brain shrinkage in alcoholics: A decade on and what have we learned? *Progress in Neurobiology* 58:381–387, 1999.

Launer, L.J.; Feskens, E.J.M.; Kalmijn, S.; and Kromhout, D. Smoking, drinking and thinking: The Zutphen elderly study. *American Journal of Epidemiology* 143:219–227, 1996.

Leibovici, D.; Ritchie, K.; Ledésert, B.; and Touchon, J. The effects of wine and tobacco consumption on cognitive performance in the elderly: A longitudinal study of relative risk. *International Journal of Epidemiology* 28:77–81, 1999.

Leon, J.; Cheng, C.K.; and Neumann, P.J. Alzheimer's disease care: Costs and potential savings. *Health Affairs* 17(6):206–216, 1998.

Little, H.J. Behavioral mechanisms underlying the link between smoking and drinking. *Alcohol Research & Health* 24(4):215–224, 2000.

Madden, P.A.F.; Bucholz, K.K.; Martin, N.G.; and Heath, A.C. Smoking and the genetic contribution to alcohol-dependence risk. *Alcohol Research & Health* 24(4):209–214, 2000.

Maelicke, A.; Samochocki, M.; Jostock, R.; et al. Allosteric sensitization of nicotinic receptors by galantamine, a new treatment strategy for Alzheimer's disease. *Biological Psychiatry* 49:279–288, 2001.

McLaughlin, J.K.; Mandel, J.S.; Mehl, E.S.; and Blot, W.J. Comparison of next-of-kin with self-respondents regarding questions on cigarette, coffee, and alcohol consumption. *Epidemiology* 1:408–412, 1990.

Meyer, J.S.; Terayama, Y.; Konno, S.; Akiyama, H.; Margishvili, G.M.; and Mortel, K.F. Risk factors for cerebral degenerative changes and dementia. *European Neurology* 39(Suppl. 1):7–16, 1998.

Morris, J.C. Clinical presentation and course of Alzheimer disease. In: Terry, R.D.; Katzman, R.; Bick, K.L.; and Sisodia, S.S., eds. *Alzheimer Disease.* Philadelphia: Lippincott Williams & Wilkins, 1999. pp. 11–24.

Newhouse, P.A.; Potter, A.; Kelton, M.; and Corwin, J. Nicotinic treatment of Alzheimer's disease. Biological Psychiatry 49:268–278, 2001.

National Institute on Alcohol Abuse and Alcoholism. Alcohol Alert No. 39: Alcohol and Tobacco. Rockville, MD: the Institute, 1998. National Institute on Alcohol Abuse and Alcoholism. Health risks and benefits of alcohol consumption. *Alcohol Research & Health* 24(1):5–11, 2000.

Orgogozo, J.M.; Dartigues, J.F.; Lafont, S.; et al. Wine consumption and dementia in the elderly: A prospective community study in the Bordeaux area. *Revue Neurologique* (Paris) 153:185–192, 1997.

Räihä, I.; Kaprio, J.; Koskenvuo, M.; Rajala, T.; and Sourander, L. Environmental differences in twin pairs discordant for Alzheimer's disease. *Journal of Neurology, Neurosurgery and Psychiatry* 65:785–787, 1998.

Reed, R.J.; Grant, I.; and Rourke, S.B. Long-term abstinent alcoholics have normal memory. *Alcoholism: Clinical and Experimental Research* 16(4):677–683, 1992.

Rosen, J.; Colantonio, A.; Becker, J.T.; Lopez, O.L.; Dekosky, S.T.; and Moss, H.B. Effects of a history of heavy alcohol consumption on Alzheimer's disease. *British Journal of Psychiatry* 163:358–363, 1993.

Saxton, J.; Munro, C.A.; Butters, M.A.; Schramke, C.; and Mcneil, M.A. Alcohol, dementia, and Alzheimer's Disease: Comparison of neuropsychological profiles. *Journal of Geriatric Psychiatry and Neurology,* 13(3):141–149, 2000.

Smith, D.M., and Atkinson, R.M. Alcoholism and dementia. In: Gurnack, A.M., ed. *Older Adults' Misuse of Alcohol, Medicines, and Other Drugs: Research and Practice Issues.* New York: Springer, 1997. pp. 132–157.

Teri, L.; Hughes, J.P.; and Larson, E.B. Cognitive deterioration in Alzheimer's disease: Behavioral and health factors. *Journal of Gerontology* 45:P58–P63, 1990.

Tyas, S.L. Are tobacco and alcohol use related to Alzheimer's disease? A critical assessment of the evidence and its implications. *Addiction Biology* 1:237–254, 1996.

Tyas, S.L.; Koval, J.J.; and Pederson, L.L. Does an interaction between smoking and drinking influence the risk of Alzheimer's disease? Results from three Canadian data sets. *Statistics in Medicine* 19:1685–1696, 2000.

Tyas, S.L.; Manfreda, J.; Strain, L.A.; and Montgomery, P.R. Risk factors for Alzheimer's disease: A population-based, longitudinal study in Manitoba, Canada. *International Journal of Epidemiology* 30:590–597, 2001.

U.S. Department of Health and Human Services. Reducing the Health Consequences of Smoking: 25 Years of Progress. A report of the Surgeon General. U.S. Department of Health and Human Services, Public Health Service, Centers for Disease Control, Center for Chronic Disease Prevention and Health Promotion, Office on Smoking and Health, 1989.

van Duijn, C.M., and Hofman, A. Risk factors for Alzheimer's disease: The EURODEM collaborative re-analysis of case-control studies. *Neuroepidemiology* 11 (Suppl. 1) 106–113, 1992.

Wang, P.N.; Wang, S.J.; Hong, C.J.; Liu, T.T.; Fuh, J.L.; Chi, C.W.; Liu, C.Y.; and Liu, H.C. Risk factors for Alzheimer's disease: A case-control study. *Neuroepidemiology* 16:234–240, 1997.

Yoshitake, T.; Kiyohara, Y.; Kato, I.; Ohmura, T.; Iwamoto, H.; Nakayama, K.; et al. Incidence and risk factors of vascular dementia and Alzheimer's disease in a defined elderly Japanese population: The Hisayama study. *Neurology* 45:1161–1168, 1995.

Section 15.2

Secondhand Smoke

A new analysis of published articles suggests smoking cigarettes may be a significant risk factor for Alzheimer's disease.

University of California at San Francisco researchers also found an association between tobacco industry affiliation and the conclusions of individual studies. Industry-affiliated studies indicated that smoking protects against the development of AD, while independent studies showed that smoking increased the risk of developing the disease.

"For many years, published studies and popular media have perpetuated the myth that smoking is protective against the development of AD. The disease's impact on quality of life and health care costs continues to rise. It is therefore critical that we better understand its causes, in particular, the role of cigarette smoking," said Janine K. Cataldo, PhD, RN, assistant professor in the UCSF School of Nursing and lead author of the study.

According to the Alzheimer's Association, 5.3 million Americans currently have the disease, and that number will escalate rapidly as the baby boom generation ages. AD also triples health care costs for Americans aged 65 and older, the organization states.

The UCSF team reviewed 43 published studies from 1984 to 2007. Authors of one-fourth of the studies had an affiliation with the tobacco industry.

The UCSF team determined that the average risk of a smoker developing AD, based on studies without tobacco industry affiliation, was estimated to be 1.72, meaning that smoking nearly doubled the risk of AD.

In contrast, the team found that studies authored by individuals with tobacco industry affiliations, showed a risk factor of .86 (less than one), suggesting that smoking protects against AD. When all studies were considered together, the risk factor for developing AD from smoking was essentially neutral at a statistically insignificant 1.05.

Previous reviews of the association between smoking and AD have not controlled for study design and author affiliation with the tobacco industry, according to Cataldo. To determine if study authors had connections to the tobacco industry, the UCSF team analyzed 877 previously secret tobacco industry documents.

The researchers used an inclusive definition of "tobacco industry affiliation" and examined authors' current or past funding, employment, paid consultation, and collaboration or co-authorship on a study with someone who had current or previous tobacco industry funding within 10 years of publication.

"We know that industry-sponsored research is more likely to reach conclusions favorable to the sponsor," said Stanton A. Glantz, PhD, of the UCSF Department of Medicine and a study co-author.

"Our findings point to the ongoing corrosive nature of tobacco industry funding and point to the need for academic institutions to decline tobacco industry funding to protect the research process."

The study is published online in the [January 2010] *Journal of Alzheimer's Disease.* Source: University of California at San Francisco.

Section 15.3

Heart Health

Study highlights:

- Keeping your heart healthy may slow down brain aging.

- Cardiac index, a measure of heart health, is linked to diminishing brain volume, a sign of brain aging.

- Brains may age faster in people whose hearts pump less blood.

Keep your heart healthy and you may slow down the aging of your brain, according to a new study reported in *Circulation: Journal of the American Heart Association* [August 17, 2010].

In the study, people whose hearts pumped less blood had brains that appeared older than the brains of those whose hearts pumped more blood. Decreased cardiac index, the amount of blood that pumps from the heart in relation to a person's body size, was associated with decreased brain volume using magnetic resonance imaging (MRI).

Researchers observed the link even in those participants who did not have cardiovascular disease, such as heart failure or coronary heart disease. As the brain ages, it begins to atrophy (shrink) and has less volume. The decrease in brain volume is considered a sign of brain aging. More severe brain atrophy occurs in those with dementia, such as Alzheimer's disease.

"The results are interesting in that they suggest cardiac index and brain health are related," said Angela L. Jefferson, PhD, the study's lead author and associate professor of neurology at the Boston University School of Medicine. "The association cannot be attributed to cardiovascular disease because the relationship also was seen when we removed those participants with known cardiovascular disease from our analyses."

In the observational study, which cannot establish cause and effect, researchers examined brain and heart MRI information on 1,504 participants of the decades-long Framingham Offspring Cohort who did not have a history of stroke, transient ischemic attack, or dementia. Participants were 34 to 84 years old and 54 percent were women.

Researchers measured cardiac output using MRI and normalized the data for each participant's body surface area. Brain volume was assessed using MRI. Participants were divided into three groups based on cardiac index values. The participants who had the lowest cardiac index, or the least amount of blood pumping from the heart for their body size, showed almost 2 years more brain aging than the people with the highest cardiac index. The participants in the middle cardiac index group, who had low but still normal levels of blood pumping from the heart, also showed almost 2 years more brain aging than the people with the highest (or healthiest) cardiac index.

"We expected an association between the lowest levels of cardiac index and smaller brain volumes, but we were surprised to find people on the lower end of normal cardiac index also have smaller brain volumes when compared to people with very healthy cardiac index," Jefferson said.

Because only 7 percent of all participants in the study had heart disease, Jefferson and her colleagues also didn't expect 30 percent of participants would have low cardiac index.

"These participants are not sick people. A very small number have heart disease. The observation that nearly a third of the entire sample has low cardiac index and that lower cardiac index is related to smaller brain volume is concerning and requires further study."

As a group, participants with smaller brain volumes did not show obvious clinical signs of diminished brain function. "We observed cardiac index is related to structural changes in the brain but not cognitive changes," Jefferson said. "The structural changes may be early evidence that something is wrong. Investigators from Framingham will continue to follow these individuals to see how structural brain changes affect memory and cognitive abilities over time."

The exact cause for a link between heart function and brain volume is still not well understood, Jefferson said. "There are several theories for why reduced cardiac index might affect brain health. For instance, a lower volume of blood pumping from the heart might reduce blood flow to the brain, providing less oxygen and fewer nutrients needed for brain cells. It is too early to dole out health advice based on this one finding but it does suggest that heart and brain health go hand in hand."

Co-authors are Jayandra J. Himali, MS; Alexa S. Beiser, PhD; Rhoda Au, PhD; Joseph M. Massaro, PhD; Sudha Seshadri, MD; Philimon

Gona, PhD; Carol J. Salton, BA; Charles DeCarli, MD; Christopher J. O'Donnell, MD, MPH; Emelia J. Benjamin, MD, ScM; Philip A. Wolf, MD; and Warren J. Manning, MD. Author disclosures are on the manuscript.

The National Institute on Aging and the National Heart, Lung, and Blood Institute funded the research.

Part Three

Other Dementia Disorders

Chapter 16

Mild Cognitive Impairment

Definition of MCI

Mild Cognitive Impairment (MCI) is a condition characterized by significant cognitive impairment in the absence of dementia. It primarily affects memory but it might cause changes in daily function in subtle ways. Memory changes from MCI are not part of normal aging and should be discussed with a physician.

MCI is different from Alzheimer's disease or other dementias. It does not typically affect a person's ability to complete daily tasks or cause general confusion.

Most people with MCI can live independently. Generally, they have no significant difficulty thinking and can carry on conversations, participate in community activities, and drive. They do tend to be forgetful and are prone to mix up the sequence of doing tasks that have multiple steps.

Recognizing Signs and Symptoms

If MCI progresses, memory problems become more noticeable. Family and friends may begin to notice signs such as:

* repeating the same question over and over again;

"Mild Cognitive Impairment (MCI): What do we do now?" © 2006 Center for Gerontology at Virginia Polytechnic Institute and State University (www.geron tology.vt.edu). Reprinted with permission.

151

- retelling the same stories or providing the same information repeatedly;
- lack of initiative in beginning or completing activities;
- trouble managing number-related tasks such as bill paying;
- lack of focus during conversations and activities;
- inability to follow multi-step directions.

Why Seek Medical Help?

Many people believe that memory loss is a normal part of aging and do not think they need to seek medical help. Others delay seeing the doctor because they want to avoid hearing the truth about their condition.

In fact, memory problems can result from a variety of medical conditions. An examination by a physician can rule out the existence of other conditions and may provide treatments and strategies to reduce non-MCI-related memory problems as well as helping with MCI.

Seeking Diagnosis

Making an appointment with a family doctor to discuss concerns about memory loss is the first step toward seeking a diagnosis.

After an initial assessment, the doctor may make a referral to a memory clinic for further evaluation. Neurologists and geriatric psychiatrists are also able to address memory-related concerns and make a referral for further testing if necessary.

Diagnosing MCI

MCI is difficult to diagnose because:

- no specific test has been developed to diagnose it;
- not everyone will exhibit all of the signs and symptoms;
- evidence of memory problems appears gradually;
- other health issues may be contributing to changes in memory;
- some people think memory loss is a normal part of aging, but it isn't.

In diagnosing MCI, the doctor may:

- ask a series of questions that test memory, language skills, recall, attention span, and visual-spatial abilities;

- review current health records and medications;
- rule out depression and other emotional health concerns;
- order additional testing and brain imaging as necessary;
- talk to family members or others close to the person to learn about changes they have noticed in memory, personality, and behavior.

During future visits, similar tests will be conducted to determine if memory loss is getting worse. Do not be surprised if your primary care doctor wants this follow-up to be done by a specialist.

Medications for MCI

At this time, there is no known cure for MCI or way of stopping or reversing its effects. However, research shows that medications prescribed for persons with Alzheimer's disease may help people with MCI focus better and think more clearly. Ask a doctor for information on current therapies.

Reactions to Having MCI

Each person responds differently to having memory loss. Some people:

- **Feel frustrated and annoyed at themselves:** A simple task now takes a great deal of time and effort to complete.

- **Respond by laughing and joking about their forgetfulness:** Making light of memory problems may disguise the true nature of memory loss and often delays recognition by doctors, friends, and family.

- **Withdraw and isolate themselves:** Withdrawal may lead to depression, which is common among individuals with memory loss. Depression is treatable and not a normal side effect of MCI.

Reactions of Family and Friends to MCI

Family and friends often have a difficult time accepting memory loss as a real medical problem.

Some people falsely believe that the person experiencing memory loss is:

- lazy and intentionally avoiding things that need to be done;

153

- purposefully trying to annoy them by pretending to forget;
- trying to get attention by claiming to have memory loss.

When family and friends spend more time with the person having MCI, they begin to understand its seriousness and how it influences daily life.

Strategies for Family and Friends

Despite having memory loss, people with MCI still want to feel useful, productive, and independent. Most report not wanting to be a burden on their families. The following approaches help promote healthy and positive relationships:

Be Supportive and Encouraging

- Accept the memory loss as real.
- Allow people with MCI to complete their daily routine at their own pace.
- Provide uninterrupted moments to allow for recalling information.
- Encourage nurturance by suggesting responsibility for caring for a pet or plants.
- Encourage usefulness by suggesting responsibility for completing household tasks.
- Promote feelings of success by giving one task to complete at a time.
- Help the person stay physically healthy.
- Avoid becoming overprotective.

Be Patient and Respectful

- Learn to recognize the signs and symptoms of MCI.
- Treat the person like an adult.
- Include the person in social events and community activities.
- Respond to the same question as if it were the first time, every time.
- Avoid beginning or ending sentences with "I already told you . . ."
- Avoid interrupting people with MCI when they are speaking.

- Avoid talking about people with MCI without including them in the conversation.

- Simplify speaking style only if those with MCI tell you that they do not understand you.

Strategies to Compensate for Memory Loss

Daily Tasks and Appointments

- Keep a pen and a calendar with large writing spaces near the telephone.

- Write medical appointments, birthdays, church services, meetings, social activities, trash pick-up, due dates for bills, and car inspections on the calendar.

- Do not agree to an appointment until you have checked it against the calendar.

- Write a daily to-do list and keep it in a visible spot.

Medication Management

- Keep daily medications organized and in a visible location.

- Use a pill box organized by days and times.

- Set pill bottles on the table or next to the bed as reminders to take the medication.

- Label pill bottle tops with different colors, each representing a different time of day.

Household Responsibilities

- Keep bills and important papers in a visible place, not tucked away in a desk, basket, or cupboard.

- Write reminder notes. Carry a pocket-sized notepad or place a notebook on the kitchen table or by a favorite chair and write down things to do or important information.

Driving

- Drive when the traffic is light and allow plenty of time to get to places.

- Drive during clear weather and during daylight hours.

- Take advantage of public transportation and people's offer to give you a ride.

Communication

- Keep using the same cell phone and small electronics, such as cameras, to eliminate confusion from switching to a new model.
- Program frequently used phone numbers into the phone's speed dial feature.
- Use a cell phone to check in with family throughout the day.
- Use a tape recorder to save important matters you want to tell others.
- Use walkie-talkies to keep track of others when shopping or spending time out in the community.

Strategies for Care Partners

Caring for Yourself

Living with a person with MCI or being a care partner can present challenges and cause stress. To maintain a positive and healthy outlook on life:

- Take one day at a time—some days are better than others.
- Pick your battles, don't sweat the small stuff.
- Use coping strategies recommended by a professional and do the best you can.
- Ask family, friends, and health professionals for help and information.
- Be willing to accept help.
- Learn to manage your feelings effectively.
- Talk to others with similar experiences or join a memory loss support group.

Looking to the Future

Memory loss associated with MCI may progress and worsen over time. To cope with and manage future needs and challenges:

- Enable the person with MCI to remain independent for as long as possible.

- Investigate housing and care options in the community that can assist in care and oversight, such as meal programs, transportation, and adult day services.

- Create a family fund into which all family members can make donations so that future uncovered expenses are not a burden on any particular family member.

- Develop strategies to prevent someone with MCI from entering into unneeded financial agreements:

  - Implement a system to block telemarketers from calling.

  - Intercept daily mail and remove special offers for merchandise.

  - Divert mail to another address and produce it only when paying bills.

- Keep current on information about MCI and treatment options.

Chapter 17

Degenerative Neurological Disease

Chapter Contents

Section 17.1

Corticobasal Degeneration

From "Corticobasal Degeneration Information Page," by the National Institute of Neurological Disorders and Stroke (NINDS, www.ninds .nih.gov), part of the National Institutes of Health, April 25, 2008.

What is corticobasal degeneration?

Corticobasal degeneration is a progressive neurological disorder characterized by nerve cell loss and atrophy (shrinkage) of multiple areas of the brain including the cerebral cortex and the basal ganglia. Corticobasal degeneration progresses gradually. Initial symptoms, which typically begin at or around age 60, may first appear on one side of the body (unilateral), but eventually affect both sides as the disease progresses. Symptoms are similar to those found in Parkinson disease, such as poor coordination, akinesia (an absence of movements), rigidity (a resistance to imposed movement), disequilibrium (impaired balance), and limb dystonia (abnormal muscle postures). Other symptoms such as cognitive and visual-spatial impairments, apraxia (loss of the ability to make familiar, purposeful movements), hesitant and halting speech, myoclonus (muscular jerks), and dysphagia (difficulty swallowing) may also occur. An individual with corticobasal degeneration eventually becomes unable to walk.

Is there any treatment?

There is no treatment available to slow the course of corticobasal degeneration, and the symptoms of the disease are generally resistant to therapy. Drugs used to treat Parkinson disease-type symptoms do not produce any significant or sustained improvement. Clonazepam may help the myoclonus. Occupational, physical, and speech therapy can help in managing disability.

What is the prognosis?

Corticobasal degeneration usually progresses slowly over the course of 6 to 8 years. Death is generally caused by pneumonia or other complications of severe debility such as sepsis or pulmonary embolism.

Section 17.2

Dementia with Lewy Bodies

This chapter contains text from "What Is LBD?", "Symptoms,"
and "Diagnosis" 2010 Lewy Body Dementia Association
(www.lbda.org). Reprinted with permission.

What Is LBD?

LBD is not a rare disease. It affects an estimated 1.3 million individuals and their families in the United States. Because LBD symptoms can closely resemble other more commonly known diseases like Alzheimer's and Parkinson's, it is currently widely underdiagnosed. Many doctors or other medical professionals still are not familiar with LBD.

LBD is an umbrella term for two related diagnoses. LBD refers to both Parkinson's disease dementia and dementia with Lewy bodies. The earliest symptoms of these two diseases differ, but reflect the same underlying biological changes in the brain. Over time, people with both diagnoses will develop very similar cognitive, physical, sleep, and behavioral symptoms.

While it may take more than a year or two for enough symptoms to develop for a doctor to diagnose LBD, it is critical to pursue a formal diagnosis. Early diagnosis allows for important early treatment that may extend quality of life and independence.

LBD is a multisystem disease and typically requires a comprehensive treatment approach. This approach involves a team of physicians from different specialties who collaborate to provide optimum treatment of each symptom without worsening other LBD symptoms. Many people with LBD enjoy significant improvement of their symptoms with a comprehensive approach to treatment, and some can have remarkably little change from year to year.

Some people with LBD are extremely sensitive or may react negatively to certain medications used to treat Alzheimer's or Parkinson's in addition to certain over-the-counter medications.

Who Was Lewy?

In the early 1900s, while researching Parkinson's disease, the scientist Friederich H. Lewy discovered abnormal protein deposits that disrupt the brain's normal functioning. These Lewy body proteins are found in an area of the brain stem where they deplete the neurotransmitter dopamine, causing Parkinsonian symptoms. In Lewy body dementia, these abnormal proteins are diffuse throughout other areas of the brain, including the cerebral cortex. The brain chemical acetylcholine is depleted, causing disruption of perception, thinking, and behavior. Lewy body dementia exists either in pure form, or in conjunction with other brain changes, including those typically seen in Alzheimer's disease and Parkinson's disease.

Symptoms

Lewy Body Dementia Symptoms and Diagnostic Criteria

Every person with LBD is different and will manifest different degrees of the following symptoms. Some will show no signs of certain features, especially in the early stages of the disease. Symptoms may fluctuate as often as moment-to-moment, hour-to-hour, or day-to-day. NOTE: Some patients meet the criteria for LBD yet score in the normal range of some cognitive assessment tools. The Mini-Mental State Examination (MMSE), for example, cannot be relied upon to distinguish LBD from other common syndromes.

LBD is an umbrella term for two related clinical diagnoses, dementia with Lewy bodies and Parkinson's disease dementia.

The latest clinical diagnostic criteria for dementia with Lewy bodies (DLB) categorize symptoms into three types, listed in the following text. A diagnosis of Parkinson's disease dementia (PDD) requires a well-established diagnosis of Parkinson's disease that later progresses into dementia, along with very similar features to DLB. A rather arbitrary time cutoff was established to differentiate between DLB and PDD. People whose dementia occurs before or within 1 year of Parkinson's symptoms are diagnosed with DLB. People who have an existing diagnosis of Parkinson's for more than a year and later develop dementia are diagnosed with PDD.

Central feature:

- Progressive dementia—deficits in attention and executive function are typical. Prominent memory impairment may not be evident in the early stages.

Core features:

- Fluctuating cognition with pronounced variations in attention and alertness
- Recurrent complex visual hallucinations, typically well-formed and detailed
- Spontaneous features of parkinsonism

Suggestive features:

- REM sleep behavior disorder (RBD), which can appear years before the onset of dementia and parkinsonism
- Severe sensitivity to neuroleptics occurs in up to 50% of LBD patients who take them.
- Low dopamine transporter uptake in the brain's basal ganglia as seen on SPECT [single photon emission computed tomography] and PET [positron emission tomography] imaging scans (These scans are not yet available outside of research settings.)

Supportive features:

- Repeated falls and syncope (fainting)
- Transient, unexplained loss of consciousness
- Autonomic dysfunction
- Hallucinations of other modalities
- Visuospatial abnormalities
- Other psychiatric disturbances

A clinical diagnosis of LBD can be probable or possible based on different symptom combinations.

A probable LBD diagnosis requires either:

- dementia plus two or more core features, or
- dementia plus one core feature and one or more suggestive features.

A possible LBD diagnosis requires:

- dementia plus one core feature, or
- dementia plus one or more suggestive features.

Symptoms Explained

In this section we'll discuss each of the symptoms, starting with the key word: dementia. Dementia is a process whereby the person becomes progressively confused. The earliest signs are usually memory problems, changes in their way of speaking, such as forgetting words, and personality problems. Cognitive symptoms of dementia include poor problem solving, difficulty with learning new skills, and impaired decision making.

Other causes of dementia should be ruled out first, such as alcoholism, overuse of medication, thyroid or metabolic problems. Strokes can also cause dementia. If these reasons are ruled out then the person is said to have a degenerative dementia. Lewy Body Dementia is second only to Alzheimer's disease as the most common form of dementia.

Fluctuations in cognition will be noticeable to those who are close to the person with LBD, such as their partner. At times the person will be alert and then suddenly have acute episodes of confusion. These may last hours or days. Because of these fluctuations, it is not uncommon for it to be thought that the person is "faking." This fluctuation is not related to the well-known "sundowning" of Alzheimer's. In other words, there is no specific time of day when confusion can be seen to occur.

Hallucinations are usually, but not always, visual and often are more pronounced when the person is most confused. They are not necessarily frightening to the person. Other modalities of hallucinations include sound, taste, smell, and touch.

Parkinsonism or Parkinson's Disease symptoms, take the form of changes in gait; the person may shuffle or walk stiffly. There may also be frequent falls. Body stiffness in the arms or legs, or tremors may also occur. Parkinson's mask (blank stare, emotionless look on face), stooped posture, drooling, and runny nose may be present.

REM Sleep Behavior Disorder (RBD) is often noted in persons with Lewy Body Dementia. During periods of REM sleep, the person will move, gesture, and/or speak. There may be more pronounced confusion between the dream and waking reality when the person awakens. RBD may actually be the earliest symptom of LBD in some patients, and is now considered a significant risk factor for developing LBD. (One recent study found that nearly two-thirds of patients diagnosed with RBD developed degenerative brain diseases, including Lewy body dementia, Parkinson's disease, and multiple system atrophy, after an average of 11 years of receiving an RBD diagnosis. All three diseases are called synucleinopathies, due to the presence of a misfolded protein in the brain called alpha-synuclein.)

Sensitivity to neuroleptic (anti-psychotic) drugs is another significant symptom that may occur. These medications can worsen the Parkinsonism and/or decrease the cognition and/or increase the hallucinations. Neuroleptic Malignancy Syndrome, a life-threatening illness, has been reported in persons with Lewy Body Dementia. For this reason, it is very important that the proper diagnosis is made and that healthcare providers are educated about the disease.

Other Symptoms

Visuospatial difficulties, including depth perception, object orientation, directional sense, and illusions, may occur.

Autonomic dysfunction includes blood pressure fluctuations (e.g., postural/orthostatic hypotension) heart rate variability (HRV), sexual disturbances/impotence, constipation, urinary problems, hyperhidrosis (excessive sweating), decreased sweating/heat intolerance, syncope (fainting), dry eyes/mouth, and difficulty swallowing which may lead to aspiration pneumonia.

Other psychiatric disturbances may include systematized delusions, aggression, and depression. The onset of aggression in LBD may have a variety of causes, including infections (e.g., UTI [urinary tract infection]), medications, misinterpretation of the environment or personal interactions, and the natural progression of the disease.

Diagnosis

An experienced clinician within the medical community should perform a diagnostic evaluation. If one is not available, the neurology department of the nearest medical university should be able to recommend appropriate resources or may even provide an experienced diagnostic team skilled in Lewy body dementia.

A thorough dementia diagnostic evaluation includes physical and neurological examinations, patient and family interviews (including a detailed lifestyle and medical history), and neuro-psychological and mental status tests. The patient's functional ability, attention, language, visuospatial skills, memory, and executive functioning are assessed. In addition, brain imaging (CT [computed tomography] or MRI [magnetic resonance imaging] scans), blood tests, and other laboratory studies may be performed. The evaluation will provide a clinical diagnosis. Currently, a conclusive diagnosis of LBD can be obtained only from a postmortem autopsy for which arrangements should be made in advance. Some research studies may offer brain autopsies as part of their protocols. Participating in research studies is a good way to benefit others with Lewy body dementia.

Medications

Medications are one of the most controversial subjects in dealing with LBD. A medication that doesn't work for one person may work for another person. Become knowledgeable about LBD treatments and medication sensitivities.

Prescribing should only be done by a physician who is thoroughly knowledgeable about LBD. With new medications and even over-the-counter drugs, the patient should be closely monitored. At the first sign of an adverse reaction, consult with the patient's physician. Consider joining the online caregiver support groups to see what others have observed with prescription and over-the-counter medicines.

Risk Factors

Advanced age is considered to be the greatest risk factor for Lewy body dementia, with onset typically, but not always, between the ages of 50 and 85. Some cases have been reported much earlier. It appears to affect slightly more men than women. Having a family member with Lewy body dementia may increase a person's risk. Observational studies suggest that adopting a healthy lifestyle (exercise, mental stimulation, nutrition) might delay age-associated dementias.

Clinical Trials

The recruitment of LBD patients for participation in clinical trials for studies on LBD, other dementias, and Parkinsonian studies is now steadily increasing.

For those interested in participating in LBD research, please check our clinical trials page (http://www.lbda.org/category/3514/clinical -trials.htm).

Prognosis and Stages

No cure or definitive treatment for Lewy body dementia has been discovered as yet. The disease has an average duration of 5 to 7 years. It is possible, though, for the time span to be anywhere from 2 to 20 years, depending on several factors, including the person's overall health, age, and severity of symptoms.

Defining the stages of disease progression for LBD is difficult. The symptoms, medicine management, and duration of LBD vary greatly from person to person. To further complicate the stages assessment, LBD has a progressive but vacillating clinical course, and one of its defining symptoms is fluctuating levels of cognitive abilities, alertness, and attention. Sudden decline is often caused by medications, infections, or other compromises to the immune system and usually the person with LBD returns to their baseline upon resolution of the problem. But for some individuals, it may also be due to the natural course of the disease.

Section 17.3

Frontotemporal Dementia

Definition

Frontotemporal Dementia (FTD) is a degenerative condition of the front (anterior) part of the brain. It differs from other causes of dementia such as Alzheimer's, Lewy body, and Creutzfeldt-Jakob diseases. FTD is currently understood as a clinical syndrome that groups together Pick's disease, primary progressive aphasia, and semantic dementia. The areas of the brain affected by FTD—the frontal and anterior temporal lobes—control reasoning, personality, movement, speech, social graces, language, and some aspects of memory.

FTD is marked by dramatic changes in personality, behavior, and some thought processes. Changes in personal and social conduct occur in early stages of the disease, including loss of inhibition, apathy, social withdrawal, hyperorality (mouthing of objects), and ritualistic compulsive behaviors. These symptoms may lead to misdiagnosis as a psychological or emotionally-based problem, or, in the elderly, be mistaken for withdrawal or eccentricity. FTD progresses to immobility and loss of speech and expression. Structural changes in the FTD patient's brain can be seen via scans or neuroimaging.

Facts

As many as seven million Americans may be afflicted with a form of dementia. Frontotemporal Dementia may account for 2–5 percent or 140,000–350,000 cases of dementia and for as many as 25 percent of pre-senile dementias.

FTD occurs predominantly after age 40 and usually before age 65, with equal incidence in men and women. In nearly half of the patients, a family history of dementia exists in a first degree relative (parent or sibling), suggesting a genetic component in these cases. Additionally, a form of dementia found in persons with motor neuron disease (amyotrophic lateral sclerosis, commonly known as Lou Gehrig's Disease) may be associated with FTD.

Symptoms

Initial symptoms of FTD are primarily changes in personality and behavior. In addition to the symptoms described below, FTD patients often present two seemingly opposite behavioral profiles in the early and middle stages of the disease. Some individuals are overactive, restless, distractible, and disinhibited. Others are apathetic, inert, aspontaneous, and emotionally blunted. These differences in outward activity disappear in the late stages of the disease.

Major symptoms of FTD are:

- Dramatic change in personal and social conduct. The individual may lack initiative, seem unconcerned, and neglect domestic, financial, and occupational responsibilities.

- Loss of empathy toward others.

- Patients may show shallow affect (flat facial expression or lack of emotional response). Or they may be inappropriately jocular and sing, dance, clap, or recite phrases repeatedly.

- Rigid and inflexible thinking and impaired judgment.

- Loss of insight into personal and social misconduct, such as small sexual or moral transgressions.

- Stereotyped (i.e., repetitive) or compulsive behavior. For example, the person with FTD may become compulsive about rituals of hygiene and dress while at the same time neglecting proper hygiene. They may echo what others say, wander restlessly over a fixed route, or adhere to a fixed daily schedule.

- Hypochondriasis, including bizarre somatic complaints.

- Excessive eating or gluttony, food fads (especially a craving for sweet foods), and even excessive alcohol consumption. (The tendency of FTD patients to consume alcohol often leads to a misdiagnosis of alcohol-related dementia.) The person may refuse to eat, however, due to a behavioral pattern called negativism or to inability to use motor skills needed for eating.

- Decreased motor skills in later stages.

- Change in sleep patterns, with prolonged sleepiness shown, especially in those that present more apathetic behaviors.

In late stage FTD symptoms include:

- a gradual reduction in speech, culminating in mutism;

- hyperoral traits;

- failure or inability to make motor responses to verbal commands;

- akinesia (loss of muscle movement) and rigidity with death due to complications of immobility.

Differences between FTD and Other Dementias

FTD differs markedly in several ways when compared to other dementias, especially Alzheimer's disease:

- FTD is characterized by cerebral atrophy in the frontal and anterior temporal lobes of the brain, while Alzheimer's affects the hippocampal, posterior temporal, and parietal regions.

- The neurofibrillary tangles, senile plaques, and Lewy bodies present in the brains of Alzheimer's and other dementia patients are absent. (Pick bodies are also usually absent.)

- Alzheimer's patients experience severe memory loss. While FTD patients exhibit memory disturbances, they remain oriented to time and place and recall information about the present and past.

- FTD patients, even in late stages of the disease, retain visuospatial orientation, and they negotiate and locate their surroundings accurately.

- Intellectual failure in FTD is distinctly different from that of Alzheimer's patients. Results of intelligence tests are normal in those with FTD until the point in the disease when disinterest results in lower scores.

169

- Life expectancy is slightly longer for FTD.

Testing and Diagnosis

FTD can be accurately diagnosed with brain scans or imaging. Computed tomography (CT scan) and magnetic resonance imaging (MRI) reveal cerebral atrophy in the frontotemporal regions. Degeneration of the corpus striatum, thalamus, and other subcortical structures occurs. Functional brain imaging and single photon emission tomography may reveal dysfunction of the frontal lobes, decreased blood flow, and a selective reduced uptake of tracer in the anterior (front) cerebral hemispheres. Electroencephalography (EEG) remains normal, however, even in advanced stages. In autopsies, brain tissue changes include large neuronal cell loss with secondary spongiform change and astrocytic gliosis.

Neuropsychological testing is useful to obtain a clinical assessment of the disease. Tests evaluate conduct, language, visuo-spatial abilities, memory, abstraction, planning and mental control, motor skills, and intelligence. Tests might show:

- An economy of mental effort and unconcern. Responses may be impulsive and tasks readily abandoned, while other patients may be slow, inert, and persistent.

- Conversation is not spontaneous; responses are brief, and one does not elaborate. Some patients may make mechanical, repetitive remarks, echo words spoken by others, or repeat responses. Apathetic patients may be hypophonic (have a weak voice) and have an odd or halting speaking pattern. Overactive patients may be the opposite, with unconstrained speech. Failure to respond or inappropriate responses should not be assumed to be incomprehension, but rather a concreteness of thinking or inattention.

- Visuo-spatial skills remain normal except for those compromised by behavioral abnormalities.

- Memory problems do not occur except as a result of ineffective use of memory.

- Thought processes show impaired powers of abstraction, verbal response, and design fluency. For example, in card and block sorting or picture arrangement, the FTD patient may abandon tasks, produce items eccentrically, not follow instructions, violate rules, etc. Comprehension is normal, however.

Duration and Treatment

The length of FTD varies, with some patients declining rapidly over 2 to 3 years and others showing only minimal changes over a decade. Studies have shown persons with FTD to live with the disease an average of 8 years, with a range from 3 years to 17 years.

No medications are known currently to treat or prevent FTD. Serotonin-boosting medications may alleviate some behaviors.

Other References

Brun, A., 1987, Frontal lobe degeneration of non-Alzheimer type I. Neuropathology. _Arch. Gerontol. Geriatr._,6:193–208.

Brun, A., 1993, Frontal Lobe Dementia of the non-Alzheimer Type Revisited. _Dementia,_ 4:126–31.

Brun, A., Englund, B., Gustafson, L., et al, 1994, Clinical and neuropathological criteria for frontotemporal dementia. _J. Neurol. Neurosurg. Psychiatry,_ 57:416–418.

Mann, D. M. A., South, P. W., Snowden, J. S., and Neary, D., 1993, Dementia of frontal lobe type: Neuropathology and immuno-histochemistry. _J. Neurol. Neurosurg. Psychiatry,_ 56:605–14.

Miller, B. L., Cummings, J. L., Villanueva-Meyer, J., et al, 1991, Frontal Lobe Degeneration: Clinical, neuropsychological and SPECT characteristics. _Neurology,_ 41:1374–1382.

Miller, B. L., Chang, L., Mena, I., Boone, K. B., Lesser, I, 1993, Clinical and imaging features of right focal lobe degenerations. _Dementia,_ 4:204–213.

Miller, B. L., Darby, A. L., Swartz, J. R., Yener, G. G., Mena, I., 1995, Dietary changes, compulsions and sexual behavior in fronto-temporal degeneration. _Dementia,_ 6:195–199.

Neary, D., Snowden, J. S., Shields, R. A., et al, 1987, Single photon emission tomography using 99mTc-HMPAO in the investigation of dementia. _J. Neurol. Neurosurg. Psychiatry,_ 50:1101–9.

Neary, D., Snowden, J. S., Northern, B., and Goulding, P. J., 1988, Dementia of frontal lobe type. _J. Neurol. Neurosurg. Psychiatry_, 51:353–61.

Orrell, M. W., Sahakian, B. J., and Bergmann, K., 1989, Self-neglect and frontal lobe dysfunction. _Br. J. Psychiatry,_ 155:101–5.

Risberg, J., 1987, Frontal lobe degeneration of non-Alzheimer type. III. Regional blood flow. *Arch. Gerontol. Geriatr.,* 6:225–33.

Snowden, J. S., Neary, D., Mann, D. M. A., 1996, Fronto-temporal lobar degeneration: Fronto-temporal dementia, progressive aphasia, semantic dementia. Churchill-Livingstone, New York, pp. 9–41.

Section 17.4

Huntington Disease

Excerpted from "Huntington's Disease: Hope Through Research," by the National Institute of Neurological Disorders and Stroke NINDS, www.ninds.nih.gov), part of the National Institutes of Health, August 13, 2010.

In 1872, the American physician George Huntington wrote about an illness that he called "an heirloom from generations away back in the dim past." He was not the first to describe the disorder, which has been traced back to the Middle Ages at least. One of its earliest names was chorea, which, as in "choreography," is the Greek word for dance. The term chorea describes how people affected with the disorder writhe, twist, and turn in a constant, uncontrollable dance-like motion. Later, other descriptive names evolved. "Hereditary chorea" emphasizes how the disease is passed from parent to child. "Chronic progressive chorea" stresses how symptoms of the disease worsen over time. Today, physicians commonly use the simple term Huntington disease (HD) to describe this highly complex disorder that causes untold suffering for thousands of families.

More than 15,000 Americans have HD. At least 150,000 others have a 50 percent risk of developing the disease and thousands more of their relatives live with the possibility that they, too, might develop HD.

Until recently, scientists understood very little about HD and could only watch as the disease continued to pass from generation to generation. Families saw the disease destroy their loved ones' ability to feel, think, and move. In the last several years, scientists working with support from the National Institute of Neurological Disorders and Stroke (NINDS) have made several breakthroughs in the area of

HD research. With these advances, our understanding of the disease continues to improve.

This text presents information about HD, and about current research progress, to health professionals, scientists, caregivers, and, most important, to those already too familiar with the disorder: The many families who are affected by HD.

What causes Huntington disease?

HD results from genetically programmed degeneration of nerve cells, called neurons, in certain areas of the brain. This degeneration causes uncontrolled movements, loss of intellectual faculties, and emotional disturbance. Specifically affected are cells of the basal ganglia, structures deep within the brain that have many important functions, including coordinating movement. Within the basal ganglia, HD especially targets neurons of the striatum, particularly those in the caudate nuclei and the pallidum. Also affected is the brain's outer surface, or cortex, which controls thought, perception, and memory.

How is HD inherited?

HD is found in every country of the world. It is a familial disease, passed from parent to child through a mutation or misspelling in the normal gene.

A single abnormal gene, the basic biological unit of heredity, produces HD. Genes are composed of deoxyribonucleic acid (DNA), a molecule shaped like a spiral ladder. Each rung of this ladder is composed of two paired chemicals called bases. There are four types of bases—adenine, thymine, cytosine, and guanine—each abbreviated by the first letter of its name: A, T, C, and G. Certain bases always "pair" together, and different combinations of base pairs join to form coded messages. A gene is a long string of this DNA in various combinations of A, T, C, and G. These unique combinations determine the gene's function, much like letters join together to form words. Each person has about 30,000 genes—a billion base pairs of DNA or bits of information repeated in the nuclei of human cells—which determine individual characteristics or traits.

Genes are arranged in precise locations along 23 rod-like pairs of chromosomes. One chromosome from each pair comes from an individual's mother, the other from the father. Each half of a chromosome pair is similar to the other, except for one pair, which determines the sex of the individual. This pair has two X chromosomes in females and one X and one Y chromosome in males. The gene that produces HD lies on chromosome 4, one of the 22 non-sex-linked, or "autosomal," pairs of chromosomes, placing men and women at equal risk of acquiring the disease.

The impact of a gene depends partly on whether it is dominant or recessive. If a gene is dominant, then only one of the paired chromosomes is required to produce its called-for effect. If the gene is recessive, both parents must provide chromosomal copies for the trait to be present. HD is called an autosomal dominant disorder because only one copy of the defective gene, inherited from one parent, is necessary to produce the disease.

The genetic defect responsible for HD is a small sequence of DNA on chromosome 4 in which several base pairs are repeated many, many times. The normal gene has three DNA bases, composed of the sequence CAG. In people with HD, the sequence abnormally repeats itself dozens of times. Over time—and with each successive generation—the number of CAG repeats may expand further.

Each parent has two copies of every chromosome but gives only one copy to each child. Each child of an HD parent has a 50-50 chance of inheriting the HD gene. If a child does not inherit the HD gene, he or she will not develop the disease and cannot pass it to subsequent generations. A person who inherits the HD gene, and survives long enough, will sooner or later develop the disease. In some families, all the children may inherit the HD gene; in others, none do. Whether one child inherits the gene has no bearing on whether others will or will not share the same fate.

A small number of cases of HD are sporadic, that is, they occur even though there is no family history of the disorder. These cases are thought to be caused by a new genetic mutation—an alteration in the gene that occurs during sperm development and that brings the number of CAG repeats into the range that causes disease.

What are the major effects of the disease?

Early signs of the disease vary greatly from person to person. A common observation is that the earlier the symptoms appear, the faster the disease progresses.

Family members may first notice that the individual experiences mood swings or becomes uncharacteristically irritable, apathetic, passive, depressed, or angry. These symptoms may lessen as the disease progresses or, in some individuals, may continue and include hostile outbursts or deep bouts of depression.

HD may affect the individual's judgment, memory, and other cognitive functions. Early signs might include having trouble driving, learning new things, remembering a fact, answering a question, or making a decision. Some may even display changes in handwriting. As the disease progresses, concentration on intellectual tasks becomes increasingly difficult.

In some individuals, the disease may begin with uncontrolled movements in the fingers, feet, face, or trunk. These movements—which are signs of chorea—often intensify when the person is anxious. HD can also begin with mild clumsiness or problems with balance. Some people develop choreic movements later, after the disease has progressed. They may stumble or appear uncoordinated. Chorea often creates serious problems with walking, increasing the likelihood of falls.

The disease can reach the point where speech is slurred and vital functions, such as swallowing, eating, speaking, and especially walking, continue to decline. Some individuals cannot recognize other family members. Many, however, remain aware of their environment and are able to express emotions.

Some physicians have employed a recently developed Unified HD Rating Scale, or UHDRS, to assess the clinical features, stages, and course of HD. In general, the duration of the illness ranges from 10 to 30 years. The most common causes of death are infection (most often pneumonia), injuries related to a fall, or other complications.

Is there a treatment for HD?

Physicians may prescribe a number of medications to help control emotional and movement problems associated with HD. It is important to remember, however, that while medicines may help keep these clinical symptoms under control, there is no treatment to stop or reverse the course of the disease.

In August 2008 the U.S. Food and Drug Administration approved tetrabenazine to treat Huntington chorea, making it the first drug approved for use in the United States to treat the disease. Antipsychotic drugs, such as haloperidol, or other drugs, such as clonazepam, may help to alleviate choreic movements and may also be used to help control hallucinations, delusions, and violent outbursts. Antipsychotic drugs, however, are not prescribed for another form of muscle contraction associated with HD, called dystonia, and may in fact worsen the condition, causing stiffness and rigidity. These medications may also have severe side effects, including sedation, and for that reason should be used in the lowest possible doses.

For depression, physicians may prescribe fluoxetine, sertraline, nortriptyline, or other compounds. Tranquilizers can help control anxiety and lithium may be prescribed to combat pathological excitement and severe mood swings. Medications may also be needed to treat the severe obsessive-compulsive rituals of some individuals with HD.

Most drugs used to treat the symptoms of HD have side effects such as fatigue, restlessness, or hyperexcitability. Sometimes it may be difficult to tell if a particular symptom, such as apathy or incontinence, is a sign of the disease or a reaction to medication.

Section 17.5

Parkinson Disease

Excerpted from "Parkinson's Disease: Hope Through Research," by the National Institute of Neurological Disorders and Stroke (NINDS, www .ninds.nih.gov), part of the National Institutes of Health, March 14, 2011.

Parkinson disease (PD) is a degenerative disorder of the central nervous system. It was first described in 1817 by James Parkinson, a British physician who published a paper on what he called "the shaking palsy." In this paper, he set forth the major symptoms of the disease that would later bear his name.

Researchers believe that at least 500,000 people in the United States currently have PD, although some estimates are much higher. Society pays an enormous price for PD. The total cost to the nation is estimated to exceed $6 billion annually. The risk of PD increases with age, so analysts expect the financial and public health impact of this disease to increase as the population gets older.

What is Parkinson disease?

Parkinson disease belongs to a group of conditions called movement disorders. The four main symptoms are tremor, or trembling in hands, arms, legs, jaw, or head; rigidity, or stiffness of the limbs and trunk; bradykinesia, or slowness of movement; and postural instability, or impaired balance. These symptoms usually begin gradually and worsen with time. As they become more pronounced, patients may have difficulty walking, talking, or completing other simple tasks. Not everyone with one or more of these symptoms has PD, as the symptoms sometimes appear in other diseases as well.

PD is both chronic, meaning it persists over a long period of time, and progressive, meaning its symptoms grow worse over time. It is not contagious. Although some PD cases appear to be hereditary, and a few can be traced to specific genetic mutations, most cases are sporadic—that is, the disease does not seem to run in families. Many researchers now believe that PD results from a combination of genetic susceptibility and exposure to one or more environmental factors that trigger the disease.

PD is the most common form of parkinsonism, the name for a group of disorders with similar features and symptoms. PD is also called primary parkinsonism or idiopathic PD. The term idiopathic means a disorder for which no cause has yet been found. Although most forms of parkinsonism are idiopathic, there are some cases where the cause is known or suspected or where the symptoms result from another disorder. For example, parkinsonism may result from changes in the brain's blood vessels.

What causes the disease?

Parkinson disease occurs when nerve cells, or neurons, in an area of the brain known as the substantia nigra die or become impaired. Normally, these neurons produce an important brain chemical known as dopamine. Dopamine is a chemical messenger responsible for transmitting signals between the substantia nigra and the next "relay station" of the brain, the corpus striatum, to produce smooth, purposeful movement. Loss of dopamine results in abnormal nerve firing patterns within the brain that cause impaired movement. Studies have shown that most Parkinson disease patients have lost 60 to 80 percent or more of the dopamine-producing cells in the substantia nigra by the time symptoms appear. Recent studies have shown that people with PD also have loss of the nerve endings that produce the neurotransmitter norepinephrine. Norepinephrine, which is closely related to dopamine, is the main chemical messenger of the sympathetic nervous system, the part of the nervous system that controls many automatic functions of the body, such as pulse and blood pressure. The loss of norepinephrine might help explain several of the non-motor features seen in PD, including fatigue and abnormalities of blood pressure regulation.

Many brain cells of people with PD contain Lewy bodies—unusual deposits or clumps of the protein alpha-synuclein, along with other proteins. Researchers do not yet know why Lewy bodies form or what role they play in development of the disease. The clumps may prevent the cell from functioning normally, or they may actually be helpful, perhaps by keeping harmful proteins "locked up" so that the cells can function.

Scientists have identified several genetic mutations associated with PD, and many more genes have been tentatively linked to the disorder. Studying the genes responsible for inherited cases of PD can help researchers understand both inherited and sporadic cases. The same genes and proteins that are altered in inherited cases may also be altered in sporadic cases by environmental toxins or other factors. Researchers also hope that discovering genes will help identify new ways of treating PD.

Although the importance of genetics in PD is increasingly recognized, most researchers believe environmental exposures increase a person's risk of developing the disease. Even in familial cases, exposure to toxins or other environmental factors may influence when symptoms of the disease appear or how the disease progresses. There are a number of toxins, such as 1-methyl-4-phenyl-1,2,3,6-tetrahydropyridine, or MPTP (found in some kinds of synthetic heroin), that can cause parkinsonian symptoms in humans. Other, still-unidentified environmental factors also may cause PD in genetically susceptible individuals.

Viruses are another possible environmental trigger for PD. People who developed encephalopathy after a 1918 influenza epidemic were later stricken with severe, progressive Parkinson-like symptoms. A group of Taiwanese women developed similar symptoms after contracting herpes virus infections. In these women, the symptoms, which later disappeared, were linked to a temporary inflammation of the substantia nigra.

Several lines of research suggest that mitochondria may play a role in the development of PD. Mitochondria are the energy-producing components of the cell and are major sources of free radicals—molecules that damage membranes, proteins, DNA [deoxyribonucleic acid], and other parts of the cell. This damage is often referred to as oxidative stress. Oxidative stress-related changes, including free radical damage to DNA, proteins, and fats, have been detected in brains of PD patients.

Other research suggests that the cell's protein disposal system may fail in people with PD, causing proteins to build up to harmful levels and trigger cell death. Additional studies have found evidence that clumps of protein that develop inside brain cells of people with PD may contribute to the death of neurons, and that inflammation or overstimulation of cells (because of toxins or other factors) may play a role in the disease. However, the precise role of the protein deposits remains unknown. Some researchers even speculate that the protein buildup is part of an unsuccessful attempt to protect the cell. Although mitochondrial dysfunction, oxidative stress, inflammation, and many other cellular processes may contribute to PD, the actual cause of the dopamine cell death is still undetermined.

What genes are linked to Parkinson disease?

Several genes have now been definitively linked to PD. The first to be identified was alpha-synuclein. In the 1990s, researchers at the National Institutes of Health (NIH) and other institutions studied the genetic profiles of a large Italian family and three Greek families with familial PD and found that their disease was related to a mutation in this gene. They found a second alpha-synuclein mutation in a German family with PD. These findings prompted studies of the role of alpha-synuclein in PD, which led to the discovery that Lewy bodies from people with the sporadic form of PD contained clumps of alpha-synuclein protein. This discovery revealed a potential link between hereditary and sporadic forms of the disease.

In 2003, researchers studying inherited PD discovered that the disease in one large family was caused by a triplication of the normal alpha-synuclein gene on one copy of chromosome 4. This triplication caused people in the affected family to produce too much of the normal alpha-synuclein. This study showed that an excess of the normal form of the protein could result in PD, just as the abnormal form does.

Other genes linked to PD include parkin, DJ-1, PINK1, and LRRK2. Parkin, DJ-1, and PINK-1 cause rare, early-onset forms of PD. The parkin gene is translated into a protein that normally helps cells break down and recycle proteins. DJ-1 normally helps regulate gene activity and protect cells from oxidative stress. PINK1 codes for a protein active in mitochondria. Mutations in this gene appear to increase susceptibility to cellular stress.

LRRK2, which is translated into a protein called dardarin, was originally identified in several English and Basque families and causes a late-onset form of PD. Subsequent studies have identified this gene in other families with PD as well as in a small percentage of people with apparently sporadic PD.

Researchers are continuing to investigate the normal functions and interactions of these genes in order to find clues about how PD develops. They also have identified a number of other genes and chromosome regions that may play a role in PD, but the nature of these links is not yet clear.

Who gets Parkinson disease?

About 50,000 Americans are diagnosed with PD each year, but getting an accurate count of the number of cases may be impossible because many people in the early stages of the disease assume their symptoms are the result of normal aging and do not seek help from a physician. Also, diagnosis is sometimes difficult and uncertain because other conditions may produce symptoms of PD and there is no definitive test for the disease. People with PD may sometimes be told by their doctors that they have other disorders, and people with PD-like diseases may be incorrectly diagnosed as having PD.

PD strikes about 50 percent more men than women, but the reasons for this discrepancy are unclear. While it occurs in people throughout the world, a number of studies have found a higher incidence in developed countries, possibly because of increased exposure to pesticides or other toxins in those countries. Other studies have found an increased risk in people who live in rural areas and in those who work in certain professions, although the studies to date are not conclusive and the reasons for the apparent risks are not clear.

One clear risk factor for PD is age. The average age of onset is 60 years, and the incidence rises significantly with increasing age. However, about 5 to 10 percent of people with PD have "early-onset" disease that begins before the age of 50. Early-onset forms of the disease are often inherited, though not always, and some have been linked to specific gene mutations. People with one or more close relatives who have PD have an increased risk of developing the disease themselves, but the total risk is still just 2 to 5 percent unless the family has a known gene mutation for the disease. An estimated 15 to 25 percent of people with PD have a known relative with the disease.

In very rare cases, parkinsonian symptoms may appear in people before the age of 20. This condition is called juvenile parkinsonism. It is most commonly seen in Japan but has been found in other countries as well. It usually begins with dystonia and bradykinesia, and the symptoms often improve with levodopa medication. Juvenile parkinsonism often runs in families and is sometimes linked to a mutated parkin gene.

What are the symptoms of the disease?

Early symptoms of PD are subtle and occur gradually. Affected people may feel mild tremors or have difficulty getting out of a chair. They may notice that they speak too softly or that their handwriting is slow and looks cramped or small. They may lose track of a word or thought, or they may feel tired, irritable, or depressed for no apparent reason. This very early period may last a long time before the more classic and obvious symptoms appear.

Friends or family members may be the first to notice changes in someone with early PD. They may see that the person's face lacks expression and animation (known as "masked face") or that the person does not move an arm or leg normally. They also may notice that the person seems stiff, unsteady, or unusually slow.

As the disease progresses, the shaking or tremor that affects the majority of Parkinson disease patients may begin to interfere with daily activities. Patients may not be able to hold utensils steady or they may find that the shaking makes reading a newspaper difficult. Tremor is usually the symptom that causes people to seek medical help.

People with PD often develop a so-called parkinsonian gait that includes a tendency to lean forward, small quick steps as if hurrying forward (called festination), and reduced swinging of the arms. They also may have trouble initiating movement (start hesitation), and they may stop suddenly as they walk (freezing).

PD does not affect everyone the same way, and the rate of progression differs among patients. Tremor is the major symptom for some patients, while for others, tremor is nonexistent or very minor.

PD symptoms often begin on one side of the body. However, as it progresses, the disease eventually affects both sides. Even after the disease involves both sides of the body, the symptoms are often less severe on one side than on the other. There are four primary symptoms of PD.

Tremor: The tremor associated with PD has a characteristic appearance. Typically, the tremor takes the form of a rhythmic back-and-forth motion at a rate of 4–6 beats per second. It may involve the thumb and forefinger and appear as a "pill rolling" tremor. Tremor often begins in a hand, although sometimes a foot or the jaw is affected first. It is most obvious when the hand is at rest or when a person is under stress. For example, the shaking may become more pronounced a few seconds after the hands are rested on a table. Tremor usually disappears during sleep or improves with intentional movement.

Rigidity: Rigidity, or a resistance to movement, affects most people with PD. A major principle of body movement is that all muscles have an opposing muscle. Movement is possible not just because one muscle becomes more active, but because the opposing muscle relaxes. In PD, rigidity comes about when, in response to signals from the brain, the delicate balance of opposing muscles is disturbed. The muscles remain constantly tensed and contracted so that the person aches or feels stiff

181

or weak. The rigidity becomes obvious when another person tries to move the patient's arm, which will move only in ratchet-like or short, jerky movements known as "cogwheel" rigidity.

Bradykinesia: Bradykinesia, or the slowing down and loss of spontaneous and automatic movement, is particularly frustrating because it may make simple tasks somewhat difficult. The person cannot rapidly perform routine movements. Activities once performed quickly and easily—such as washing or dressing—may take several hours.

Postural instability: Postural instability, or impaired balance, causes patients to fall easily. Affected people also may develop a stooped posture in which the head is bowed and the shoulders are drooped.

A number of other symptoms may accompany PD. Some are minor; others are not. Many can be treated with medication or physical therapy. No one can predict which symptoms will affect an individual patient, and the intensity of the symptoms varies from person to person.

Depression: This is a common problem and may appear early in the course of the disease, even before other symptoms are noticed. Fortunately, depression usually can be successfully treated with anti-depressant medications.

Emotional changes: Some people with PD become fearful and insecure. Perhaps they fear they cannot cope with new situations. They may not want to travel, go to parties, or socialize with friends. Some lose their motivation and become dependent on family members. Others may become irritable or uncharacteristically pessimistic.

Difficulty with swallowing and chewing: Muscles used in swallowing may work less efficiently in later stages of the disease. In these cases, food and saliva may collect in the mouth and back of the throat, which can result in choking or drooling. These problems also may make it difficult to get adequate nutrition. Speech-language therapists, occupational therapists, and dieticians can often help with these problems.

Speech changes: About half of all PD patients have problems with speech. They may speak too softly or in a monotone, hesitate before speaking, slur or repeat their words, or speak too fast. A speech therapist may be able to help patients reduce some of these problems.

Urinary problems or constipation: In some patients, bladder and bowel problems can occur due to the improper functioning of the autonomic nervous system, which is responsible for regulating smooth muscle activity. Some people may become incontinent, while others have trouble urinating. In others, constipation may occur because the intestinal tract operates more slowly. Constipation can also be caused by inactivity, eating a poor diet, or drinking too little fluid. The medications used to treat PD also can contribute to constipation. It can be a persistent problem and, in rare cases, can be serious enough to require hospitalization.

Skin problems: In PD, it is common for the skin on the face to become very oily, particularly on the forehead and at the sides of the nose. The scalp may become oily too, resulting in dandruff. In other cases, the skin can become very dry. These problems are also the result of an improperly functioning autonomic nervous system. Standard treatments for skin problems can help. Excessive sweating, another common symptom, is usually controllable with medications used for PD.

Sleep problems: Sleep problems common in PD include difficulty staying asleep at night, restless sleep, nightmares and emotional dreams, and drowsiness or sudden sleep onset during the day. Patients with PD should never take over-the-counter sleep aids without consulting their physicians.

Dementia or other cognitive problems: Some, but not all, people with PD may develop memory problems and slow thinking. In some of these cases, cognitive problems become more severe, leading to a condition called Parkinson dementia late in the course of the disease. This dementia may affect memory, social judgment, language, reasoning, or other mental skills. There is currently no way to halt PD dementia, but studies have shown that a drug called rivastigmine may slightly reduce the symptoms. The drug donepezil also can reduce behavioral symptoms in some people with PD-related dementia.

Orthostatic hypotension: Orthostatic hypotension is a sudden drop in blood pressure when a person stands up from a lying-down position. This may cause dizziness, lightheadedness, and, in extreme cases, loss of balance or fainting. Studies have suggested that, in PD, this problem results from a loss of nerve endings in the sympathetic nervous system that controls heart rate, blood pressure, and other automatic functions in the body. The medications used to treat PD also may contribute to this symptom.

Muscle cramps and dystonia: The rigidity and lack of normal movement associated with PD often causes muscle cramps, especially in the legs and toes. Massage, stretching, and applying heat may help

183

with these cramps. PD also can be associated with dystonia—sustained muscle contractions that cause forced or twisted positions. Dystonia in PD is often caused by fluctuations in the body's level of dopamine. It can usually be relieved or reduced by adjusting the person's medications.

Pain: Many people with PD develop aching muscles and joints because of the rigidity and abnormal postures often associated with the disease. Treatment with levodopa and other dopaminergic drugs often alleviates these pains to some extent. Certain exercises also may help. People with PD also may develop pain due to compression of nerve roots or dystonia-related muscle spasms. In rare cases, people with PD may develop unexplained burning, stabbing sensations. This type of pain, called "central pain," originates in the brain. Dopaminergic drugs, opiates, antidepressants, and other types of drugs may all be used to treat this type of pain.

Fatigue and loss of energy: The unusual demands of living with PD often lead to problems with fatigue, especially late in the day. Fatigue may be associated with depression or sleep disorders, but it also may result from muscle stress or from overdoing activity when the person feels well. Fatigue also may result from akinesia—trouble initiating or carrying out movement. Exercise, good sleep habits, staying mentally active, and not forcing too many activities in a short time may help to alleviate fatigue.

Sexual dysfunction: PD often causes erectile dysfunction because of its effects on nerve signals from the brain or because of poor blood circulation. PD-related depression or use of antidepressant medication also may cause decreased sex drive and other problems. These problems are often treatable.

What other diseases resemble Parkinson disease?

A number of disorders can cause symptoms similar to those of PD. People with symptoms that resemble PD but that result from other causes are sometimes said to have parkinsonism. Some of these disorders are listed in the following text.

Postencephalitic parkinsonism: Just after the first World War, a viral disease, encephalitis lethargica, attacked almost 5 million people throughout the world, and then suddenly disappeared in the 1920s. Known as sleeping sickness in the United States, this disease killed one third of its victims and led to post-encephalitic parkinsonism in many others. This resulted in a particularly severe form of movement disorder that appeared sometimes years after the initial illness. (In 1973, neurologist Oliver Sacks published *Awakenings,* an account of his work in the late 1960s with surviving post-encephalitic patients in a New York hospital. Using the then-experimental drug levodopa, Dr. Sacks was able to temporarily "awaken" these patients from their statue-like state). In rare cases, other viral infections, including western equine encephalomyelitis, eastern equine encephalomyelitis, and Japanese B encephalitis, have caused parkinsonian symptoms.

Drug-induced parkinsonism: A reversible form of parkinsonism sometimes results from use of certain drugs, such as chlorpromazine and haloperidol, which are prescribed for patients with psychiatric disorders. Some drugs used for stomach disorders (metoclopramide), high blood pressure (reserpine), and epilepsy (valproate) may also produce parkinsonian symptoms. Stopping the medication or lowering the dosage of these medications usually causes the symptoms to go away.

Toxin-induced parkinsonism: Some toxins—such as manganese dust, carbon disulfide, and carbon monoxide—can cause parkinsonism. The chemical MPTP also causes a permanent form of parkinsonism that closely resembles PD. Investigators discovered this reaction in the 1980s when heroin addicts in California who had taken an illicit street drug contaminated with MPTP began to develop severe parkinsonism. This discovery, which showed that a toxic substance could damage the brain and produce parkinsonian symptoms, caused a dramatic breakthrough in Parkinson disease research: For the first time, scientists were able to simulate PD in animals and conduct studies to increase understanding of the disease.

Arteriosclerotic parkinsonism: Sometimes known as pseudoparkinsonism, vascular parkinsonism, or atherosclerotic parkinsonism, arteriosclerotic parkinsonism involves damage to the brain due to multiple small strokes. Tremor is rare in this type of parkinsonism, whereas dementia—the loss of mental skills and abilities—is common. Antiparkinsonian drugs are of little help to patients with this form of parkinsonism.

Parkinsonism-dementia complex of Guam: This disease occurs among the Chamorro populations of Guam and the Mariana Islands and may be accompanied by a motor neuron disease resembling amyotrophic lateral sclerosis (Lou Gehrig disease). The course of the disease is rapid, with death typically occurring within 5 years.

Post-traumatic parkinsonism: Also known as post-traumatic encephalopathy or "punch-drunk syndrome," parkinsonian symptoms can sometimes develop after a severe head injury or frequent head trauma that results from boxing or other activities. This type of trauma also can cause a form of dementia called dementia pugilistica.

Essential tremor: Essential tremor, sometimes called benign essential tremor or familial tremor, is a common condition that tends to run in families and progresses slowly over time. The tremor is usually equal in both hands and increases when the hands are moving. The tremor may involve the head but usually spares the legs. Patients with essential tremor have no other parkinsonian features. Essential tremor is not the same as PD, and usually does not lead to it, although in some cases the two conditions may overlap in one person. Essential tremor does not respond to levodopa or most other PD drugs, but it can be treated with other medications.

Normal pressure hydrocephalus: Normal pressure hydrocephalus (NPH) is an abnormal increase of cerebrospinal fluid (CSF) in the brain's ventricles, or cavities. It occurs if the normal flow of CSF throughout the brain and spinal cord is blocked in some way. This causes the ventricles to enlarge, putting pressure on the brain. Symptoms include problems with walking, impaired bladder control leading to urinary frequency or incontinence, and progressive mental impairment and dementia. The person also may have a general slowing of movements or may complain that his or her feet feel "stuck." These symptoms may sometimes be mistaken for PD. Brain scans, intracranial pressure monitoring, and other tests can help to distinguish NPH from PD and other disorders. NPH can sometimes be treated by surgically implanting a CSF shunt that drains excess cerebrospinal fluid into the abdomen, where it is absorbed.

Progressive supranuclear palsy: Progressive supranuclear palsy (PSP), sometimes called Steele-Richardson-Olszewski syndrome, is a rare, progressive brain disorder that causes problems with control of gait and balance. People often tend to fall early in the course of PSP. One of the most obvious signs of the disease is an inability to move the eyes properly. Some patients describe this effect as a blurring. PSP patients often show alterations of mood and behavior, including depression and apathy as well as mild dementia. The symptoms of PSP are caused by a gradual deterioration of brain cells in the brainstem. It is often misdiagnosed because some of its symptoms are very much like those of PD, Alzheimer disease, and other brain disorders. PSP symptoms usually do not respond to medication.

Corticobasal degeneration: Corticobasal degeneration results from atrophy of multiple areas of the brain, including the cerebral cortex and the basal ganglia. Initial symptoms may first appear on one side of the body, but eventually affect both sides. Symptoms are similar to those found in PD, including rigidity, impaired balance and coordination, and dystonia. Other symptoms may include cognitive and visual-spatial impairments, apraxia (loss of the ability to make familiar, purposeful movements), hesitant and halting speech, myoclonus (muscular jerks), and dysphagia (difficulty swallowing). Unlike PD, corticobasal degeneration usually does not respond to medication.

Multiple system atrophy: Multiple system atrophy (MSA) refers to a set of slowly progressive disorders that affect the central and autonomic nervous systems. MSA may have symptoms that resemble PD. It also may take a form that primarily produces poor coordination and slurred speech, or it may have a mixture of these symptoms. Other symptoms may include breathing and swallowing difficulties, male impotence, constipation, and urinary difficulties. The disorder previously called Shy-Drager syndrome refers to MSA with prominent orthostatic hypotension—a fall in blood pressure every time the person stands up. MSA with parkinsonian symptoms is sometimes referred to as striatonigral degeneration, whereas MSA with poor coordination and slurred speech is sometimes called olivopontocerebellar atrophy.

Dementia with Lewy bodies: Dementia with Lewy bodies is a neurodegenerative disorder associated with abnormal protein deposits (Lewy bodies) found in certain areas of the brain. Symptoms can range from traditional parkinsonian symptoms, such as bradykinesia, rigidity, tremor, and shuffling gait, to symptoms similar to those of Alzheimer disease. These symptoms may fluctuate, or wax and wane dramatically. Visual hallucinations may be one of the first symptoms, and patients may suffer from other psychiatric disturbances such as delusions and depression. Cognitive problems also occur early in the course of the disease. Levodopa and other antiparkinsonian medications can help with the motor symptoms of dementia with Lewy bodies, but they may make hallucinations and delusions worse.

Parkinsonism accompanying other conditions: Parkinsonian symptoms may also appear in patients with other, clearly distinct neurological disorders such as Wilson disease, Huntington disease, Alzheimer disease, spinocerebellar ataxias, and Creutzfeldt-Jakob disease. Each of these disorders has specific features that help to distinguish them from PD.

MSA, corticobasal degeneration, and progressive supranuclear palsy are sometimes referred to as "Parkinson-plus" diseases because they have the symptoms of PD plus additional features.

How is Parkinson disease diagnosed?

There are currently no blood or laboratory tests that have been proven to help in diagnosing sporadic PD. Therefore the diagnosis is based on medical history and a neurological examination. The disease can be difficult to diagnose accurately. Early signs and symptoms of PD may sometimes be dismissed as the effects of normal aging. The physician may need to observe the person for some time until it is apparent that the symptoms are consistently present. Doctors may sometimes request brain scans or laboratory tests in order to rule out other diseases. However, CT [computed tomography] and MRI [magnetic resonance imaging] brain scans of people with PD usually appear normal. Since many other diseases have similar features but require different treatments, making a precise diagnosis as soon as possible is essential so that patients can receive the proper treatment.

What is the prognosis?

PD is not by itself a fatal disease, but it does get worse with time. The average life expectancy of a PD patient is generally the same as for people who do not have the disease. However, in the late stages of the disease, PD may cause complications such as choking, pneumonia, and falls that can lead to death. Fortunately, there are many treatment options available for people with PD.

The progression of symptoms in PD may take 20 years or more. In some people, however, the disease progresses more quickly. There is no way to predict what course the disease will take for an individual person. One commonly used system for describing how the symptoms of PD progress is called the Hoehn and Yahr scale.

Another commonly used scale is the Unified Parkinson disease Rating Scale (UPDRS). This much more complicated scale has multiple ratings that measure mental functioning, behavior, and mood; activities of daily living; and motor function. Both the Hoehn and Yahr scale and the UPDRS are used to measure how individuals are faring and how much treatments are helping them.

With appropriate treatment, most people with PD can live productive lives for many years after diagnosis.

How is the disease treated?

At present, there is no cure for PD. But medications or surgery can sometimes provide dramatic relief from the symptoms.

Drug Treatments

Medications for PD fall into three categories. The first category includes drugs that work directly or indirectly to increase the level of dopamine in the brain. The most common drugs for PD are dopamine precursors—substances such as levodopa that cross the blood-brain barrier and are then changed into dopamine. Other drugs mimic dopamine or prevent or slow its breakdown.

The second category of PD drugs affects other neurotransmitters in the body in order to ease some of the symptoms of the disease. For example, anticholinergic drugs interfere with production or uptake of the neurotransmitter acetylcholine. These drugs help to reduce tremors and muscle stiffness, which can result from having more acetylcholine than dopamine.

The third category of drugs prescribed for PD includes medications that help control the non-motor symptoms of the disease, that is, the symptoms that don't affect movement. For example, people with PD-related depression may be prescribed antidepressants.

Levodopa: The cornerstone of therapy for PD is the drug levodopa (also called L-dopa). Levodopa (from the full name L-3,4-dihydroxyphenylalanine) is a simple chemical found naturally in plants and animals. Levodopa is the generic name used for this chemical when it is formulated for drug use in patients. Nerve cells can use levodopa to make dopamine and replenish the brain's dwindling supply. People cannot simply take dopamine pills because dopamine does not easily pass through the blood-brain barrier, a lining of cells inside blood vessels that regulates the transport of oxygen, glucose, and other substances into the brain. Usually, patients are given levodopa combined with another substance called carbidopa. When added to levodopa, carbidopa delays the conversion of levodopa into dopamine until it reaches the brain, preventing or diminishing some of the side effects that often accompany levodopa therapy. Carbidopa also reduces the amount of levodopa needed.

Levodopa is very successful at reducing the tremors and other symptoms of PD during the early stages of the disease. It allows the majority of people with PD to extend the period of time in which they can lead relatively normal, productive lives.

Although levodopa helps most people with PD, not all symptoms respond equally to the drug. Levodopa usually helps most with bradykinesia and rigidity. Problems with balance and other non-motor symptoms may not be alleviated at all.

People who have taken other medications before starting levodopa therapy may have to cut back or eliminate these drugs in order to feel the full benefit of levodopa. People often see dramatic improvement in their symptoms after starting levodopa therapy. However, they may need to increase the dose gradually for maximum benefit. A high-protein diet can interfere with the absorption of levodopa, so some physicians recommend that patients taking the drug restrict their protein consumption during the early parts of the day or avoid taking their medications with protein-rich meals.

Levodopa is often so effective that some people may temporarily forget they have PD during the early stages of the disease. But levodopa is not a cure. Although it can reduce the symptoms of PD, it does not replace lost nerve cells and it does not stop the progression of the disease.

Levodopa can have a variety of side effects. The most common initial side effects include nausea, vomiting, low blood pressure, and restlessness. The drug also can cause drowsiness or sudden sleep onset, which can make driving and other activities dangerous. Long-term use of levodopa sometimes causes hallucinations and psychosis. The nausea and vomiting caused by levodopa are greatly reduced by combining levodopa and carbidopa, which enhances the effectiveness of a lower dose.

Dyskinesias, or involuntary movements such as twitching, twisting, and writhing, commonly develop in people who take large doses of levodopa over an extended period. These movements may be either mild or severe and either very rapid or very slow. The dose of levodopa is often reduced in order to lessen these drug-induced movements. However, the PD symptoms often reappear even with lower doses of medication. Doctors and patients must work together closely to find a tolerable balance between the drug's benefits and side effects. If dyskinesias are severe, surgical treatment may be considered. Because dyskinesias tend to occur with long-term use of levodopa, doctors often start younger PD patients on other dopamine-increasing drugs and switch to levodopa only when those drugs become ineffective.

Other troubling and distressing problems may occur with long-term levodopa use. Patients may begin to notice more pronounced symptoms before their first dose of medication in the morning, and they may develop muscle spasms or other problems when each dose begins to wear off. The period of effectiveness after each dose may begin to shorten, called the wearing-off effect. Another potential problem is referred to as the on-off effect—sudden, unpredictable changes in movement, from normal to parkinsonian movement and back again. These effects probably indicate that the patient's response to the drug is changing or that the disease is progressing.

One approach to alleviating these side effects is to take levodopa more often and in smaller amounts. People with PD should never stop taking levodopa without their physician's knowledge or consent because rapidly withdrawing the drug can have potentially serious side effects, such as immobility or difficulty breathing.

Fortunately, physicians have other treatment choices for some symptoms and stages of PD. These therapies include the following medications.

Dopamine agonists: These drugs, which include bromocriptine, apomorphine, pramipexole, and ropinirole, mimic the role of dopamine in the brain. They can be given alone or in conjunction with levodopa. They may be used in the early stages of the disease, or later on in order to lengthen the duration of response to levodopa in patients who experience wearing off or on-off effects. They are generally less effective than levodopa in controlling rigidity and bradykinesia. Many of the potential side effects are similar to those associated with the use of levodopa, including drowsiness, sudden sleep onset, hallucinations, confusion, dyskinesias, edema (swelling due to excess fluid in body tissues), nightmares, and vomiting. In rare cases, they can cause compulsive behavior, such as an uncontrollable desire to gamble, hypersexuality, or compulsive shopping. Bromocriptine can also cause fibrosis, or a buildup of fibrous tissue, in the heart valves or the chest cavity. Fibrosis usually goes away once the drugs are stopped.

MAO-B inhibitors: These drugs inhibit the enzyme monoamine oxidase B, or MAO-B, which breaks down dopamine in the brain. MAO-B inhibitors cause dopamine to accumulate in surviving nerve cells and reduce the symptoms of PD. Selegiline, also called deprenyl, is an MAO-B inhibitor that is commonly used to treat PD. Studies supported by the NINDS have shown that selegiline can delay the need for levodopa therapy by up to a year or more. When selegiline is given with levodopa, it appears to enhance and prolong the response to levodopa and thus may reduce wearing-off fluctuations. Selegiline is usually well-tolerated, although side effects may include nausea, orthostatic hypotension, or insomnia. It should not be taken with the antidepressant fluoxetine or the sedative meperidine, because combining selegiline with these drugs can be harmful. An NINDS-sponsored study of selegiline in the late 1980s suggested that it might help to slow the loss of nerve cells in PD. However, follow-up studies cast doubt on this finding. Another MAO-B inhibitor, rasagiline, was approved by the FDA in May 2006 for use in treating PD.

COMT inhibitors: COMT stands for catechol-O-methyltransferase, another enzyme that helps to break down dopamine. Two COMT inhibitors are approved to treat PD in the United States—entacapone and tolcapone. These drugs prolong the effects of levodopa by preventing the breakdown of dopamine. COMT inhibitors can decrease the duration of "off" periods, and they usually make it possible to reduce the person's dose of levodopa. The most common side effect is diarrhea. The drugs may also cause nausea, sleep disturbances, dizziness, urine discoloration, abdominal pain, low blood pressure, or hallucinations. In a few rare cases, tolcapone has caused severe liver disease. Because of this, patients taking tolcapone need regular monitoring of their liver function.

Amantadine: An antiviral drug, amantadine, can help reduce symptoms of PD and levodopa-induced dyskinesia. It is often used alone in the early stages of the disease. It also may be used with an anticholinergic drug or levodopa. After several months, amantadine's effectiveness wears off in up to half of the patients taking it. Amantadine's side effects may include insomnia, mottled skin, edema, agitation, or hallucinations. Researchers are not certain how amantadine works in PD, but it may increase the effects of dopamine.

Anticholinergics: These drugs, which include trihexyphenidyl, benztropine, and ethopropazine, decrease the activity of the neurotransmitter acetylcholine and help to reduce tremors and muscle rigidity. Only about half the patients who receive anticholinergics are helped by it, usually for a brief period and with only a 30 percent improvement. Side effects may include dry mouth, constipation, urinary retention, hallucinations, memory loss, blurred vision, and confusion.

When recommending a course of treatment, a doctor will assess how much the symptoms disrupt the patient's life and then tailor therapy to the person's particular condition. Since no two patients will react the same way to a given drug, it may take time and patience to get the dose just right. Even then, symptoms may not be completely alleviated.

Medications for Non-Motor Symptoms

Doctors may prescribe a variety of medications to treat the non-motor symptoms of PD, such as depression and anxiety. For example, depression can be treated with standard anti-depressant drugs such as amitriptyline or fluoxetine (however, as stated earlier, fluoxetine should not be combined with MAO-B inhibitors). Anxiety can sometimes be treated with drugs called benzodiazepines. Orthostatic hypotension may be helped by increasing salt intake, reducing antihypertension drugs, or prescribing medications such as fludrocortisone.

Hallucinations, delusions, and other psychotic symptoms are often caused by the drugs prescribed for PD. Therefore reducing or stopping PD medications may alleviate psychosis. If such measures are not effective, doctors sometimes prescribe drugs called atypical antipsychotics, which include clozapine and quetiapine. Clozapine also may help to control dyskinesias. However, clozapine also can cause a serious blood disorder called agranulocytosis, so people who take it must have their blood monitored frequently.

What surgeries are used to treat PD?

Treating PD with surgery was once a common practice. But after the discovery of levodopa, surgery was restricted to only a few cases. Studies in the past few decades have led to great improvements in surgical techniques, and surgery is again being used in people with advanced PD for whom drug therapy is no longer sufficient.

Pallidotomy and thalamotomy: The earliest types of surgery for PD involved selectively destroying specific parts of the brain that contribute to the symptoms of the disease. Investigators have now greatly refined the use of these procedures. The most common of these procedures is called pallidotomy. In this procedure, a surgeon selectively destroys a portion of the brain called the globus pallidus. Pallidotomy can improve symptoms of tremor, rigidity, and bradykinesia, possibly by interrupting the connections between the globus pallidus and the striatum or thalamus. Some studies have also found that pallidotomy can improve gait and balance and reduce the amount of levodopa patients require, thus reducing drug-induced dyskinesias and dystonia. A related procedure, called thalamotomy, involves surgically destroying part of the brain's thalamus. Thalamotomy is useful primarily to reduce tremor.

Because these procedures cause permanent destruction of brain tissue, they have largely been replaced by deep brain stimulation for treatment of PD.

Deep brain stimulation: Deep brain stimulation, or DBS, uses an electrode surgically implanted into part of the brain. The electrodes are connected by a wire under the skin to a small electrical device called a pulse generator that is implanted in the chest beneath the collarbone. The pulse generator and electrodes painlessly stimulate the brain in a way that helps to stop many of the symptoms of PD. DBS has now been approved by the U.S. Food and Drug Administration, and it is widely used as a treatment for PD.

DBS can be used on one or both sides of the brain. If it is used on just one side, it will affect symptoms on the opposite side of the body. DBS is primarily used to stimulate one of three brain regions: the subthalamic nucleus, the globus pallidus, or the thalamus. However, the subthalamic nucleus, a tiny area located beneath the thalamus, is the most common target. Stimulation of either the globus pallidus or the subthalamic nucleus can reduce tremor, bradykinesia, and rigidity. Stimulation of the thalamus is useful primarily for reducing tremor.

DBS usually reduces the need for levodopa and related drugs, which in turn decreases dyskinesias. It also helps to relieve on-off fluctuation of symptoms.

People who initially responded well to treatment with levodopa tend to respond well to DBS. While the benefits of DBS can be substantial, it usually does not help with speech problems, "freezing," posture, balance, anxiety, depression, or dementia.

One advantage of DBS compared to pallidotomy and thalamotomy is that the electrical current can be turned off using a handheld device. The pulse generator also can be externally programmed.

Patients must return to the medical center frequently for several months after DBS surgery in order to have the stimulation adjusted by trained doctors or other medical professionals. The pulse generator must be programmed very carefully to give the best results. Doctors also must supervise reductions in patients' medications. After a few months, the number of medical visits usually decreases significantly, though patients may occasionally need to return to the center to have their stimulator checked. Also, the battery for the pulse generator must be surgically replaced every 3 to 5 years, though externally rechargeable batteries may eventually become available. Long-term results of DBS are still being determined. DBS does not stop PD from progressing, and some problems may gradually return. However, studies up to several years after surgery have shown that many people's symptoms remain significantly better than they were before DBS.

DBS is not a good solution for everyone. It is generally used only in people with advanced, levodopa-responsive PD who have developed dyskinesias or other disabling "off" symptoms despite drug therapy. It is not normally used in people with memory problems, hallucinations, a poor response to levodopa, severe depression, or poor health. DBS generally does not help people with "atypical" parkinsonian syndromes such as multiple system atrophy, progressive supranuclear palsy, or post-traumatic parkinsonism. Younger people generally do better than older people after DBS, but healthy older people can undergo DBS and they may benefit a great deal.

As with any brain surgery, DBS has potential complications, including stroke or brain hemorrhage. These complications are rare, however. There is also a risk of infection, which may require antibiotics or even replacement of parts of the DBS system. The stimulator may sometimes cause speech problems, balance problems, or even dyskinesias. However, those problems are often reversible if the stimulation is modified.

Researchers are continuing to study DBS and to develop ways of improving it. They are conducting clinical studies to determine the best part of the brain to receive stimulation and to determine the long-term effects of this therapy. They also are working to improve the technology used in DBS.

What complementary and supportive therapies are used for PD?

A wide variety of complementary and supportive therapies may be used for PD. Among these therapies are standard physical, occupational, and speech therapy techniques, which can help with such problems as gait and voice disorders, tremors and rigidity, and cognitive decline. Other types of supportive therapies include the following:

Diet: At this time there are no specific vitamins, minerals, or other nutrients that have any proven therapeutic value in PD. Some early reports have suggested that dietary supplements might be protective in PD. In addition, a phase II clinical trial of a supplement called co-enzyme Q10 suggested that large doses of this substance might slow disease progression in patients with early-stage PD.

The NINDS and other components of the National Institutes of Health are funding research to determine if caffeine, antioxidants, and other dietary factors may be beneficial for preventing or treating PD. While there is currently no proof that any specific dietary factor is beneficial, a normal, healthy diet can promote overall well-being for PD patients just as it would for anyone else. Eating a fiber-rich diet and drinking plenty of fluids also can help alleviate constipation. A high protein diet, however, may limit levodopa's effectiveness.

Exercise: Exercise can help people with PD improve their mobility and flexibility. Some doctors prescribe physical therapy or muscle-strengthening exercises to tone muscles and to put underused and rigid muscles through a full range of motion. Exercises will not stop disease progression, but they may improve body strength so that the person is less disabled. Exercises also improve balance, helping people minimize gait problems, and can strengthen certain muscles so that people can speak and swallow better. Exercise can also improve the emotional well-being of people with PD, and it may improve the brain's dopamine synthesis or increase levels of beneficial compounds called neurotrophic factors in the brain. Although structured exercise programs help many patients, more general physical activity, such as walking, gardening, swimming, calisthenics, and using exercise machines, also is beneficial. People with PD should always check with their doctors before beginning a new exercise program.

Other complementary therapies that are used by some individuals with PD include massage therapy, yoga, tai chi, hypnosis, acupuncture, and the Alexander technique, which optimizes posture and muscle activity. There have been limited studies suggesting mild benefits with some of these therapies, but they do not slow PD and there is no convincing evidence that they are beneficial.

How can people cope with Parkinson disease?

While PD usually progresses slowly, eventually the most basic daily routines may be affected—from socializing with friends and enjoying normal relationships with family members to earning a living and taking care of a home. These changes can be difficult to accept. Support groups can help people cope with the disease emotionally. These groups can also provide valuable information, advice, and experience to help people with PD, their families, and their caregivers deal with a wide range of issues, including locating doctors familiar with the disease and coping with physical limitations. Individual or family counseling also may help people find ways to cope with PD.

People with PD also can benefit from being proactive and finding out as much as possible about the disease in order to alleviate fear of the unknown and to take a positive role in maintaining their health. Many people with PD continue to work either full- or part-time, although eventually they may need to adjust their schedule and working environment to cope with the disease.

Can scientists predict or prevent Parkinson disease?

In most cases, there is no way to predict or prevent sporadic PD. However, researchers are looking for a biomarker—a biochemical abnormality that all patients with PD might share—that could be picked up by screening techniques or by a simple chemical test given to people who do not have any parkinsonian symptoms. This could help doctors identify people at risk of the disease. It also might allow them to find treatments that will stop the disease process in the early stages.

Positron emission tomography (PET) scanning may lead to important advances in our knowledge about PD. PET scans of the brain produce pictures of chemical changes as they occur. Using PET, research scientists can study the brain's dopamine receptors (the sites on nerve cells that bind with dopamine) to determine if the loss of dopamine activity follows or precedes degeneration of the neurons that make this chemical. This information could help scientists better understand the disease process and may potentially lead to improved treatments.

In rare cases, where people have a clearly inherited form of PD, researchers can test for known gene mutations as a way of determining an individual's risk of the disease. However, this genetic testing can have far-reaching implications and people should carefully consider whether they want to know the results of such tests. Genetic testing is currently available only as a part of research studies.

Chapter 18

Vascular Dementia

Chapter Contents

Section 18.1

What Is Vascular Dementia?

"Vascular Dementia and Stroke," © 2009 National Stroke
Association (www.stroke.org). Reprinted with permission.

A common complication resulting from stroke is loss of cognitive function, or intellectual abilities, often called vascular dementia.

Vascular dementia (VaD) is a decline in intellectual abilities as a result of a stroke. It occurs when brain tissue is damaged because of reduced blood flow to the brain, most commonly by a stroke or series of strokes. The brain cells, in effect, have difficulty working together to process information. This can lead to memory loss, confusion, and decreased attention span, in addition to problems with activities of daily living.

It is estimated that nearly a fifth of people who suffer a stroke will develop problems involving their mental abilities.

Approximately 10 to 20 percent of Americans over age 65 experiencing dementia have VaD, making it second only to Alzheimer's disease as a leading cause of dementia.

The occurrence of VaD increases with age, and the number of Americans age 65 and older is expected to increase to nearly 70 million by 2030.

Some of the risk factors for VaD are the same as for stroke, including high blood pressure, history of previous stroke, diabetes, heart disease, and high cholesterol levels.

Vascular Dementia (VaD) Diagnosis

Your healthcare provider should conduct a complete medical and patient history evaluation in order to determine the presence of VaD. Diagnostic tests may be used to exclude other possible causes of cognitive decline. Clinical tools are available to assist healthcare professionals in diagnosing VaD, including brain imaging techniques (CT [computed tomography] or MRI [magnetic resonance imaging]) and tests of cognitive functioning.

Symptoms of vascular dementia (VaD) include:

- memory loss;

- confusion;

- mood swings and personality changes;

- language problems;

- difficulty paying attention or following a conversation;

- impaired motor skills;

- difficulty planning and organizing tasks;

- visual orientation problems;

- difficulty with calculations, making decisions, solving problems;

- depression-like behavior.

Patients with VaD often deteriorate in a step-wise manner, with symptoms becoming greater with each new stroke. Sometimes, however, dementia can come on abruptly as the result of a single stroke, depending on the location and size of the damaged brain area.

In some instances, the onset of VaD is so gradual that healthcare providers have difficulty distinguishing it from Alzheimer's disease. The dementia in these cases is likely the result of chronic inadequate blood circulation in the brain that can cause small, silent strokes, or TIAs [transient ischemic attacks].

Patients with VaD may become more dependent upon family members or caregivers for assistance with activities of daily living due to physical and behavioral changes.

Vascular Dementia (VaD) Treatments

There are currently no therapies or drugs approved by the U.S. Food and Drug Administration (FDA) available for the treatment of VaD. Recently, an existing drug was submitted to the FDA for review as a potential treatment for VaD.

The current treatment strategies focus on reducing the risk of additional strokes, or prevention of stroke.

Other clinical trials are currently underway to test drugs that may treat patients with VaD.

Section 18.2

Binswanger Disease (Subcortical Vascular Dementia)

From "Binswanger's Disease Information Page," by the National Institute of Neurological Disorders and Stroke (NINDS, www.ninds.nih .gov), part of the National Institutes of Health, November 19, 2010.

What is Binswanger disease?

Binswanger disease (BD), also called subcortical vascular dementia, is a type of dementia caused by widespread, microscopic areas of damage to the deep layers of white matter in the brain. The damage is the result of the thickening and narrowing (atherosclerosis) of arteries that feed the subcortical areas of the brain. Atherosclerosis (commonly known as "hardening of the arteries") is a systemic process that affects blood vessels throughout the body. It begins late in the fourth decade of life and increases in severity with age. As the arteries become more and more narrowed, the blood supplied by those arteries decreases and brain tissue dies. A characteristic pattern of BD-damaged brain tissue can be seen with modern brain imaging techniques such as CT (computed tomography) scans or magnetic resonance imaging (MRI). The symptoms associated with BD are related to the disruption of subcortical neural circuits that control what neuroscientists call executive cognitive functioning—short-term memory, organization, mood, the regulation of attention, the ability to act or make decisions, and appropriate behavior. The most characteristic feature of BD is psychomotor slowness—an increase in the length of time it takes, for example, for the fingers to turn the thought of a letter into the shape of a letter on a piece of paper. Other symptoms include forgetfulness (but not as severe as the forgetfulness of Alzheimer disease), changes in speech, an unsteady gait, clumsiness or frequent falls, changes in personality or mood (most likely in the form of apathy, irritability, and depression), and urinary symptoms that aren't caused by urological disease. Brain imaging, which reveals the characteristic brain lesions of BD, is essential for a positive diagnosis.

202

Is there any treatment?

There is no specific course of treatment for BD. Treatment is symptomatic. People with depression or anxiety may require antidepressant medications such as the serotonin-specific reuptake inhibitors (SSRI) sertraline or citalopram.

Atypical antipsychotic drugs, such as risperidone and olanzapine, can be useful in individuals with agitation and disruptive behavior. Recent drug trials with the drug memantine have shown improved cognition and stabilization of global functioning and behavior. The successful management of hypertension and diabetes can slow the progression of atherosclerosis, and subsequently slow the progress of BD. Because there is no cure, the best treatment is preventive, early in the adult years, by controlling risk factors such as hypertension, diabetes, and smoking.

What is the prognosis?

BD is a progressive disease; there is no cure. Changes may be sudden or gradual and then progress in a stepwise manner. BD can often coexist with Alzheimer disease. Behaviors that slow the progression of high blood pressure, diabetes, and atherosclerosis—such as eating a healthy diet and keeping healthy wake/sleep schedules, exercising, and not smoking or drinking too much alcohol—can also slow the progression of BD.

Section 18.3

Cerebral Autosomal Dominant Arteriopathy with Subcortical Infarcts and Leukoencephalopathy (CADASIL)

From "CADASIL Information Page," by the National Institute of Neurological Disorders and Stroke (NINDS, www.ninds.nih.gov), part of the National Institutes of Health, October 13, 2009.

What is CADASIL?

CADASIL (cerebral autosomal dominant arteriopathy with subcortical infarcts and leukoencephalopathy) is an inherited form of cerebrovascular disease that occurs when the thickening of blood vessel walls blocks the flow of blood to the brain.

The disease primarily affects small blood vessels in the white matter of the brain. A mutation in the Notch3 gene alters the muscular walls in these small arteries. CADASIL is characterized by migraine headaches and multiple strokes progressing to dementia. Other symptoms include white matter lesions throughout the brain, cognitive deterioration, seizures, vision problems, and psychiatric problems such as severe depression and changes in behavior and personality.

Individuals may also be at higher risk of heart attack. Symptoms and disease onset vary widely, with signs typically appearing in the mid-30s. Some individuals may not show signs of the disease until later in life. CADASIL—formerly known by several names, including hereditary multi-infarct dementia—is one cause of multi-infarct dementia (dementia caused by lack of blood to several areas of the brain). It is an autosomal dominant inheritance disorder, meaning that one parent carries and passes on the defective gene. Most individuals with CADASIL have a family history of the disorder.

Is there any treatment?

There is no treatment to halt this genetic disorder. Individuals are given supportive care. Migraine headaches may be treated by different drugs and a daily aspirin may reduce stroke and heart attack risk.

Drug therapy for depression may be given. Affected individuals who smoke should quit as it can increase the risk of stroke in CADASIL.

What is the prognosis?

Symptoms usually progress slowly. By age 65, the majority of persons with CADASIL have severe cognitive problems and dementia. Some people lose the ability to walk and most become completely dependent due to multiple strokes.

Section 18.4

Multi-Infarct Dementia

From "Multi-Infarct Dementia Information Page," by the National Institute of Neurological Disorders and Stroke (NINDS, www.ninds.nih .gov), part of the National Institutes of Health, November 19, 2010.

What is multi-infarct dementia?

Multi-infarct dementia (MID) is a common cause of memory loss in the elderly. MID is caused by multiple strokes (disruption of blood flow to the brain). Disruption of blood flow leads to damaged brain tissue. Some of these strokes may occur without noticeable clinical symptoms. Doctors refer to these as silent strokes. An individual having a silent stroke may not even know it is happening, but over time, as more areas of the brain are damaged and more small blood vessels are blocked, the symptoms of MID begin to appear. MID can be diagnosed by MRI (magnetic resonance imaging) or CT (computed tomography) of the brain, along with a neurological examination.

Symptoms include confusion or problems with short-term memory; wandering, or getting lost in familiar places; walking with rapid, shuffling steps; losing bladder or bowel control; laughing or crying inappropriately; having difficulty following instructions; and having problems counting money and making monetary transactions. MID, which typically begins between the ages of 60 and 75, affects men more often than women. Because the symptoms of MID are so similar to Alzheimer disease, it can be difficult for a doctor to make a firm diagnosis. Since the diseases often occur together, making a single diagnosis of one or the other is even more problematic.

Is there any treatment?

There is no treatment available to reverse brain damage that has been caused by a stroke. Treatment focuses on preventing future strokes by controlling or avoiding the diseases and medical conditions that put people at high risk for stroke, including high blood pressure, diabetes, high cholesterol, and cardiovascular disease. The best treatment for MID is prevention early in life—eating a healthy diet, exercising, not smoking, moderately using alcohol, and maintaining a healthy weight.

What is the prognosis?

The prognosis for individuals with MID is generally poor. The symptoms of the disorder may begin suddenly, often in a step-wise pattern after each small stroke. Some people with MID may even appear to improve for short periods of time, then decline after having more silent strokes. The disorder generally takes a downward course with intermittent periods of rapid deterioration. Death may occur from stroke, heart disease, pneumonia, or other infection.

Chapter 19

Dementia Caused by Infection

Chapter Contents

Section 19.1

Creutzfeldt-Jakob Disease

From "Creutzfeldt-Jakob Disease Fact Sheet," by the National Institute of Neurological Disease and Stroke (NINDS, www.ninds.nih.gov), part of the National Institutes of Health, November 19, 2010.

What is Creutzfeldt-Jakob disease?

Creutzfeldt-Jakob disease (CJD) is a rare, degenerative, invariably fatal brain disorder. It affects about one person in every 1 million people per year worldwide; in the United States there are about 200 cases per year. CJD usually appears in later life and runs a rapid course. Typically, onset of symptoms occurs about age 60, and about 90 percent of individuals die within 1 year. In the early stages of disease, people may have failing memory, behavioral changes, lack of coordination, and visual disturbances. As the illness progresses, mental deterioration becomes pronounced and involuntary movements, blindness, weakness of extremities, and coma may occur.

There are three major categories of CJD:

- In sporadic CJD, the disease appears even though the person has no known risk factors for the disease. This is by far the most common type of CJD and accounts for at least 85 percent of cases.

- In hereditary CJD, the person has a family history of the disease and/or tests positive for a genetic mutation associated with CJD. About 5 to 10 percent of cases of CJD in the United States are hereditary.

- In acquired CJD, the disease is transmitted by exposure to brain or nervous system tissue, usually through certain medical procedures. There is no evidence that CJD is contagious through casual contact with a CJD patient.

Since CJD was first described in 1920, fewer than 1 percent of cases have been acquired CJD.

CJD belongs to a family of human and animal diseases known as the transmissible spongiform encephalopathies (TSEs). Spongiform refers to the characteristic appearance of infected brains, which become filled with holes until they resemble sponges under a microscope. CJD is the most common of the known human TSEs. Other human TSEs include kuru, fatal familial insomnia (FFI), and Gerstmann-Straussler-Scheinker disease (GSS). Kuru was identified in people of an isolated tribe in Papua New Guinea and has now almost disappeared. FFI and GSS are extremely rare hereditary diseases, found in just a few families around the world. Other TSEs are found in specific kinds of animals. These include bovine spongiform encephalopathy (BSE), which is found in cows and is often referred to as "mad cow" disease; scrapie, which affects sheep and goats; mink encephalopathy; and feline encephalopathy. Similar diseases have occurred in elk, deer, and exotic zoo animals.

What are the symptoms of the disease?

CJD is characterized by rapidly progressive dementia. Initially, individuals experience problems with muscular coordination; personality changes, including impaired memory, judgment, and thinking; and impaired vision. People with the disease also may experience insomnia, depression, or unusual sensations. CJD does not cause a fever or other flu-like symptoms. As the illness progresses, mental impairment becomes severe. Individuals often develop involuntary muscle jerks called myoclonus, and they may go blind. They eventually lose the ability to move and speak and enter a coma. Pneumonia and other infections often occur in these individuals and can lead to death.

There are several known variants of CJD. These variants differ somewhat in the symptoms and course of the disease. For example, a variant form of the disease—called new variant or variant (nv-CJD, v-CJD), described in Great Britain and France—begins primarily with psychiatric symptoms, affects younger individuals than other types of CJD, and has a longer than usual duration from onset of symptoms to death. Another variant, called the panencephalopathic form, occurs primarily in Japan and has a relatively long course, with symptoms often progressing for several years. Scientists are trying to learn what causes these variations in the symptoms and course of the disease.

Some symptoms of CJD can be similar to symptoms of other progressive neurological disorders, such as Alzheimer or Huntington disease. However, CJD causes unique changes in brain tissue, which can be seen at autopsy. It also tends to cause more rapid deterioration of a person's abilities than Alzheimer disease or most other types of dementia.

How is CJD diagnosed?

There is currently no single diagnostic test for CJD. When a doctor suspects CJD, the first concern is to rule out treatable forms of dementia such as encephalitis (inflammation of the brain) or chronic meningitis. A neurological examination will be performed and the doctor may seek consultation with other physicians. Standard diagnostic tests will include a spinal tap to rule out more common causes of dementia and an electroencephalogram (EEG) to record the brain's electrical pattern, which can be particularly valuable because it shows a specific type of abnormality in CJD. Computerized tomography of the brain can help rule out the possibility that the symptoms result from other problems such as stroke or a brain tumor. Magnetic resonance imaging (MRI) brain scans also can reveal characteristic patterns of brain degeneration that can help diagnose CJD.

The only way to confirm a diagnosis of CJD is by brain biopsy or autopsy. In a brain biopsy, a neurosurgeon removes a small piece of tissue from the patient's brain so that it can be examined by a neuropathologist. This procedure may be dangerous for the individual, and the operation does not always obtain tissue from the affected part of the brain. Because a correct diagnosis of CJD does not help the person, a brain biopsy is discouraged unless it is needed to rule out a treatable disorder. In an autopsy, the whole brain is examined after death. Both brain biopsy and autopsy pose a small, but definite, risk that the surgeon or others who handle the brain tissue may become accidentally infected by self-inoculation. Special surgical and disinfection procedures can minimize this risk.

Scientists are working to develop laboratory tests for CJD. One such test is performed on a person's cerebrospinal fluid and detects a protein marker that indicates neuronal degeneration. This can help diagnose CJD in people who already show the clinical symptoms of the disease. This test is much easier and safer than a brain biopsy. The false positive rate is about 5 to 10 percent. Scientists are working to develop this test for use in commercial laboratories. They are also working to develop other tests for this disorder.

What causes Creutzfeldt-Jakob disease?

Some researchers believe an unusual "slow virus" or another organism causes CJD. However, they have never been able to isolate a virus or other organism in people with the disease. Furthermore, the agent that causes CJD has several characteristics that are unusual for known organisms such as viruses and bacteria. It is difficult to

210

kill, it does not appear to contain any genetic information in the form of nucleic acids (DNA or RNA), and it usually has a long incubation period before symptoms appear. In some cases, the incubation period may be as long as 50 years. The leading scientific theory at this time maintains that CJD and the other TSEs are caused by a type of protein called a prion.

Prion proteins occur in both a normal form, which is a harmless protein found in the body's cells, and in an infectious form, which causes disease. The harmless and infectious forms of the prion protein have the same sequence of amino acids (the "building blocks" of proteins) but the infectious form of the protein takes a different folded shape than the normal protein. Sporadic CJD may develop because some of a person's normal prions spontaneously change into the infectious form of the protein and then alter the prions in other cells in a chain reaction.

Once they appear, abnormal prion proteins aggregate, or clump together. Investigators think these protein aggregates may lead to the neuron loss and other brain damage seen in CJD. However, they do not know exactly how this damage occurs.

About 5 to 10 percent of all CJD cases are inherited. These cases arise from a mutation, or change, in the gene that controls formation of the normal prion protein. While prions themselves do not contain genetic information and do not require genes to reproduce themselves, infectious prions can arise if a mutation occurs in the gene for the body's normal prion protein. If the prion protein gene is altered in a person's sperm or egg cells, the mutation can be transmitted to the person's offspring. All mutations in the prion protein gene are inherited as dominant traits. Therefore, family history is helpful in considering the diagnosis. Several different mutations in the prion gene have been identified. The particular mutation found in each family affects how frequently the disease appears and what symptoms are most noticeable. However, not all people with mutations in the prion protein gene develop CJD.

How is CJD transmitted?

CJD cannot be transmitted through the air or through touching or most other forms of casual contact. Spouses and other household members of sporadic CJD patients have no higher risk of contracting the disease than the general population. However, exposure to brain tissue and spinal cord fluid from infected individuals should be avoided to prevent transmission of the disease through these materials.

In some cases, CJD has spread to other people from grafts of dura mater (a tissue that covers the brain), transplanted corneas, implantation of inadequately sterilized electrodes in the brain, and injections of contaminated pituitary growth hormone derived from human pituitary glands taken from cadavers. Doctors call these cases that are linked to medical procedures iatrogenic cases. Since 1985, all human growth hormone used in the United States has been synthesized by recombinant DNA procedures, which eliminates the risk of transmitting CJD by this route.

The appearance of the new variant of CJD (nv-CJD or v-CJD) in several younger than average people in Great Britain and France has led to concern that BSE may be transmitted to humans through consumption of contaminated beef. Although laboratory tests have shown a strong similarity between the prions causing BSE and v-CJD, there is no direct proof to support this theory.

Many people are concerned that it may be possible to transmit CJD through blood and related blood products such as plasma. Some animal studies suggest that contaminated blood and related products may transmit the disease, although this has never been shown in humans. If there are infectious agents in these fluids, they are probably in very low concentrations. Scientists do not know how many abnormal prions a person must receive before he or she develops CJD, so they do not know whether these fluids are potentially infectious or not. They do know that, even though millions of people receive blood transfusions each year, there are no reported cases of someone contracting CJD from a transfusion. Even among people with hemophilia, who sometimes receive blood plasma concentrated from thousands of donors, there are no reported cases of CJD.

While there is no evidence that blood from people with sporadic CJD is infectious, studies have found that infectious prions from BSE and v-CJD may accumulate in the lymph nodes (which produce white blood cells), the spleen, and the tonsils. These findings suggest that blood transfusions from people with v-CJD might transmit the disease. The possibility that blood from people with v-CJD may be infectious has led to a policy preventing people in the United States from donating blood if they have resided for more than 3 months in a country or countries where BSE is common.

What research is taking place?

Many researchers are studying CJD. They are examining whether the transmissible agent is, in fact, a prion or a product of the infection, and are trying to discover factors that influence prion infectivity and how the disorder damages the brain. Using rodent models of the disease and brain tissue from autopsies, they are also trying to identify factors that influence susceptibility to the disease and that govern when in life the disease appears. They hope to use this knowledge to develop improved tests for CJD and to learn what changes ultimately kill the neurons so that effective treatments can be developed.

Section 19.2

Acquired Immunodeficiency Syndrome (AIDS) Dementia Complex

"AIDS Dementia Complex," © 2010 Project Inform. Reprinted with permission. For more information, contact the National HIV/AIDS Treatment Hotline, 1-800-822-7422, or visit www.projectinform.org.

Dementia is a brain disorder that affects a person's ability to think clearly and can impact his or her daily activities. AIDS [acquired immunodeficiency syndrome] dementia complex (ADC)—dementia caused by HIV [human immunodeficiency virus] infection—is a complicated syndrome of different nervous system and mental symptoms. These are somewhat common in people with HIV disease.

The frequency of ADC increases with advancing HIV disease and as CD4 counts decline. It's fairly uncommon in people with early HIV disease, and more common in people with severely weakened immune systems. Severe ADC is almost exclusively seen in advanced HIV disease.

ADC consists of many conditions. These can easily be mistaken for symptoms of other common problems including depression, drug side effects, or infections like toxo [toxoplasmosis] or lymphoma. Because ADC varies so much from person to person, it's poorly understood and there's no way to tell how a person will progress with ADC.

What Is ADC?

ADC is characterized by severe changes in four areas: A person's ability to understand and remember information (cognition); behavior;

ability to move their bodies (motor coordination); or emotions (mood). These changes are called ADC when they're believed to be related to HIV itself rather than other factors. Cognitive impairment often appears as memory loss, speech problems, inability to concentrate, and poor judgment. These are often the first symptoms a person will notice. They include the need to make lists in order to remember routine tasks or forgetting, in mid-sentence, what one was talking about.

Behavioral changes are the least understood. They can be described as impairments in one's ability to perform common tasks and activities of daily living. These changes are found in 30–40% of people with early ADC.

Motor impairment is often characterized by a loss of control of the bladder; loss of feeling in and loss of control of the legs; and stiff, awkward, or obviously slowed movements. It's not common in early ADC. A change in handwriting may be an early sign.

Mood impairments are defined as changes in emotional responses. In ADC, this is associated with several conditions, such as severe depression, severe personality changes (psychosis), and, less commonly, intense excitability (mania).

The Symptoms of ADC

Diagnosing ADC is heavily dependent on the keen judgment of doctors, often together with psychiatric, brain, or neurology experts. It's difficult to determine impairments in mood and behavior since there's no standard course of ADC. In one person it may be very mild with periods of varying severity of symptoms. In another it can be abrupt, severe, and progressive.

Sometimes symptoms are overlooked or dismissed by caregivers, who may believe the symptoms are due to advanced HIV disease or depression. ADC symptoms may include poor concentration, forgetfulness, loss of short- or long-term memory, social withdrawal, slowed thinking, short attention span, irritability, apathy (lack of caring or concern for oneself or others), weakness, poor coordination, impaired judgment, vision problems, and personality change.

ADC occurs more commonly in children with HIV than adults. It presents similarly and is often more severe and progressive.

Possible Early Stage Symptoms

- Difficulty concentrating
- Difficulty remembering phone numbers or appointments

- Slowed thinking
- Longer time needed to complete tasks
- Reliance on keeping lists
- Mental status tests and other mental capabilities may be normal
- Irritability
- Unsteady gait (walk) or difficulty keeping balance
- Poor hand coordination or writing
- Depression

Possible Middle Stage Symptoms

- Symptoms of muscle weakness
- Poor performance on regular tasks
- More concentration and attention required
- Slow responses and frequently dropping objects
- Feelings of indifference or apathy
- Slowness in normal activities, like eating and writing
- Walking, balance, and coordination require a great deal of effort

Possible Late Stage Symptoms

- Loss of bladder or bowel control
- Difficulty walking
- Loss of initiative or interest
- Withdrawing from life
- Psychosis or mania
- Confinement to bed

How Does HIV Cause ADC?

While it is clear that HIV can cause serious disease in the nervous system, how it causes ADC is unclear. In general, nervous system and mental disorders are caused by the death of nerve cells. While HIV does not directly infect nerve cells, it's thought it can somehow kill them indirectly.

Macrophages—white blood cells that are common in the brain and act as large reservoirs for HIV—appear to be HIV's first target in the central nervous system. Infected macrophages can carry HIV into the brain from the bloodstream. From there, these cells likely cause damage in many different ways.

What If You Think You Have ADC?

- Don't be afraid to tell your doctor or any other providers that you suspect something is wrong. Find a second opinion if you need one.

- Keep a notepad with you and write down your symptoms whenever they occur. This will greatly help your doctor to help you.

- Build as much support as possible, including friends, family, and professionals. Although it's possible to treat ADC, it may take a while for some symptoms to go away.

Incidence

Anecdotal reports indicate that there are fewer people with ADC since HIV therapy became standard. People who develop ADC today tend to be "sicker" than those before the use of HIV therapy. The rate of ADC dropped from 53% in 1987 to 3% in 1988 (after the first HIV drug was approved).

Early in the epidemic, many new AIDS cases were attributed to ADC. Many doctors now report that they're no longer seeing people who have just ADC. It has increasingly become a disease of late-stage AIDS when people suffer from multiple infections.

Diagnosing ADC

Three tests are required to diagnose ADC accurately: A mental status exam, one of the standard scans (CT [computed tomography] and/or MRI [magnetic resonance imaging]), and a spinal tap. These may also help tell ADC apart from other brain diseases like toxo, PML [progressive multifocal leukoencephalopathy], or lymphoma. However, ADC can occur along with these other brain diseases, so diagnosing multiple conditions can be more difficult.

A mental status exam helps reveal problems like short- or long-term memory loss, difficulty concentrating and abstract thinking, as well as swings in mood. Imaging scans of the brain are also used. Certain lab tests can examine cerebrospinal fluid (CSF) that's been obtained by a spinal tap. CT scans are x-rays that can show signs of destroyed brain tissue. MRI, or Magnetic Resonance Imaging, is a more sensitive scan. Results from both tests can help rule out other causes for the symptoms.

Testing CSF may help determine ADC, but they're not conclusive. Mostly they're used to rule out other causes of the symptoms. Many people with ADC have higher levels of certain proteins or white blood cells in their CSF. However, not everyone with these levels turn out to have ADC. Also, people with advanced ADC are more likely to have higher HIV levels in their CSF, though this is also not conclusive.

Treating ADC

The best therapies to treat ADC appear to be HIV drugs, and high-dose Retrovir (zidovudine, AZT) is the most studied drug for it. However, many specialists contend that how well a potent regimen controls HIV overall is more important than the actual drugs used. This may or may not include using standard, or even high-dose, Retrovir as part of the regimen.

Generally speaking, creating an HIV regimen to treat ADC follows three principles:

- start a potent regimen (usually three drugs) to decrease viral load to undetectable levels;
- in people on HIV therapy, consider their drug history and resistance test results; and
- if possible, use HIV drugs that cross the blood-brain barrier as part of the new regimen.

It's believed that an HIV drug that crosses the blood-brain barrier might help prevent or treat ADC. Findings from earlier in the epidemic show that high-dose Retrovir (1,000–1,200mg/day) can cross the blood-brain barrier and effectively treat it. Several researchers have reported improvements in symptoms. However, many with HIV are often unable to tolerate its side effects.

While Retrovir may be the most researched drug, other HIV drugs that cross the blood-brain barrier may be equally useful. These include Zerit, Ziagen, Viramune, Agenerase, and to a lesser degree, Crixivan and Epivir. Sustiva does not cross it to a significant degree, but some experts speculate it may be useful in treating ADC.

Treating the Symptoms

Psychoactive drugs are often used to treat ADC symptoms: Antipsychotics, anti-depressants, anxiolytics, psycho-stimulants, anti-manics, and anti-convulsants. These drugs do not treat the underlying cause of ADC, or even stop its progression. However, they may ease some of its symptoms. Haldol (haloperidol) is often used though it has many side effects, so smaller doses of 5–10mg daily should be used.

Ritalin (methylphenidate) has been used successfully in people with ADC to ease apathy and to increase energy, concentration, and appetite. Daily doses of 5–10mg are often enough.

In cases of severe behavior disorders, drugs like Thorazine and Mellaril can be used to control agitation. Ativan (lorazepam) and Valium (diazepam) may also be used for sedation and controlling anxiety. Others include Trilafon (perphenazine), Navane (thiothixene), Moban (molindone), and Prozac (fluoxetine) with Wellbutrin (bupropion).

Chapter 20

Other Health Conditions That Cause Dementia

Chapter Contents

Section 20.1

Cancer, Delirium, and Dementia

PDQ® Cancer Information Summary. National Cancer Institute; Bethesda, MD. Cognitive Disorders and Dementia (PDQ®): Patient Version. Updated 06/2010. Available at: http://cancer.gov. Accessed February 18, 2011.

Cognitive disorders and delirium are conditions in which the patient experiences a confused mental state and changes in behavior.

People who have cognitive disorders or delirium may fall in and out of consciousness and may have problems with the following:

- Attention
- Thinking
- Awareness
- Emotion
- Memory
- Muscle control
- Sleeping and waking

Delirium occurs frequently in patients with cancer, especially in patients with advanced cancer.

Delirium usually occurs suddenly and the patient's symptoms may come and go during the day. This condition can be treated and is often temporary, even in people with advanced illness. In the last 24 to 48 hours of life, however, delirium may be permanent due to problems such as organ failure.

Causes of Cognitive Disorders and Delirium

Cognitive disorders and delirium may be complications of cancer and cancer treatment, especially in people with advanced cancer.

In patients with cancer, cognitive disorders and delirium may be due to the direct effects that cancer has on the brain, such as the pressure of a growing tumor. Cognitive disorders and delirium may also be caused by indirect effects of cancer or its treatment, including the following:

- Organ failure

- Electrolyte imbalances (Electrolytes are important minerals [including salt, potassium, calcium, and phosphorous] that are needed to keep the heart, kidneys, nerves, and muscles working correctly.)

- Infection

- Symptoms caused by the cancer but that occur apart from the local or distant spread of the tumor (paraneoplastic syndromes), such as inflammation of the brain

- Medication side effects (Patients with cancer usually take many medications. Some drugs have side effects that include delirium and confusion. The effects of these drugs usually go away after the drug is stopped.)

- Withdrawal from drugs that depress (slow down) the central nervous system (brain and spinal cord)

Risk factors for delirium include having a serious disease and having more than one disease.

Other conditions besides having cancer may place a patient at risk for developing delirium. Risk factors include the following:

- Advanced cancer or other serious illness

- Having more than one disease

- Older age

- Previous mental disorder, such as dementia

- Low levels of albumin (protein) in the blood

- Infection

- Taking medications that affect the mind or behavior

- Taking high doses of pain medication

Early identification of risk factors may help prevent the onset of delirium or may reduce the length of time it takes to correct it.

Effects of Cognitive Disorders and Delirium on the Patient, Family, and Health Care Providers

Cognitive disorders and delirium can be upsetting to the family and caregivers, and may be dangerous to the patient if judgment is affected.

These conditions can cause the patient to act unpredictably and sometimes violently. Even a quiet or calm patient can suddenly experience a change in mood or become agitated, requiring increased care. The safety of the patient, family, and caregivers is most important.

Cognitive disorders and delirium may affect physical health and communication. Patients with cognitive disorders or delirium are more likely to fall, be incontinent (unable to control bladder and/or bowels), and become dehydrated (drink too little water to maintain health). They often require a longer hospital stay than patients without cognitive disorders or delirium.

The confused mental state of these patients may hinder their communication with family members and the health care providers. Assessment of the patient's symptoms becomes difficult and the patient may be unable to make decisions regarding care. Agitation in these patients may be mistaken as an expression of pain. Conflict can arise among the patient, family, and staff concerning the level of pain medication needed.

Diagnosis of Cognitive Disorders and Delirium

Possible signs of cognitive disorders and delirium include sudden personality changes, impaired thinking, or unusual anxiety or depression. A patient who suddenly becomes agitated or uncooperative, experiences personality or behavior changes, has impaired thinking, decreased attention span, or intense, unusual anxiety or depression, may be experiencing cognitive disorders or delirium. Patients who develop these symptoms need to be assessed completely.

Early symptoms of delirium are similar to symptoms of anxiety, anger, depression, and dementia. Delirium that causes the patient to be very inactive may appear to be depression. Delirium and dementia are difficult to tell apart, since both may cause disorientation and impair memory, thinking, and judgment. Dementia may be caused by a number of medical conditions, including Alzheimer disease. Some differences in the symptoms of delirium and dementia include the following:

- Patients with delirium often go in and out of consciousness. Patients who have dementia usually remain alert.

- Delirium may occur suddenly. Dementia appears gradually and gets worse over time.

- Sleeping and waking problems are more common with delirium than with dementia.

In elderly patients who have cancer, dementia is often present along with delirium, making diagnosis difficult. The diagnosis is more likely dementia if symptoms continue after treatment for delirium is given.

In patients aged 65 or older who have survived cancer for more than 5 years, the risk for cognitive disorders and dementia is increased, apart from the risk for delirium.

Regular screening of the patient and monitoring of the patient's symptoms can help in the diagnosis of delirium.

Treatment of Delirium

Patient and family concerns are addressed when deciding the treatment of delirium. Deciding if, when, and how to treat a person with delirium depends on the setting, how advanced the cancer is, the wishes of the patient and family, and how the delirium symptoms are affecting the patient.

Monitoring alone may be all that is necessary for patients who are not dangerous to themselves. In other cases, symptoms may be treated or causes of the delirium may be identified and treated.

Treatment of the Symptoms of Delirium by Changing the Patient's Surroundings

Controlling the patient's surroundings may help reduce mild symptoms of delirium. The following changes may be effective:

• Putting the patient in a quiet, well-lit room with familiar objects

• Placing a clock or calendar where the patient can see it

• Reducing noise

• Having family present

• Limiting changes in caregivers

To prevent a patient from harming himself or herself or others, physical restraints also may be necessary.

Treatment of the Causes of Delirium

The standard approach to managing delirium is to find and treat the causes. Symptoms may be treated at the same time. Identifying the causes of delirium will include a physical examination to check general signs of health, including checking for signs of disease. A medical history of the patient's past illnesses and treatments will also be taken. In a terminally ill delirious patient being cared for at home, the doctor may do a limited assessment to determine the cause or may treat just the symptoms.

Treatment may include the following:

- Stopping or reducing medications that cause delirium
- Giving fluids into the bloodstream to correct dehydration
- Giving drugs to correct hypercalcemia (too much calcium in the blood)
- Giving antibiotics for infections

Treatment of the Symptoms of Delirium with Medication

Drugs called antipsychotics may be used to treat the symptoms of delirium. Drugs that sedate (calm) the patient may also be used, especially if the patient is near death. All of these drugs have side effects and the patient will be monitored closely by a doctor. The decision to use drugs that sedate the patient will be made in cooperation with family members after efforts have been made to reverse the delirium.

Delirium and Sedation

The decision to use drugs to sedate the patient who is near death and has symptoms of delirium, pain, and difficult breathing presents ethical and legal issues for both the doctor and the family. When the symptoms of delirium are not relieved with standard treatment approaches and the patient is experiencing severe distress and suffering, the doctor may discuss the option to give drugs that will sedate the patient.

Section 20.2

Dementia:
A Symptom of Normal
Pressure Hydrocephalus

Excerpted from "Hydrocephalus Fact Sheet," by the National
Institute of Neurological Disorders and Stroke (NINDS, www
.ninds.nih.gov), part of the National Institutes of Health, July
1, 2010.

What is hydrocephalus?

The term hydrocephalus is derived from the Greek words "hydro"
meaning water and "cephalus" meaning head. As the name implies,
it is a condition in which the primary characteristic is excessive accumulation of fluid in the brain. Although hydrocephalus was once
known as "water on the brain," the "water" is actually cerebrospinal
fluid (CSF)—a clear fluid that surrounds the brain and spinal cord.
The excessive accumulation of CSF results in an abnormal widening of
spaces in the brain called ventricles. This widening creates potentially
harmful pressure on the tissues of the brain.

The ventricular system is made up of four ventricles connected by
narrow passages. Normally, CSF flows through the ventricles, exits
into cisterns (closed spaces that serve as reservoirs) at the base of the
brain, bathes the surfaces of the brain and spinal cord, and then reab-
sorbs into the bloodstream. CSF has three important life-sustaining
functions: 1) to keep the brain tissue buoyant, acting as a cushion or
"shock absorber"; 2) to act as the vehicle for delivering nutrients to the
brain and removing waste; and 3) to flow between the cranium and
spine and compensate for changes in intracranial blood volume (the
amount of blood within the brain).

The balance between production and absorption of CSF is critically
important. Because CSF is made continuously, medical conditions that
block its normal flow or absorption will result in an over accumulation
of CSF. The resulting pressure of the fluid against brain tissue is what
causes hydrocephalus.

What are the different types of hydrocephalus?

Hydrocephalus may be congenital or acquired. Congenital hydrocephalus is present at birth and may be caused by either events or influences that occur during fetal development, or genetic abnormalities. Acquired hydrocephalus develops at the time of birth or at some point afterward. This type of hydrocephalus can affect individuals of all ages and may be caused by injury or disease.

Hydrocephalus may also be communicating or non-communicating. Communicating hydrocephalus occurs when the flow of CSF is blocked after it exits the ventricles. This form is called communicating because the CSF can still flow between the ventricles, which remain open. Non-communicating hydrocephalus—also called obstructive hydrocephalus—occurs when the flow of CSF is blocked along one or more of the narrow passages connecting the ventricles. One of the most common causes of hydrocephalus is aqueductal stenosis. In this case, hydrocephalus results from a narrowing of the aqueduct of Sylvius, a small passage between the third and fourth ventricles in the middle of the brain.

There are two other forms of hydrocephalus that do not fit exactly into the categories mentioned above and primarily affect adults—hydrocephalus ex-vacuo and normal pressure hydrocephalus.

Hydrocephalus ex-vacuo occurs when stroke or traumatic injury cause damage to the brain. In these cases, brain tissue may actually shrink. Normal pressure hydrocephalus can happen to people at any age, but it is most common among the elderly. It may result from a subarachnoid hemorrhage, head trauma, infection, tumor, or complications of surgery. However, many people develop normal pressure hydrocephalus even when none of these factors are present for reasons that are unknown.

Who gets this disorder?

The number of people who develop hydrocephalus or who are currently living with it is difficult to establish since there is no national registry or database of people with the condition. However, experts estimate that hydrocephalus affects approximately one in every 500 children.

What causes hydrocephalus?

The causes of hydrocephalus are still not well understood. Hydrocephalus may result from inherited genetic abnormalities (such as the genetic defect that causes aqueductal stenosis) or developmental

disorders (such as those associated with neural tube defects including spina bifida and encephalocele). Other possible causes include
complications of premature birth such as intraventricular hemorrhage, diseases such as meningitis, tumors, traumatic head injury,
or subarachnoid hemorrhage, which block the exit of CSF from the
ventricles to the cisterns or eliminate the passageway for CSF into
the cisterns.

What are the symptoms?

Symptoms of hydrocephalus vary with age, disease progression, and
individual differences in tolerance to the condition. For example, an infant's ability to compensate for increased CSF pressure and enlargement
of the ventricles differs from an adult's. The infant skull can expand to
accommodate the buildup of CSF because the sutures (the fibrous joints
that connect the bones of the skull) have not yet closed.

In infancy, the most obvious indication of hydrocephalus is often a
rapid increase in head circumference or an unusually large head size.
Other symptoms may include vomiting, sleepiness, irritability, downward deviation of the eyes (also called sunsetting), and seizures.

Older children and adults may experience different symptoms because their skulls cannot expand to accommodate the buildup of CSF.
Symptoms may include headache followed by vomiting, nausea, papille-
dema (swelling of the optic disk that is part of the optic nerve), blurred
or double vision, sunsetting of the eyes, problems with balance, poor
coordination, gait disturbance, urinary incontinence, slowing or loss
of developmental progress, lethargy, drowsiness, irritability, or other
changes in personality or cognition including memory loss.

Symptoms of normal pressure hydrocephalus include problems with
walking, impaired bladder control leading to urinary frequency and/or
incontinence, and progressive mental impairment and dementia. An
individual with this type of hydrocephalus may have a general slowing
of movements or may complain that his or her feet feel stuck. Because
some of these symptoms may also be experienced in other disorders
such as Alzheimer disease, Parkinson disease, and Creutzfeldt-Jakob
disease, normal pressure hydrocephalus is often incorrectly diagnosed
and never properly treated. Doctors may use a variety of tests, including brain scans (CT [computed tomography] and/or MRI [magnetic
resonance imaging]), a spinal tap or lumbar catheter, intracranial
pressure monitoring, and neuropsychological tests, to help them accurately diagnose normal pressure hydrocephalus and rule out any
other conditions.

The symptoms described in this text account for the most typical ways in which progressive hydrocephalus manifests itself, but it is important to remember that symptoms vary significantly from one person to the next.

Part Four

Recognizing, Diagnosing, and Treating Symptoms of AD and Dementias

Chapter 21

Forgetfulness: Knowing When to Ask for Help

Maria has been a teacher for 35 years. Teaching fills her life and gives her a sense of accomplishment, but recently she has begun to forget details and has become more and more disorganized. At first, she laughed it off, but her memory problems have worsened. Her family and friends have been sympathetic but are not sure what to do. Parents and school administrators are worried about Maria's performance in the classroom. The principal has suggested she see a doctor. Maria is angry with herself and frustrated, and she wonders whether these problems are signs of Alzheimer disease or just forgetfulness that comes with getting older.

Many people worry about becoming forgetful. They think forgetfulness is the first sign of Alzheimer disease. Over the past few years, scientists have learned a lot about memory and why some kinds of memory problems are serious but others are not.

Age-Related Changes in Memory

Forgetfulness can be a normal part of aging. As people get older, changes occur in all parts of the body, including the brain. As a result, some people may notice that it takes longer to learn new things, they don't remember information as well as they did, or they lose things like their glasses. These usually are signs of mild forgetfulness, not serious memory problems.

From "Forgetfulness: Knowing When to Ask For Help," by the National Institute on Aging (NIA, www.nia.nih.gov), part of the National Institutes of Health, February 2010.

Some older adults also find that they don't do as well as younger people on complex memory or learning tests. Scientists have found, though, that given enough time, healthy older people can do as well as younger people do on these tests. In fact, as they age, healthy adults usually improve in areas of mental ability such as vocabulary.

Keeping Your Memory Sharp

People with some forgetfulness can use a variety of techniques that may help them stay healthy and maintain their memory and mental skills. Here are some tips that can help:

- Plan tasks, make to-do lists, and use memory aids like notes and calendars. Some people find they remember things better if they mentally connect them to other meaningful things, such as a familiar name, song, book, or TV show.

- Develop interests or hobbies and stay involved in activities that can help both the mind and body.

- Engage in physical activity and exercise. Several studies have associated exercise (such as walking) with better brain function, although more research is needed to say for sure whether exercise can help to maintain brain function or prevent or delay symptoms of Alzheimer disease.

- Limit alcohol use. Although some studies suggest that moderate alcohol use has health benefits, heavy or binge drinking over time can cause memory loss and permanent brain damage.

- Find activities, such as exercise or a hobby, to relieve feelings of stress, anxiety, or depression. If these feelings last for a long time, talk with your doctor.

Other Causes of Memory Loss

Some memory problems are related to health issues that may be treatable. For example, medication side effects, vitamin B12 deficiency, chronic alcoholism, tumors or infections in the brain, or blood clots in the brain can cause memory loss or possibly dementia. Some thyroid, kidney, or liver disorders also can lead to memory loss. A doctor should treat serious medical conditions like these as soon as possible.

Emotional problems, such as stress, anxiety, or depression, can make a person more forgetful and can be mistaken for dementia. For instance, someone who has recently retired or who is coping with the death of a spouse, relative, or friend may feel sad, lonely, worried, or bored. Trying to deal with these life changes leaves some people confused or forgetful.

The confusion and forgetfulness caused by emotions usually are temporary and go away when the feelings fade. The emotional problems can be eased by supportive friends and family, but if these feelings last for a long time, it is important to get help from a doctor or counselor. Treatment may include counseling, medication, or both.

More Serious Memory Problems

For some older people, memory problems are a sign of a serious problem, such as mild cognitive impairment or dementia. People who are worried about memory problems should see a doctor. The doctor might conduct or order a thorough physical and mental health evaluation to reach a diagnosis. Often, these evaluations are conducted by a neurologist, a physician who specializes in problems related to the brain and central nervous system.

A complete medical exam for memory loss should review the person's medical history, including the use of prescription and over-the-counter medicines, diet, past medical problems, and general health. A correct diagnosis depends on accurate details, so in addition to talking with the patient, the doctor might ask a family member, caregiver, or close friend for information.

Blood and urine tests can help the doctor find the cause of the memory problems or dementia. The doctor also might do tests for memory loss and test the person's problem-solving and language abilities. A computed tomography (CT) or magnetic resonance imaging (MRI) brain scan may help rule out some causes of the memory problems.

Amnestic mild cognitive impairment (MCI): Some people with memory problems have a condition called amnestic mild cognitive impairment, or amnestic MCI. People with this condition have more memory problems than normal for people their age, but their symptoms are not as severe as those of Alzheimer disease, and they are able to carry out their normal daily activities.

Signs of MCI include misplacing things often, forgetting to go to important events and appointments, and having trouble coming up with desired words. Family and friends may notice memory lapses, and the person with MCI may worry about losing his or her memory. These worries may prompt the person to see a doctor for diagnosis.

Researchers have found that more people with MCI than those without it go on to develop Alzheimer disease within a certain timeframe.

However, not everyone who has MCI develops AD. Studies are underway to learn why some people with MCI progress to AD and others do not.

There currently is no standard treatment for MCI. Typically, the doctor will regularly monitor and test a person diagnosed with MCI to detect any changes in memory and thinking skills over time. There are no medications approved for use for MCI.

Dementia: Dementia is the loss of thinking, memory, and reasoning skills to such an extent that it seriously affects a person's ability to carry out daily activities. Dementia is not a disease itself but a group of symptoms caused by certain diseases or conditions such as Alzheimer disease. People with dementia lose their mental abilities at different rates.

Symptoms may include the following:

• Being unable to remember things

• Asking the same question or repeating the same story over and over

• Becoming lost in familiar places

• Being unable to follow directions

• Getting disoriented about time, people, and places

• Neglecting personal safety, hygiene, and nutrition

Two of the most common forms of dementia in older people are Alzheimer disease and vascular dementia. These types of dementia cannot be cured at present.

In Alzheimer disease, changes to nerve cells in certain parts of the brain result in the death of a large number of cells. Symptoms of Alzheimer disease begin slowly and worsen steadily as damage to nerve cells spreads throughout the brain. As time goes by, forgetfulness gives way to serious problems with thinking, judgment, recognizing family and friends, and the ability to perform daily activities like driving a car or handling money. Eventually, the person needs total care.

In vascular dementia, a series of strokes or changes in the brain's blood supply leads to the death of brain tissue. Symptoms of vascular dementia can vary but usually begin suddenly, depending on where in the brain the strokes occurred and how severe they were. The person's memory, language, reasoning, and coordination may be affected. Mood and personality changes are common as well.

It's not possible to reverse damage already caused by a stroke, so it's very important to get medical care right away if someone has signs of a stroke. It's also important to take steps to prevent further strokes, which worsen vascular dementia symptoms. Some people have both Alzheimer disease and vascular dementia.

Treatment for Dementia

A person with dementia should be under a doctor's care. The doctor might be a neurologist, family doctor, internist, geriatrician, or psychiatrist. He or she can treat the patient's physical and behavioral problems (such as aggression, agitation, or wandering) and answer the many questions that the person or family may have.

People with dementia caused by Alzheimer disease may be treated with medications. Four medications are approved by the U.S. Food and Drug Administration to treat Alzheimer disease. Donepezil (Aricept®), rivastigmine (Exelon®), and galantamine (Razadyne®) are used to treat mild to moderate Alzheimer disease (donepezil has been approved to treat severe Alzheimer disease as well). Memantine (Namenda®) is used to treat moderate to severe Alzheimer disease. These drugs may help maintain thinking, memory, and speaking skills, and may lessen certain behavioral problems for a few months to a few years in some people. However, they don't stop Alzheimer disease from progressing. Studies are underway to investigate medications to slow cognitive decline and to prevent the development of Alzheimer disease.

People with vascular dementia should take steps to prevent further strokes. These steps include controlling high blood pressure, monitoring and treating high blood cholesterol and diabetes, and not smoking. Studies are underway to develop medicines to reduce the severity of memory and thinking problems that come with vascular dementia. Other studies are looking at the effects of drugs to relieve certain symptoms of this type of dementia.

Family members and friends can help people in the early stages of dementia to continue their daily routines, physical activities, and social contacts. People with dementia should be kept up to date about the details of their lives, such as the time of day, where they live, and what is happening at home or in the world. Memory aids may help. Some families find that a big calendar, a list of daily plans, notes about simple safety measures, and written directions describing how to use common household items are useful aids.

What You Can Do

If you're concerned that you or someone you know has a serious memory problem, talk with your doctor. He or she may be able to diagnose the problem or refer you to a specialist in neurology or geriatric psychiatry.

Healthcare professionals who specialize in Alzheimer disease can recommend ways to manage the problem or suggest treatment or services that might help.

Chapter 22

Talking with Your Doctor

How well you and your doctor talk to each other is one of the most important parts of getting good health care. But, talking to your doctor isn't always easy. It takes time and effort on your part as well as your doctor's.

In the past, the doctor typically took the lead and the patient followed. Today, a good patient-doctor relationship is more of a partnership. You and your doctor can work as a team, along with nurses, physician assistants, pharmacists, and other health care providers, to solve your medical problems and keep you healthy.

This means asking questions if the doctor's explanations or instructions are unclear, bringing up problems even if the doctor doesn't ask, and letting the doctor know if you have concerns about a particular treatment or change in your daily life. Taking an active role in your health care puts the responsibility for good communication on both you and your doctor.

All of this is true at any age. But when you're older, it becomes even more important to talk often and comfortably with your doctor. That's partly because you may have more health conditions and treatments to discuss. It's also because your health has a big impact on other parts of your life, and that needs to be talked about, too.

Excerpted from "Talking with Your Doctor: A Guide for Older People," by the National Institute on Aging (NIA, www.nia.nih.gov), part of the National Institutes of Health, April 2010.

Choosing a Doctor You Can Talk To

Finding a main doctor (often called your primary doctor or primary care doctor) that you feel comfortable talking to is the first step in good communication. It is also a way to ensure your good health. This doctor gets to know you and what your health is normally like. He or she can help you make medical decisions that suit your values and daily habits and can keep in touch with the other medical specialists and health care providers you may need.

If you don't have a primary doctor or are not at ease with the one you currently see, now may be the time to find a new doctor. Whether you just moved to a new city, changed insurance providers, or had a bad experience with your doctor or medical staff, it is worthwhile to spend time finding a doctor you can trust.

People sometimes hesitate to change doctors because they worry about hurting their doctor's feelings. But doctors understand that different people have different needs. They know it is important for everyone to have a doctor with whom they are comfortable.

Primary care doctors frequently are family practitioners, internists, or geriatricians. A geriatrician is a doctor who specializes in older people, but family practitioners and internists may also have a lot of experience with older patients.

The following suggestions can help you find a doctor who meets your needs:

Decide what you are looking for in a doctor: A good first step is to make a list of qualities that matter to you. Do you care if your doctor is a man or a woman? Is it important that your doctor has evening office hours, is associated with a specific hospital or medical center, or speaks your language? Do you prefer a doctor who has an individual practice or one who is part of a group so you can see one of your doctor's partners if your doctor is not available? After you have made your list, go back over it and decide which qualities are most important and which are nice, but not essential.

Identify several possible doctors: Once you have a general sense of what you are looking for, ask friends and relatives, medical specialists, and other health professionals for the names of doctors with whom they have had good experiences. Rather than just getting a name, ask about the person's experiences. For example: say, "What do you like about Dr. Smith?" and "Does this doctor take time to answer questions?" A doctor whose name comes up often may be a strong possibility.

If you belong to a managed care plan—a health maintenance organization (HMO) or preferred provider organization (PPO)—you may be required to choose a doctor in the plan or else you may have to pay extra to see a doctor outside the network. Most managed care plans will provide information on their doctors' backgrounds and credentials. Some plans have websites with lists of participating doctors from which you can choose.

It may be helpful to develop a list of a few names you can choose from. As you find out more about the doctors on this list, you may rule out some of them. In some cases, a doctor may not be taking new patients and you may have to make another choice.

Consult reference sources: The *Directory of Physicians in the United States* and the *Official American Board of Medical Specialties Directory of Board Certified Medical Specialists* are available at many libraries. These books don't recommend individual doctors but they do provide a list of doctors you may want to consider. MedlinePlus, a website from the National Library of Medicine, has a comprehensive list of directories (www.nlm.nih.gov/medlineplus/directories.html) which may also be helpful.

There are plenty of other internet resources, too—for example, you can find doctors through the American Medical Association's website at www.ama-assn.org (click on "Doctor Finder"). For a list of doctors who participate in Medicare, visit www.medicare.gov (click on "Search Tools" then "Find a Doctor"). WebMD also provides a list of doctors at www.webmd.com (click on "Doctors").

Don't forget to call your local or state medical society to check if complaints have been filed against any of the doctors you are considering.

Learn more about the doctors you are considering: Once you have narrowed your list to two or three doctors, call their offices. The office staff is a good source of information about the doctor's education and qualifications, office policies, and payment procedures. Pay attention to the office staff—you will have to deal with them often!

You may want to set up an appointment to meet and talk with a doctor you are considering. He or she is likely to charge you for such a visit. After the appointment, ask yourself whether this doctor is a person with whom you could work well. If you are not satisfied, schedule a visit with one of your other candidates.

When learning about a doctor, consider asking questions like the following:

• Do you have many older patients?

- How do you feel about involving my family in care decisions?
- Can I call or e-mail you or your staff when I have questions?
- Do you charge for telephone or e-mail time?
- What are your thoughts about complementary or alternative treatments?

When making a decision about which doctor to choose, you might want to ask yourself questions like the following:

- Did the doctor give me a chance to ask questions?
- Was the doctor really listening to me?
- Could I understand what the doctor was saying? Was I comfortable asking him or her to say it again?

Make a choice: Once you've chosen a doctor, make your first actual health care appointment. This visit may include a medical history and a physical exam. Be sure to bring your medical records, or have them sent from your former doctor. Bring a list of your current medicines or put the medicines in a bag and take them with you. If you haven't already met the doctor, ask for extra time during this visit to ask any questions you have about the doctor or the practice.

Getting Ready for an Appointment

A basic plan can help you make the most of your appointment whether you are starting with a new doctor or continuing with the doctor you've seen for years. The following tips will make it easier for you and your doctor to cover everything you need to talk about.

Make a list of your concerns and prioritize them: Make a list of what you want to discuss. For example, do you have a new symptom you want to ask the doctor about? Do you want to get a flu shot? Are you concerned about how a treatment is affecting your daily life? If you have more than a few items to discuss, put them in order and ask about the most important ones first. Don't put off the things that are really on your mind until the end of your appointment—bring them up right away!

Take information with you: Some doctors suggest you put all your prescription drugs, over-the-counter medicines, vitamins, and herbal remedies or supplements in a bag and bring them with you.

Others recommend you bring a list of everything you take. You should also take your insurance cards, names, and phone numbers of other doctors you see, and your medical records if the doctor doesn't already have them.

Make sure you can see and hear as well as possible: Many older people use glasses or need aids for hearing. Remember to take your eyeglasses to the doctor's visit. If you have a hearing aid, make sure that it is working well and wear it. Let the doctor and staff know if you have a hard time seeing or hearing. For example, you may want to say: "My hearing makes it hard to understand everything you're saying. It helps a lot when you speak slowly."

Consider bringing a family member or friend: Sometimes it is helpful to bring a family member or close friend with you. Let your family member or friend know in advance what you want from your visit. Your companion can remind you what you planned to discuss with the doctor if you forget, she or he can take notes for you, and can help you remember what the doctor said.

Find an interpreter if you know you'll need one: If the doctor you selected or were referred to doesn't speak your language, consider bringing an interpreter with you. Sometimes community groups can help find an interpreter. Or you can call the doctor's office ahead of time to see if one can be provided for you. Sometimes doctors ask a staff member to help with interpretation. Even though some English-speaking doctors know basic medical terms in Spanish or other languages, you may feel more comfortable speaking in your own language, especially when it comes to sensitive subjects, such as sexuality or depression.

You can also ask a family member who speaks English to go with you. This person should be someone you trust with knowing your symptoms or condition. Finally, let the doctor, your interpreter, or the staff know if you do not understand your diagnosis or the instructions the doctor gives you. Don't let language barriers stop you from asking questions or voicing your concerns.

Plan to update the doctor: Let your doctor know what has happened in your life since your last visit. If you have been treated in the emergency room or by a specialist, tell the doctor right away. Mention any changes you have noticed in your appetite, weight, sleep, or energy level. Also tell the doctor about any recent changes in any medications you take or the effects they have had on you.

Giving Information

Talking about your health means sharing information about how you feel physically, emotionally, and mentally. Knowing how to describe your symptoms and bring up other concerns will help you become a partner in your health care.

Share any symptoms: A symptom is evidence of a disease or disorder in the body. Examples of symptoms include pain, fever, a lump or bump, unexplained weight loss or gain, or having a hard time sleeping. Be clear and concise when describing your symptoms. Your description helps the doctor identify the problem. A physical exam and medical tests provide valuable information, but it is your symptoms that point the doctor in the right direction.

Questions to ask yourself about your symptoms include the following:

- What exactly are my symptoms?
- Are the symptoms constant? If not, when do I experience them?
- Does anything I do make the symptoms better? Or worse?
- Do the symptoms affect my daily activities? Which ones? How?

Your doctor will ask when your symptoms started, what time of day they happen, how long they last (seconds? days?), how often they occur, if they seem to be getting worse or better, and if they keep you from going out or doing your usual activities.

Take the time to make some notes about your symptoms before you call or visit the doctor. Worrying about your symptoms is not a sign of weakness. Being honest about what you are experiencing doesn't mean that you are complaining. The doctor needs to know how you feel.

Give information about your medications: It is possible for medicines to interact causing unpleasant and sometimes dangerous side effects. Your doctor needs to know about all of the medicines you take, including over-the-counter (nonprescription) drugs and herbal remedies or supplements, so bring everything with you to your visit—don't forget about eyedrops, vitamins, and laxatives. Tell the doctor how often you take each. Describe any drug allergies or reactions you have had. Say which medications work best for you. Be sure your doctor has the phone number of the pharmacy you use.

Tell the doctor about your habits: To provide the best care, your doctor must understand you as a person and know what your life is like. The doctor may ask about where you live, what you eat, how you sleep, what you do each day, what activities you enjoy, what your sex life is like, and if you smoke or drink. Be open and honest with your doctor. It will help him or her to understand your medical conditions fully and recommend the best treatment choices for you.

Voice other concerns: Your doctor may ask you how your life is going. This isn't being impolite or nosy. Information about what's happening in your life may be useful medically. Let the doctor know about any major changes or stresses in your life, such as a divorce or the death of a loved one. You don't have to go into detail; you may want to say something like: "It might be helpful for you to know that my sister passed away since my last visit with you." or "I recently had to sell my home and move in with my daughter."

Getting Information

Asking questions is key to good communication with your doctor. If you don't ask questions, he or she may assume you already know the answer or that you don't want more information. Don't wait for the doctor to raise a specific question or subject because he or she may not know it's important to you. Be proactive. Ask questions when you don't know the meaning of a word (like aneurysm, hypertension, or infarct) or when instructions aren't clear (for example, does taking medicine with food mean before, during, or after a meal?).

Learn about medical tests: Sometimes doctors need to do blood tests, x-rays, or other procedures to find out what is wrong or to learn more about your medical condition. Some tests, such as Pap smears, mammograms, glaucoma tests, and screenings for prostate and colorectal cancer, are done regularly to check for hidden medical problems.

Before having a medical test, ask your doctor to explain why it is important, what it will show, and what it will cost. Ask what kind of things you need to do to prepare for the test. For example, you may need to have an empty stomach, or you may have to provide a urine sample. Ask how you will be notified of the test results and how long they will take to come in.

Questions to ask about medical tests include the following:

- Why is the test being done?

- What steps does the test involve? How should I get ready?

- Are there any dangers or side effects?

243

- How will I find out the results? How long will it take to get the results?

- What will we know after the test?

When the results are ready, make sure the doctor tells you what they are and explains what they mean. You may want to ask your doctor for a written copy of the test results. If the test is done by a specialist, ask to have the results sent to your primary doctor.

Discuss your diagnosis and what you can expect: A diagnosis identifies your disease or physical problem. The doctor makes a diagnosis based on the symptoms you are experiencing and the results of the physical exam, laboratory work, and other tests.

If you understand your medical condition, you can help make better decisions about treatment. If you know what to expect, it may be easier for you to deal with the condition.

Ask the doctor to tell you the name of the condition and why he or she thinks you have it. Ask how it may affect you and how long it might last. Some medical problems never go away completely. They can't be cured, but they can be treated or managed.

Questions to ask about your diagnosis include the following:

- What may have caused this condition? Will it be permanent?

- How is this condition treated or managed?

- What will be the long-term effects on my life?

- How can I learn more about my condition?

Find out about your medications: Your doctor may prescribe a drug for your condition. Make sure you know the name of the drug and understand why it has been prescribed for you. Ask the doctor to write down how often and for how long you should take it.

Make notes about any other special instructions. There may be foods or drinks you should avoid while you are taking the medicine. Or you may have to take the medicine with food or a whole glass of water. If you are taking other medications, make sure your doctor knows, so he or she can prevent harmful drug interactions.

Sometimes medicines affect older people differently than younger people. Let the doctor know if your medicine doesn't seem to be working or if it is causing problems. It is best not to stop taking the medicine on your own. If you want to stop taking your medicine, check with your doctor first.

If another doctor (for example, a specialist) prescribes a medication for you, call your primary doctor's office and leave a message letting him or her know. Also call to check with your doctor's office before taking any over-the-counter medications. You may find it helpful to keep a chart of all the medicines you take and when you take them.

The pharmacist is also a good source of information about your medicines. In addition to answering questions and helping you select over-the-counter medications, the pharmacist keeps records of all the prescriptions you get filled at that pharmacy. Because your pharmacist keeps these records, it is helpful to use the same store regularly. At your request, the pharmacist can fill your prescriptions in easy-to-open containers and may be able to provide large-print prescription labels.

Questions to ask about medications include the following:

- What are the common side effects? What should I pay attention to?

- When will the medicine begin to work?

- What should I do if I miss a dose?

- Should I take it at meals or between meals? Do I need to drink a whole glass of water with it?

- Are there foods, drugs, or activities I should avoid while taking this medicine?

- Will I need a refill? How do I arrange that?

Understand your prescriptions: When the doctor writes you a prescription, it is important that you are able to read and understand the directions for taking the medication. Doctors and pharmacists often use abbreviations or terms that may not be familiar. Here is an explanation of some of the most common abbreviations you will see on the labels of your prescription medications:

- p.r.n.—as needed

- q.d.—every day

- b.i.d.—twice a day

- t.i.d.—three times a day

- q.i.d.—four times a day

- a.c.—before meals

- p.c.—after meals

245

- h.s.—at bedtime

- p.o.—by mouth

- ea.—each

If you have questions about your prescription or how you should take the medicine, ask your doctor or pharmacist. If you do not understand the directions, make sure you ask someone to explain them. It is important to take the medicine as directed by your doctor.

Keeping a record of the medications you take and the instructions for taking them can help you get the most benefit from them.

Making Decisions with Your Doctor

Giving and getting information are two important steps in talking with your doctor. The third big step is making decisions about your care.

Ask about different treatments: You will benefit most from a treatment when you know what is happening and are involved in making decisions. Make sure you understand what your treatment involves and what it will or will not do. Have the doctor give you directions in writing and feel free to ask questions. For example: "What are the pros and cons of having surgery at this stage?" or "Do I have any other choices?"

If your doctor suggests a treatment that makes you uncomfortable, ask if there are other treatments that might work. If cost is a concern, ask the doctor if less expensive choices are available. The doctor can work with you to develop a treatment plan that meets your needs.

Here are some things to remember when deciding on a treatment:

- Discuss choices. There are different ways to manage many health conditions, especially chronic conditions like high blood pressure and cholesterol. Ask what your options are.

- Discuss risks and benefits. Once you know your options, ask about the pros and cons of each one. Find out what side effects might occur, how long the treatment would continue, and how likely it is that the treatment will work for you.

- Consider your own values and circumstances. When thinking about the pros and cons of a treatment, don't forget to consider its impact on your overall life. For instance, will one of the side effects interfere with a regular activity that means a lot to you?

Is one treatment choice expensive and not covered by your insurance? Doctors need to know about these practical matters and can work with you to develop a treatment plan that meets your needs.

Ask about prevention: Doctors and other health professionals may suggest you change your diet, activity level, or other aspects of your life to help you deal with medical conditions. Research has shown that these changes, particularly an increase in exercise, have positive effects on overall health.

Until recently, preventing disease in older people received little attention. But things are changing. We now know that it's never too late to stop smoking, improve your diet, or start exercising. Getting regular checkups and seeing other health professionals such as dentists and eye specialists helps promote good health. Even people who have chronic diseases, like arthritis or diabetes, can prevent further disability and, in some cases, control the progress of the disease.

If a certain disease or health condition runs in your family, ask your doctor if there are steps you can take to help prevent it. If you have a chronic condition, ask how you can manage it and if there are things you can do to prevent it from getting worse. If you want to discuss health and disease prevention with your doctor, say so when you make your next appointment. This lets the doctor plan to spend more time with you.

It is just as important to talk with your doctor about lifestyle changes as it is to talk about treatment. For example: "I know that you've told me to eat more dairy products, but they really disagree with me. Is there something else I could eat instead?" or "Maybe an exercise class would help, but I have no way to get to the senior center. Is there something else you could suggest?"

Just as with treatments, consider all the alternatives, look at pros and cons, and remember to take into account your own point of view. Tell your doctor if you feel his or her suggestions won't work for you and explain why. Keep talking with your doctor to come up with a plan that works.

Chapter 23

Diagnosing AD

Chapter Contents

Section 23.1

How Is AD Diagnosed?

Excerpted from "Alzheimer's Disease: Unraveling the Mystery,"
by the National Institute on Aging (NIA, www.nia.nih.gov), part
of the National Institutes of Health, September 2008.

A man in his mid-60s begins to notice that his memory isn't as good as it used to be. More and more often, a word will be on the tip of his tongue but he just can't remember it. He forgets appointments, makes mistakes when paying his bills, and finds that he's often confused or anxious about the normal hustle and bustle of life around him. One evening, he suddenly finds himself walking in a neighborhood he doesn't recognize. He has no idea how he got there or how to get home.

Not so long ago, this man's condition would have been swept into a broad catch-all category called senile dementia or senility. Although we now know that Alzheimer disease (AD) and other causes of dementia are distinct diseases, in the early stages it is difficult to differentiate between the onset of AD and other types of age-related cognitive decline. We have improved our ability to diagnose AD correctly, and doctors experienced in AD can diagnose the disease with up to 90 percent accuracy. A definitive diagnosis of AD, however, is still only possible after death, during an autopsy, and we are still far from the ultimate goal—a reliable, valid, inexpensive, and early diagnostic marker that can be used in any doctor's office.

Early diagnosis has several advantages. For example, many conditions cause symptoms that mimic those of AD. Finding out early that the observed changes in cognitive abilities are not AD but something else is almost always a relief and may be just the prod needed to seek appropriate medical treatment. For the small percentage of dementias that are treatable or even reversible, early diagnosis increases the chances of successful treatment.

Even when the cause of a loved one's dementia turns out to be AD, it is best to find out sooner rather than later. One benefit of knowing is medical. The drugs now available to treat AD can help some people maintain their mental abilities for months to years, although they do not change the underlying course of the disease.

Other benefits are practical. The sooner the person with AD and the family have a firm diagnosis, the more time they have to make future living arrangements, handle financial matters, establish a durable power of attorney and advance directives, deal with other legal issues, create a support network, and even consider joining a clinical trial or other research study. Being able to participate for as long as possible in making personal decisions is important to many people with AD.

Early diagnosis also gives families time to recognize that life does not stop with a diagnosis of AD. The person is still able to participate in many of the daily activities he or she has always enjoyed, and families can encourage the person to continue with them for as long as possible. Finally, early diagnosis gives family caregivers the opportunity to learn how to recognize and cope with changes over time in their loved one as well as to develop strategies that support their own physical, emotional, and financial health.

Scientists also see advantages to early diagnosis. Developing tests that can reveal what is happening in the brain in the early stages of AD will help them understand more about the cause and development of the disease. It also will help scientists learn when and how to prescribe the use of drugs and other treatments so they can be most effective.

Current Tools for Diagnosing AD

With the tools now available, experienced physicians can be reasonably confident about making an accurate diagnosis of AD in a living person. Here is how they do it.

They take a detailed patient history, including the following:

- A description of how and when symptoms developed
- A description of the person's and his or her family's overall medical condition and history
- An assessment of the person's emotional state and living environment

They get information from family members or close friends:

- People close to the person can provide valuable insights into how behavior and personality have changed; many times, family and friends know something is wrong even before changes are evident on tests.

They conduct physical and neurological examinations and laboratory tests:

- Blood and other medical tests help determine neurological functioning and identify possible non-AD causes of dementia.

They conduct neuropsychological testing:

- Question-and-answer tests or other tasks that measure memory, language skills, ability to do arithmetic, and other abilities related to brain functioning help show what kind of cognitive changes are occurring.

They may do a computed tomography (CT) scan or a magnetic resonance imaging (MRI) test:

- CT and MRI scans can detect strokes or tumors or can reveal changes in the brain's structure that indicate early AD.

Exams and tests may be repeated every so often to give physicians information about how the person's memory and other symptoms are changing over time.

Based on findings from these exams and tests, experienced physicians can diagnose or rule out other causes of dementia, or determine whether the person has mild cognitive impairment (MCI), possible AD (the symptoms may be due to another cause), or probable AD (no other cause for the symptoms can be found).

New Developments in AD Diagnosis

Scientists are now exploring ways to help physicians diagnose AD earlier and more accurately. For example, some studies are focusing on changes in mental functioning. These changes can be measured through memory and recall tests. Tests that measure a person's abilities in areas such as abstract thinking, planning, and language can help pinpoint changes in these areas of cognitive function. Researchers are working to improve standardized tests that might be used to point to early AD or predict which individuals are at higher risk of developing AD in the future.

Other studies are examining the relationship between early damage to brain tissue and outward clinical signs. Still others are looking for changes in biomarkers in the blood or cerebrospinal fluid that may indicate the progression of AD.

One of the most exciting areas of ongoing research in this area is neuroimaging. Over the past decade, scientists have developed several highly sophisticated imaging systems that have been used in many areas of medicine, including AD. PET (positron emission tomography) scans, single photon emission computed tomography (SPECT), and MRI are all examples. These windows on the living brain may help scientists measure the earliest changes in brain function or structure in order to identify people who are at the very first stages of the disease—well before they develop clinically apparent signs and symptoms.

To help advance this area of research, NIA launched the multi-year AD Neuroimaging Initiative (ADNI) in 2004. This project is following about 200 cognitively healthy individuals and 400 people with MCI for 3 years and 200 people with early AD for 2 years. Over the course of this study, participants undergo multiple MRI and PET scans so that study staff can assess how the brain changes in the course of normal aging and MCI, and with the progression of AD. By using MRI and PET scans at regularly scheduled intervals, study investigators hope to learn when and where in the brain degeneration occurs as memory problems develop.

Another innovative aspect of ADNI is that scientists are correlating the participants' imaging information with information from clinical, memory, and other cognitive function tests, and with information from blood, cerebrospinal fluid, and urine samples. Results from these samples may provide valuable biomarkers of disease progress, such as changing levels of beta-amyloid and tau, indicators of inflammation, measures of oxidative stress, and changing cognitive abilities.

An important ADNI achievement is the creation of a publicly accessible database of images, biomarker data, and clinical information available to qualified researchers worldwide. Biological samples also are available for approved biomarker projects. NIA hopes that this initiative will help create rigorous imaging and biomarker standards that will provide measures for the success of potential treatments. This would substantially increase the pace and decrease the cost of developing new treatments. The ADNI study is being replicated in similar studies by researchers in Europe, Japan, and Australia.

These types of neuroimaging scans are still primarily research tools, but one day they may be used more commonly to help physicians diagnose AD at very early stages. It is conceivable that these tools also may someday be used to monitor the progress of the disease and to assess responses to drug treatment.

Section 23.2

AD Guidelines Updated for First Time in Decades

"Alzheimer's Diagnostic Guidelines Updated for First Time in Decades,"
a press release from the National Institute on Aging (NIA, www.nia
.nih.gov), part of the National Institutes of Health, April 19, 2011.

For the first time in 27 years, clinical diagnostic criteria for Alzheimer disease dementia have been revised, and research guidelines for earlier stages of the disease have been characterized to reflect a deeper understanding of the disorder. The National Institute on Aging/Alzheimer's Association Diagnostic Guidelines for Alzheimer's Disease outline some new approaches for clinicians and provide scientists with more advanced guidelines for moving forward with research on diagnosis and treatments. They mark a major change in how experts think about and study Alzheimer disease. Development of the new guidelines was led by the National Institutes of Health and the Alzheimer's Association.

The original criteria were the first to address the disease and described only later stages, when symptoms of dementia are already evident. The updated guidelines announced on April 19, 2011 cover the full spectrum of the disease as it gradually changes over many years. They describe the earliest preclinical stages of the disease, mild cognitive impairment, and dementia due to Alzheimer disease pathology. Importantly, the guidelines now address the use of imaging and biomarkers in blood and spinal fluid that may help determine whether changes in the brain and those in body fluids are due to Alzheimer disease. Biomarkers are increasingly employed in the research setting to detect onset of the disease and to track progression, but cannot yet be used routinely in clinical diagnosis without further testing and validation.

"Alzheimer's research has greatly evolved over the past quarter of a century. Bringing the diagnostic guidelines up to speed with those advances is both a necessary and rewarding effort that will benefit patients and accelerate the pace of research," said National Institute on Aging Director Richard J. Hodes, MD.

"We believe that the publication of these articles is a major milestone for the field," said William Thies, PhD, chief medical and scientific officer at the Alzheimer's Association. "Our vision is that this process will result in improved diagnosis and treatment of Alzheimer's, and will drive research that ultimately will enable us to detect and treat the disease earlier and more effectively. This would allow more people to live full, rich lives without—or with a minimum of—Alzheimer's symptoms."

The new guidelines appear online April 19, 2011 in *Alzheimer's & Dementia: The Journal of the Alzheimer's Association*. They were developed by expert panels convened last year by the National Institute on Aging (NIA), part of the National Institutes of Health, and the Alzheimer's Association. Preliminary recommendations were announced at the Association's International Conference on Alzheimer's Disease in July 2010, followed by a comment period.

Guy M. McKhann, MD, Johns Hopkins University School of Medicine, Baltimore, and David S. Knopman, MD, Mayo Clinic, Rochester, Minnesota, co-chaired the panel that revised the 1984 clinical Alzheimer dementia criteria. Marilyn Albert, PhD, Johns Hopkins University School of Medicine, headed the panel refining the mild cognitive impairment criteria. Reisa A. Sperling, MD, Brigham and Women's Hospital, Harvard Medical School, Boston, led the panel tasked with defining the preclinical stage. The journal also includes a paper by Clifford Jack, MD, Mayo Clinic, Rochester, Minnesota, as senior author, on the need for and concept behind the new guidelines.

The original 1984 clinical criteria for Alzheimer disease, reflecting the limited knowledge of the day, defined Alzheimer disease as having a single stage, dementia, and based diagnosis solely on clinical symptoms. It assumed that people free of dementia symptoms were disease-free. Diagnosis was confirmed only at autopsy, when the hallmarks of the disease, abnormal amounts of amyloid proteins forming plaques and tau proteins forming tangles, were found in the brain.

Since then, research has determined that Alzheimer disease may cause changes in the brain a decade or more before symptoms appear and that symptoms do not always directly relate to abnormal changes in the brain caused by Alzheimer disease. For example, some older people are found to have abnormal levels of amyloid plaques in the brain at autopsy yet never showed signs of dementia during life. It also appears that amyloid deposits begin early in the disease process but that tangle formation and loss of neurons occur later and may accelerate just before clinical symptoms appear.

To reflect what has been learned, the National Institute on Aging/ Alzheimer's Association Diagnostic Guidelines for Alzheimer's Disease cover three distinct stages of Alzheimer disease:

- **Preclinical:** The preclinical stage, for which the guidelines only apply in a research setting, describes a phase in which brain changes, including amyloid buildup and other early nerve cell changes, may already be in process. At this point, significant clinical symptoms are not yet evident. In some people, amyloid buildup can be detected with positron emission tomography (PET) scans and cerebrospinal fluid (CSF) analysis, but it is unknown what the risk for progression to Alzheimer dementia is for these individuals. However, use of these imaging and bio-marker tests at this stage are recommended only for research. These biomarkers are still being developed and standardized and are not ready for use by clinicians in general practice.

- **Mild cognitive impairment (MCI):** The guidelines for the MCI stage are also largely for research, although they clarify existing guidelines for MCI for use in a clinical setting. The MCI stage is marked by symptoms of memory problems, enough to be noticed and measured, but not compromising a person's independence. People with MCI may or may not progress to Alzheimer dementia. Researchers will particularly focus on standardizing biomark-ers for amyloid and for other possible signs of injury to the brain. Currently, biomarkers include elevated levels of tau or decreased levels of beta-amyloid in the CSF, reduced glucose uptake in the brain as determined by PET, and atrophy of certain areas of the brain as seen with structural magnetic resonance imaging (MRI). These tests will be used primarily by researchers, but may be ap-plied in specialized clinical settings to supplement standard clini-cal tests to help determine possible causes of MCI symptoms.

- **Alzheimer dementia:** These criteria apply to the final stage of the disease, and are most relevant for doctors and patients. They outline ways clinicians should approach evaluating causes and progression of cognitive decline. The guidelines also expand the concept of Alzheimer dementia beyond memory loss as its most central characteristic. A decline in other aspects of cognition, such as word-finding, vision/spatial issues, and impaired reasoning or judgment may be the first symptom to be noticed. At this stage, biomarker test results may be used in some cases to increase or decrease the level of certainty about a diagnosis of

Alzheimer dementia and to distinguish Alzheimer dementia from other dementias, even as the validity of such tests is still under study for application and value in everyday clinical practice.

The panels purposefully left the guidelines flexible to allow for changes that could come from emerging technologies and advances in understanding of biomarkers and the disease process itself.

"The guidelines discuss biomarkers currently known, and mention others that may have future applications," said Creighton H. Phelps, PhD, of the NIA Alzheimer's Disease Centers Program. "With researchers worldwide striving to develop, validate and standardize the application of biomarkers at every stage of Alzheimer disease, we devised a framework flexible enough to incorporate new findings."

References

Clifford R. Jack Jr., et al. "Introduction to Revised Criteria for the Diagnosis of Alzheimer's Disease: National Institute on Aging and the Alzheimer's Association Workgroups."

Guy M. McKhann and David S. Knopman, et al. "The Diagnosis of Dementia due to Alzheimer's Disease: Recommendations from the National Institute on Aging and the Alzheimer's Association Workgroup."

Marilyn S. Albert, et al. "The Diagnosis of Mild Cognitive Impairment due to Alzheimer's Disease: Recommendations from the National Institute on Aging and Alzheimer's Association Workgroup."

Reisa A. Sperling, et al. "Toward Defining the Preclinical Stages of Alzheimer's Disease: Recommendations from the National Institute on Aging and the Alzheimer's Association Workgroup."

Chapter 24

Testing for AD

Chapter Contents

Section 24.1

Mental Status Tests

"Neurocognitive Testing," © 2010 A.D.A.M., Inc.
Reprinted with permission.

Neurocognitive testing is used to find out about a person's thinking abilities, and to determine whether these problems are improving or getting worse.

How the Test Is Performed

A nurse, physician, physician assistant, or mental health worker will ask a number of questions. The test can be performed in the home, in an office, nursing home, or hospital. Occasionally, a psychologist with special training will do more extensive tests.

Most of the time, the provider will use neurocognitive tests that are also used by many other providers, which gives a score at the end. The most common test used is called the Mini-Mental state examination (MMSE) or Folstein test.

The following areas may be tested:

Appearance

The health care provider will check the person's physical appearance, including:

- age;
- dress;
- general level of comfort;
- gender;
- grooming;
- height/weight.

Orientation

The health care provider will ask questions that may include:

- the person's name, age, and job;

- the place where the person lives, type of building, city, and state, or the hospital or facility they are currently in;

- the time, date, and season.

Attention Span

Attention span may be tested earlier, because this fundamental skill can influence the rest of the tests.

The provider will want to test:

- the person's ability to complete a thought;

- the person's ability to think and problem solve;

- whether the person is easily distracted.

A person may be asked to do the following:

- Start at a certain number, and then begin to subtract backwards by sevens.

- Spell a word such as "WORLD" forward, and then backward.

- Repeat up to seven numbers forward, and up to five numbers in reverse order.

Recent and Past Memory

The provider will ask questions related to recent people, places, and events in the person's life or in the world.

Three items may be presented, and the person may then be asked to repeat them, and then recall them after 5 minutes.

The provider will ask about the person's childhood, school, or events that occurred earlier in life.

Language Function

The provider will point to everyday items in the room and ask the person to name them, and possibly to name less common items.

The person may be asked to follow a 1-step, 2-step, and 3-step instruction.

The provider may ask the person to say as many words as possible that start with a certain letter, or that are part of a certain category, in 1 minute.

The person may be asked to read or write a sentence.

Judgment

To test the person's judgment and ability to solve a problem or situation, the provider might ask questions such as:

- "If you found a driver's license on the ground, what would you do?"
- "If a police officer approached you from behind in a car with lights flashing, what would you do?"

How to Prepare for the Test

No preparation is necessary for these tests.

How the Test Will Feel

There is no physical discomfort. Some people might find it stressful to answer all of the questions. Difficulties answering could lead to frustration.

Normal Results

The most commonly used test, the Mini-Mental state examination (MMSE) or Folstein test, is scored from 0 to 30. The test is also divided up into sections, each one with its own smaller score. These results may help show which part of someone's thinking and memory may be affected.

What Abnormal Results Mean

A number of conditions or problems can affect mental status:

- Alcohol intoxication
- Certain drugs and medications
- Encephalopathy, either chronic or acute
- Head trauma or concussion
- Many psychiatric conditions
- Many neurologic conditions
- Withdrawal from narcotics and barbiturates

Risks

There are no risks with these tests.

Considerations

Some tests that screen for language problems using reading or writing do not account for people who may never have been able to read or write.

If you know that the person being tested has never been able to read or write, tell the health care provider in advance.

If your child is having any of these tests performed, it is important to help him or her understand the reasons for the tests.

Section 24.2

Positron Emission Tomography (PET) and Single Photon Emission Computed Tomography (SPECT)

Excerpted from "Nuclear Imaging (PET and SPECT)," by the National Cancer Institute (NCI, www.cancer.gov), part of the National Institutes of Health. This document is undated. Reviewed by David A. Cooke, MD, FACP, February 17, 2011.

Nuclear imaging uses low doses of radioactive substances linked to compounds used by the body's cells or compounds that attach to tumor cells. Using special detection equipment, the radioactive substances can be traced in the body to see where and when they concentrate. Two major instruments of nuclear imaging are PET and SPECT scanners.

PET Scan

The positron emission tomography (PET) scan creates computerized images of chemical changes, such as sugar metabolism, that take place in tissue. Typically, the patient is given an injection of a substance that consists of a combination of a sugar and a small amount of radioactively labeled sugar. The radioactive sugar can help in locating a tumor, because cancer cells take up or absorb sugar more avidly than other tissues in the body.

After receiving the radioactive sugar, the patient lies still for about 60 minutes while the radioactively labeled sugar circulates throughout the body. If a tumor is present, the radioactive sugar will accumulate in the tumor. The patient then lies on a table, which gradually moves through the PET scanner six to seven times during a 45–60-minute period. The PET scanner is used to detect the distribution of the sugar in the tumor and in the body. By the combined matching of a CT [computed tomography] scan with PET images, there is an improved capacity to discriminate normal from abnormal tissues. A computer translates this information into the images that are interpreted by a radiologist.

SPECT Scan

Similar to PET, single photon emission computed tomography (SPECT) uses radioactive tracers and a scanner to record data that a computer constructs into two- or three-dimensional images. A small amount of a radioactive drug is injected into a vein and a scanner is used to make detailed images of areas inside the body where the radioactive material is taken up by the cells. SPECT can give information about blood flow to tissues and chemical reactions (metabolism) in the body.

In this procedure, antibodies (proteins that recognize and stick to tumor cells) can be linked to a radioactive substance. If a tumor is present, the antibodies will stick to it. Then a SPECT scan can be done to detect the radioactive substance and reveal where the tumor is located.

Section 24.3

Magnetic Resonance Imaging (MRI)

"MRI," © 2010 A.D.A.M., Inc.
Reprinted with permission.

Magnetic resonance imaging (MRI) is a noninvasive way to take pictures of the body.

Unlike x-rays and computed tomographic (CT) scans, which use radiation, MRI uses powerful magnets and radio waves. The MRI scanner contains the magnet. The magnetic field produced by an MRI is about 10,000 times greater than the earth's.

The magnetic field forces hydrogen atoms in the body to line up in a certain way (similar to how the needle on a compass moves when you hold it near a magnet). When radio waves are sent toward the lined-up hydrogen atoms, they bounce back, and a computer records the signal. Different types of tissues send back different signals.

Single MRI images are called slices. The images can be stored on a computer or printed on film. One exam produces dozens or sometimes hundreds of images.

How the Test Is Performed

You may be asked to wear a hospital gown or clothing without metal fasteners (such as sweatpants and a t-shirt). Certain types of metal can cause inaccurate images.

You will lie on a narrow table, which slides into the middle of the MRI machine. If you fear confined spaces (have claustrophobia), tell your doctor before the exam. You may be prescribed a mild sedative, or your doctor may recommend an "open" MRI, in which the machine is not as close to the body.

Small devices, called coils, may be placed around the head, arm, or leg, or other areas to be studied. These devices help send and receive the radio waves, and improve the quality of the images.

Some exams require a special dye (contrast). The dye is usually given before the test through a vein (IV) in your hand or forearm. The dye helps the radiologist see certain areas more clearly.

During the MRI, the person who operates the machine will watch you from another room. Several sets of images are usually needed, each taking 2–15 minutes. Depending on the areas being studied and type of equipment, the exam may take 1 hour or longer.

How to Prepare for the Test

Depending on the area being studied, you may be asked not to eat or drink anything for 4–6 hours before the scan. Other preparations are usually not needed.

The strong magnetic fields created during an MRI can interfere with certain implants, particularly pacemakers. Persons with cardiac pacemakers cannot have an MRI and should not enter an MRI area.

You may not be able to have an MRI if you have any of the following metallic objects in your body:

- Brain aneurysm clips

- Certain artificial heart valves

- Inner ear (cochlear) implants

- Recently placed artificial joints

- Some older types of vascular stents

Tell your health care provider if you have one of these devices when scheduling the test, so the exact type of metal can be determined.

Before an MRI, sheet metal workers or any person that may have been exposed to small metal fragments should receive a skull x-ray to check for metal in the eyes.

Because the MRI contains a magnet, metal-containing objects such as pens, pocketknives, and eyeglasses may fly across the room. This can be dangerous, so they are not allowed into the scanner area.

Other metallic objects are also not allowed into the room:

- Items such as jewelry, watches, credit cards, and hearing aids can be damaged.

- Pins, hairpins, metal zippers, and similar metallic items can distort the images.

- Removable dental work should be taken out just before the scan.

How the Test Will Feel

An MRI exam causes no pain. Some people may become anxious inside the scanner. If you have difficulty lying still or are very anxious, you may be given a mild sedative. Excessive movement can blur MRI images and cause errors.

The table may be hard or cold, but you can request a blanket or pillow. The machine produces loud thumping and humming noises when turned on. You can wear ear plugs to help reduce the noise.

An intercom in the room allows you to speak to the person operating the scanner at any time. Some MRIs have televisions and special headphones that you can use to help the time pass.

There is no recovery time, unless you need sedation. After an MRI scan, you can resume your normal diet, activity, and medications.

Why the Test Is Performed

Combining MRIs with other imaging methods can often help the doctor make a more definitive diagnosis.

MRI images taken after a special dye (contrast) is delivered into the body may provide additional information about the blood vessels.

MRA, or magnetic resonance angiogram, is a form of magnetic resonance imaging, that creates three-dimensional pictures of blood vessels. It is often used when traditional angiography cannot be done.

Normal Values

Results are considered normal if the organs and structures being examined are normal in appearance.

What Abnormal Results Mean

Results depend on the part of the body being examined and the nature of the problem. Different types of tissues send back different MRI signals. For example, healthy tissue sends back a slightly different signal than cancerous tissue. Consult your health care provider with any questions and concerns.

Risks

MRI contains no ionizing radiation. To date, there have been no documented significant side effects of the magnetic fields and radio waves used on the human body.

The most common type of contrast (dye) used is gadolinium. It is very safe. Allergic reactions to the substance rarely occur. The person operating the machine will monitor your heart rate and breathing as needed.

MRI is usually not recommended for acute trauma situations, because traction and life-support equipment cannot safely enter the scanner area and the exam can take quite a bit of time.

People have been harmed in MRI machines when they did not remove metal objects from their clothes or when metal objects were left in the room by others.

Section 24.4

ApoE Genotyping

How is it used?

In cardiovascular disease (CVD): The test for ApoE is not widely used and its clinical usefulness is still being researched. When it is ordered, it may be used in combination with other lipid tests that evaluate risk for CVD, such as cholesterol levels and lipoprotein electrophoresis. It may sometimes be used to check for and help diagnose a genetic component to a lipid abnormality.

Testing for ApoE may sometimes be ordered to help guide lipid treatment. In cases of high cholesterol and triglyceride levels, statins are usually considered the treatment of choice to decrease the risk of developing CVD. However, there is a wide variability in the response to these lipid-lowering drugs that is in part influenced by the ApoE genotype. Though appropriately responsive to a low-fat diet, people with ApoE e4 may be less likely than those with ApoE e2 to respond to statins by decreasing their levels of LDL-C and may require adjustments to their treatment plans. At present, the clinical utility of this type of information is yet to be totally understood. Dietary adjustment and statin drugs are the preferred agents for lipid-lowering therapy. ApoE genotyping may be used to provide supplemental information.

ApoE testing may also be ordered occasionally to help diagnose type III hyperlipoproteinemia in a person with symptoms that suggest the disorder and to evaluate the potential for the condition in other family members.

In Alzheimer's disease: ApoE genotyping is also sometimes used as an adjunct test to help in the diagnosis of probable late onset Alzheimer's disease (AD) in symptomatic adults. It is called susceptibility or risk factor testing because it indicates whether there is an increased risk of AD but is not specifically diagnostic of AD. If a patient has dementia, the presence of ApoE4 may increase the likelihood that the dementia is due to AD, but does not prove that it is. There are no clear-cut tests to diagnose Alzheimer's disease during life. Physicians can, however, make a reasonably accurate clinical diagnosis of AD by ruling out other potential causes of dementia and checking for a genetic predisposition to AD with ApoE genotyping as supplemental information in conjunction with Tau/Alpha-tau 42 testing.

When is it ordered?

- ApoE genotyping is sometimes ordered when a patient has significantly elevated cholesterol and triglyceride levels that do not respond to dietary and exercise lifestyle changes.

- When family members have ApoE e2/e2 and a doctor wants to see if the person might be at a higher risk for early heart disease

- When someone has yellowish skin lesions called xanthomas and the doctor suspects Type III hyperlipoproteinemia

ApoE genotyping is also sometimes ordered as an adjunct test when patients have symptoms of progressive dementia, such as decreasing intellectual ability and language and speech skills, memory loss, and personality and behavioral changes that are starting to interfere with daily living. After non-AD causes, such as overmedication, vascular dementia (caused by strokes), and thyroid disease, have been ruled out, ApoE genotyping may help determine the probability that dementia is due to Alzheimer's disease.

What does the test result mean?

People with ApoE e2/e2 alleles are at a higher risk of premature vascular disease, but they may never develop disease. Likewise, they may have the disease and not have e2/e2 alleles because it is only one of the factors involved. ApoE genotyping adds additional information and, if symptoms are present, e2/e2 can help confirm type III hyperlipoproteinemia.

Those who have ApoE e4/e4 are more likely to have atherosclerosis. People who have symptoms of late onset Alzheimer's disease (AD) **and** have one or more ApoE e4 copies of the e4 gene are more likely to have AD. However, it is not diagnostic of AD and should **not** be used to screen asymptomatic people or their family members. Many of those who have e4 alleles will never develop AD. Even in symptomatic people, only about 60% of those with late onset AD will have ApoE e4 alleles.

ApoE e3 has "normal" lipid metabolism, thus may not have any genotype impact.

Is there anything else I should know?

Although ApoE genotyping is being used clinically by Alzheimer's experts, the most it can provide at this time is additional information about a patient with dementia. A definite diagnosis of Alzheimer's disease can only be made by examining a patient's brain tissue after their death. ApoE genotyping is not available in every laboratory. If your doctor recommends this test, your specimen will need to be sent to a reference lab, and results may take longer to return than they would from a local laboratory.

Alterations in lipid concentrations do not lead directly to vascular disease or atherosclerosis. Other factors, such as obesity, diabetes, and hypothyroidism, also play a role in whether a person actually develops disease.

Section 24.5

Biomarker Testing for AD: Checking for Tau Protein and Amyloid Beta 42 in Cerebrospinal Fluid

From "Scientists Report Important Step in Biomarker Testing for Alzheimer's Disease," by the National Institute on Aging (NIA, www.nia.nih.gov), part of the National Institutes of Health, March 17, 2009.

Scientists have made a significant step forward in developing a test to help diagnose the early stages of Alzheimer disease sooner and more accurately by measuring two biomarkers—tau and beta-amyloid proteins—in cerebrospinal fluid. Researchers from the Alzheimer's Disease Neuroimaging Initiative (ADNI) not only confirmed that certain changes in biomarker levels in cerebrospinal fluid may signal the onset of mild Alzheimer disease, but also established a method and standard of testing for these biomarkers. ADNI is a research partnership supported primarily by the National Institute on Aging (NIA), part of the National Institutes of Health, with private sector support through the Foundation for NIH, seeking to find neuroimaging and biomarker tests that can detect Alzheimer disease progression and measure the effectiveness of potential therapies.

These are the first cerebrospinal fluid biomarker findings to be reported by ADNI, a $60-million, 5-year research program launched in 2004 to observe and track changes in some 800 older people in the United States and Canada with normal cognition, mild cognitive impairment (MCI)—a condition that often precedes Alzheimer disease—or the early stages of Alzheimer disease. The ADNI Biomarker Core at the University of Pennsylvania's School of Medicine in Philadelphia, headed by Leslie M. Shaw, PhD, and John Q. Trojanowski, MD, PhD, led the study, which was reported online March 17 [2009] in the *Annals of Neurology*.

"Research indicates that Alzheimer's pathology causes changes in the brain some 10 to 20 years before any symptoms appear," said NIA Director Richard J. Hodes, MD. "This work gives researchers a systematic and reliable method to measure changes in cerebrospinal

271

fluid biomarkers that may herald the onset of Alzheimer's disease. More research is needed to validate these findings, but this study takes us one step closer to providing researchers and clinicians with tools to detect and understand the very early signs of the disease."

The researchers collected cerebrospinal fluid from 410 ADNI volunteers at 56 different sites, tested the samples for the tau and beta-amyloid protein biomarkers associated with Alzheimer disease pathology, and then retested the volunteers a year later to track changes in cognition. The scientists also compared the ADNI cerebrospinal fluid samples to those collected from an independent group of 56 people who were later confirmed in autopsy to have had Alzheimer disease and from 52 older people with normal cognition.

This comprehensive analysis allowed the scientists to systematically confirm earlier studies on cerebrospinal fluid findings and to develop biomarker profiles that may signal the onset of the disease.

Their findings include the following:

- Levels of beta-amyloid protein, in particular beta-amyloid 1-42, were lower among ADNI volunteers with MCI compared to those with normal cognition, and lower still among those diagnosed with mild Alzheimer disease. Decreased levels of this biomarker in the cerebrospinal fluid may indicate that this least soluble form of amyloid is forming sticky plaques between neurons, a hallmark of Alzheimer disease.

- Levels of beta-amyloid 1-42 proved to be the most sensitive biomarker, with an overall test accuracy rate of 87 percent in detecting Alzheimer disease pathology in the ADNI volunteers and in people with autopsy-confirmed Alzheimer disease.

- Levels of tau were higher among ADNI volunteers with MCI than among people with normal cognition, and even higher among the volunteers diagnosed with mild Alzheimer disease. Tau, a protein released by damaged and dying brain cells, can form tangles within cells and may prevent neurons from communicating with each other.

In addition to cerebrospinal fluid biomarker levels, the researchers factored in a known genetic risk factor for Alzheimer disease—the gene APOE-e4—into their analysis. The gene occurs in about 40 percent of all people who develop Alzheimer disease at age 65 or later, but how it increases risk is not yet known. ADNI volunteers with APOE-e4 genes, high levels of tau, and low levels of amyloid were most likely to have mild Alzheimer disease.

The scientists noted that all 37 ADNI volunteers diagnosed with MCI at the start of the study were documented as having probable Alzheimer disease a year later. That conversion could be predicted by their cerebrospinal fluid biomarkers, since their baseline profiles were similar to ADNI volunteers already diagnosed with the disease. Conversely, three ADNI volunteers with MCI at the start of the study, but whose cerebrospinal fluid biomarker levels were similar to volunteers free of the disease, reverted back to normal cognition by the end of the study.

"This effort may open the door to the discovery of an entire panel of cerebrospinal fluid biomarkers that will not only predict those at risk of developing Alzheimer disease, but also reveal how the disease is responding to therapies," said Neil Buckholtz, PhD, of the NIA Division of Neuroscience. "Like all ADNI results, these findings have been posted to a publicly accessible database available to qualified researchers worldwide."

Chapter 25

Overview of AD Interventions

How is AD treated?

Alzheimer disease (AD) is a complex disease, and no single "magic bullet" is likely to prevent or cure it. That's why current treatments focus on several different issues, including helping people maintain mental function, managing behavioral symptoms, and slowing AD.

AD research has developed to a point where scientists can look beyond treating symptoms to think about delaying or preventing AD by addressing the underlying disease process. Scientists are looking at many possible interventions, such as treatments for heart disease and type 2 diabetes, immunization therapy, cognitive training, changes in diet, and physical activity.

What drugs are currently available to treat AD?

No treatment has been proven to stop AD. The U.S. Food and Drug Administration has approved four drugs to treat AD. For people with mild or moderate AD, donepezil (Aricept®), rivastigmine (Exelon®), or galantamine (Razadyne®) may help maintain cognitive abilities and help control certain behavioral symptoms for a few months to a few years. Donepezil can be used for severe AD, too. Another drug, memantine (Namenda®), is used to treat moderate to severe AD. However,

---

Excerpted from "Treatment," by the National Institute on Aging (NIA, www .nia.nih.gov), part of the National Institutes of Health, December 8, 2010.

these drugs don't stop or reverse AD and appear to help patients only for months to a few years.

These drugs work by regulating neurotransmitters, the chemicals that transmit messages between neurons. They may help maintain thinking, memory, and speaking skills and may help with certain behavioral problems.

Other medicines may ease the behavioral symptoms of AD—sleeplessness, agitation, wandering, anxiety, anger, and depression. Treating these symptoms often makes patients more comfortable and makes their care easier for caregivers.

No published study directly compares the four approved AD drugs. Because they work in a similar way, it is not expected that switching from one of these drugs to another will produce significantly different results. However, an AD patient may respond better to one drug than another.

What potential new treatments are being researched?

NIA, part of the National Institutes of Health, is the lead federal agency for AD research. NIA-supported scientists are testing a number of drugs and other interventions to see if they prevent AD, slow the disease, or help reduce symptoms.

Beta-amyloid: Scientists are very interested in the toxic effects of beta-amyloid—a part of amyloid precursor protein found in deposits (plaques) in the brains of people with AD. Studies have moved forward to the point that researchers are carrying out preliminary tests in humans of potential therapies aimed at removing beta-amyloid, halting its formation, or breaking down early forms before they can become harmful. For example, in a clinical trial sponsored by NIA, scientists are testing whether "passive" immunization with an FDA-approved drug called IGIV [immune globulin (intravenous)] can successfully treat people with Alzheimer disease.

The aging process: Some age-related changes may make AD damage in the brain worse. Researchers think that inflammation may play a role in AD. Studies have suggested that common nonsteroidal anti-inflammatory drugs (NSAIDs) might help slow the progression of AD, but clinical trials so far have not shown a benefit from these drugs. Researchers are continuing to look at how other NSAIDs might affect the development or progression of AD.

Scientists are also looking at free radicals, which are oxygen or nitrogen molecules that combine easily with other molecules. The production of free radicals can damage nerve cells. The discovery that beta-amyloid generates free radicals in some AD plaques is a potentially significant finding in the quest to understand AD better.

Heart disease and diabetes: Research has begun to tease out relationships between AD and vascular diseases, which affect the body's blood vessels. Some scientists have found that some chronic conditions that affect the vascular system, such as heart disease and diabetes, have been tied to declines in cognitive function or increased AD risk. Several clinical trials are studying whether treatments for these diseases can improve memory and thinking skills in people with AD or mild cognitive impairment.

Lifestyle factors: A number of studies suggest that factors such as a healthy diet, exercise, and social engagement may be related to the risk of cognitive decline and AD. For example, emerging evidence suggests that physical activity might be good for our brains as well as our hearts and waistlines. Some studies in older people have shown that higher levels of physical activity or exercise are associated with a reduced risk of AD. Clinical trials are underway to study the relationship of exercise to healthy brain aging and the development of AD.

Scientists have also studied whether diet may help preserve cognitive function or reduce AD risk. Some studies have found that a "Mediterranean diet" was associated with a reduced risk of AD. To confirm the results, scientists are conducting clinical trials to examine the relationship between specific dietary components and cognitive function and AD.

Studies are looking into many other possible treatments, including hormones and cognitive training, to see if they might improve thinking skills in people with AD or even prevent AD in people who are at risk.

Chapter 26

AD Medications

Several prescription drugs are currently approved by the U.S. Food and Drug Administration (FDA) to treat people who have been diagnosed with Alzheimer disease. Treating the symptoms of Alzheimer disease can provide patients with comfort, dignity, and independence for a longer period of time and can encourage and assist their caregivers as well.

It is important to understand that none of these medications stops the disease itself.

Dosage and Side Effects

Doctors usually start patients at low drug doses and gradually increase the dosage based on how well a patient tolerates the drug. There is some evidence that certain patients may benefit from higher doses of the cholinesterase inhibitors. However, the higher the dose, the more likely are side effects. The recommended effective dosages of drugs prescribed to treat the symptoms of Alzheimer disease and the drugs' possible side effects are summarized below. However, the list provided does not include all information important for patient use and should not be used as a substitute for professional medical advice. Consult the prescribing doctor and read the package insert before using these or any other medications or supplements. Drugs are listed in order of FDA approval, starting with the most recent.

Excerpted from "Alzheimer's Disease Medications Fact Sheet," from the National Institute on Aging (NIA, www.nia.nih.gov), part of the National Institutes of Health, July 2010.

Patients should be monitored when a drug is started. Report any unusual symptoms to the prescribing doctor right away. It is important to follow the doctor's instructions when taking any medication, including vitamins and herbal supplements. Also, let the doctor know before adding or changing any medications.

Namenda® (memantine)

- **Drug Type and Use:** N-methyl D-aspartate (NMDA) antagonist prescribed to treat symptoms of moderate to severe Alzheimer disease

- **Manufacturer's Recommended Dosage:** *Tablet:* Initial dose of 5 mg once a day; may increase dose to 10 mg/day (5 mg twice a day), 15 mg/day (5 mg and 10 mg as separate doses), and 20 mg/day (10 mg twice a day) at minimum 1-week intervals if well tolerated; *Oral solution:* Same dosage as tablet; *Extended-release tablet:* Initial dose of 7 mg once a day; may increase dose to 14 mg/day, 21 mg/day, and 28 mg/day at minimum 1-week intervals if well tolerated.

- **How It Works:** Blocks the toxic effects associated with excess glutamate and regulates glutamate activation

- **Common Side Effects:** Dizziness, headache, constipation, confusion

Razadyne® (galantamine)

- **Drug Type and Use:** Cholinesterase inhibitor prescribed to treat symptoms of mild to moderate Alzheimer disease

- **Manufacturer's Recommended Dosage:** *Tablet (available as a generic):* Initial dose of 8 mg/day (4 mg twice a day); may increase dose to 16 mg/day (8 mg twice a day) and 24 mg/day (12 mg twice a day) at minimum 4-week intervals if well tolerated; *Oral solution (available as a generic):* Same dosage as tablet; *Extended-release capsule (available as a generic):* Same dosage as tablet but taken once a day

- **How It Works:** Prevents the breakdown of acetylcholine and stimulates nicotinic receptors to release more acetylcholine in the brain

- **Common Side Effects:** Nausea, vomiting, diarrhea, weight loss, loss of appetite

Exelon® (rivastigmine)

- **Drug Type and Use:** Cholinesterase inhibitor prescribed to treat symptoms of mild to moderate Alzheimer disease

- **Manufacturer's Recommended Dosage:** *Capsule (available as a generic):* Initial dose of 3 mg/day (1.5 mg twice a day); may increase dose to 6 mg/day (3 mg twice a day), 9 mg (4.5 mg twice a day), and 12 mg/day (6 mg twice a day) at minimum 2-week intervals if well tolerated; *Patch:* Initial dose of 4.6 mg once a day; may increase to 9.5 mg once a day after minimum of 4 weeks if well tolerated; *Oral solution:* Same dosage as capsule.

- **How It Works:** Prevents the breakdown of acetylcholine and butyrylcholine (a brain chemical similar to acetylcholine) in the brain

- **Common Side Effects:** Nausea, vomiting, diarrhea, weight loss, loss of appetite, muscle weakness

Aricept® (donepezil)

- **Drug Type and Use:** Cholinesterase inhibitor prescribed to treat symptoms of mild to moderate, and moderate to severe Alzheimer disease

- **Manufacturer's Recommended Dosage:** *Tablet (available as a generic):* Initial dose of 5 mg once a day; may increase dose to 10 mg/day after 4–6 weeks if well tolerated, then to 23 mg/day after at least 3 months; *Orally disintegrating tablet (available as a generic):* Same dosage as tablet; 23 mg dose available as brand-name tablet only.

- **How It Works:** Prevents the breakdown of acetylcholine in the brain

- **Common Side Effects:** Nausea, vomiting, diarrhea

Treatment for Mild to Moderate Alzheimer Disease

Medications called cholinesterase inhibitors are prescribed for mild to moderate Alzheimer disease. These drugs may help delay or prevent symptoms from becoming worse for a limited time and may help control some behavioral symptoms. The medications include: Razadyne® (galantamine), Exelon® (rivastigmine), and Aricept® (donepezil). Another drug, Cognex® (tacrine), was the first approved cholinesterase inhibitor but is rarely prescribed today due to safety concerns.

Scientists do not yet fully understand how cholinesterase inhibitors work to treat Alzheimer disease, but research indicates that they prevent the breakdown of acetylcholine, a brain chemical believed to be important for memory and thinking. As Alzheimer disease progresses, the brain produces less and less acetylcholine; therefore, cholinesterase inhibitors may eventually lose their effect.

No published study directly compares these drugs. Because they work in a similar way, switching from one of these drugs to another probably will not produce significantly different results. However, an Alzheimer disease patient may respond better to one drug than another.

Treatment for Moderate to Severe Alzheimer Disease

A medication known as Namenda® (memantine), an N-methyl D-aspartate (NMDA) antagonist, is prescribed to treat moderate to severe Alzheimer disease. This drug's main effect is to delay progression of some of the symptoms of moderate to severe Alzheimer disease. It may allow patients to maintain certain daily functions a little longer than they would without the medication. For example, Namenda® may help a patient in the later stages of the disease maintain his or her ability to use the bathroom independently for several more months, a benefit for both patients and caregivers. Namenda® is believed to work by regulating glutamate, an important brain chemical. When produced in excessive amounts, glutamate may lead to brain cell death. Because NMDA antagonists work very differently from cholinesterase inhibitors, the two types of drugs can be prescribed in combination.

The FDA has also approved Aricept® for the treatment of moderate to severe Alzheimer disease.

Chapter 27

Medications for Cognitive Changes

Although current medications cannot cure Alzheimer's or stop it from progressing, they may help lessen symptoms, such as memory loss and confusion, for a limited time. See Table 27.1 for a summary of available medications.

Types of Drugs

The U.S. Food and Drug Administration (FDA) has approved two types of medications—cholinesterase inhibitors (Aricept, Exelon, Razadyne, Cognex) and memantine (Namenda)—to treat the cognitive symptoms (memory loss, confusion, and problems with thinking and reasoning) of Alzheimer's disease.

As Alzheimer's progresses, brain cells die and connections among cells are lost, causing cognitive symptoms to worsen. While current medications cannot stop the damage Alzheimer's causes to brain cells, they may help lessen or stabilize symptoms for a limited time by affecting certain chemicals involved in carrying messages among the brain's nerve cells. Doctors sometimes prescribe both types of medications together. Some doctors also prescribe high doses of vitamin E for cognitive changes of Alzheimer's disease.

Medication Safety

Before beginning a new medication, make sure your physician and pharmacist are aware of all medications currently being taken (including over-the-counter and alternative preparations). This is important to make certain medications will not interact with one another, causing side effects.

Table 27.1. Treatments-at-a-Glance

Generic	Brand	Approved For	Side Effects
donepezil	Aricept	All stages	Nausea, vomiting, loss of appetite, and increased frequency of bowel movements.
galantamine	Razadyne	Mild to moderate	Nausea, vomiting, loss of appetite, and increased frequency of bowel movements.
memantine	Namenda	Moderate to severe	Headache, constipation, confusion, and dizziness.
rivastigmine	Exelon	Mild to moderate	Nausea, vomiting, loss of appetite, and increased frequency of bowel movements.
tacrine	Cognex	Mild to moderate	Possible liver damage, nausea, and vomiting.
vitamin E	Not applicable	Not approved	Can interact with medications prescribed to lower cholesterol or prevent blood clots; may slightly increase risk of death.

Medications for Early to Moderate Stages

All of the prescription medications currently approved to treat Alzheimer's symptoms in early to moderate stages are from a class of drugs called cholinesterase inhibitors. Cholinesterase inhibitors are prescribed to treat symptoms related to memory, thinking, language, judgment, and other thought processes.

Cholinesterase inhibitors:

- prevent the breakdown of acetylcholine (a-SEA-til-KOH-lean), a chemical messenger important for learning and memory. This supports communication among nerve cells by keeping acetylcholine levels high.

- delay worsening of symptoms for 6 to 12 months, on average, for about half the people who take them.

- are generally well tolerated. If side effects occur, they commonly include nausea, vomiting, loss of appetite, and increased frequency of bowel movements.

Three cholinesterase inhibitors are commonly prescribed:

- Donepezil (Aricept) is approved to treat all stages of Alzheimer's.

- Rivastigmine (Exelon) is approved to treat mild to moderate Alzheimer's.

- Galantamine (Razadyne) is approved to treat mild to moderate Alzheimer's.

Tacrine (Cognex) was the first cholinesterase inhibitor approved. Doctors rarely prescribe it today because it's associated with more serious side effects than the other three drugs in this class.

Medication for Moderate to Severe Stages

A second type of medication, memantine (Namenda) is approved by the FDA for treatment of moderate to severe Alzheimer's.

Memantine is prescribed to improve memory, attention, reason, language, and the ability to perform simple tasks. It can be used alone or with other Alzheimer's disease treatments. There is some evidence that individuals with moderate to severe Alzheimer's who are taking a cholinesterase inhibitor might benefit by also taking memantine. Donepezil (Aricept) is the only cholinesterase inhibitor approved to treat all stages of Alzheimer's disease, including moderate to severe.

Memantine:

- regulates the activity of glutamate, a different messenger chemical involved in learning and memory.

- delays worsening of symptoms for some people temporarily. Many experts consider its benefits similar to those of cholinesterase inhibitors.

- can cause side effects, including headache, constipation, confusion, and dizziness.

Vitamin E

Doctors sometimes prescribe vitamin E to treat cognitive Alzheimer's symptoms. No one should take vitamin E to treat Alzheimer's disease except under the supervision of a physician.

Vitamin E is an antioxidant, a substance that may protect brain cells and other body tissues from certain kinds of chemical wear and tear. Its use in Alzheimer's disease is based chiefly on a 1997 study showing that high doses delayed loss of ability to carry out daily activities and placement in residential care for several months. That study was conducted by the Alzheimer's Disease Cooperative Study (ADCS), the clinical research consortium of the National Institute on Aging (NIA). Since the ADCS study was carried out, scientists have found evidence in other studies that high-dose vitamin E may slightly increase the risk of death, especially for those with coronary artery disease.

No one should take vitamin E to treat Alzheimer's disease except under the supervision of a physician. Vitamin E—especially at the high doses used in the ADCS study—can negatively interact with other medications, including those prescribed to keep blood from clotting or to lower cholesterol.

Tomorrow's Treatments

Ultimately, the path to effective new treatments is through clinical trials. Right now, at least 50,000 volunteers are urgently needed to participate in more than 100 actively enrolling clinical trials about Alzheimer's and related dementias. Trials are recruiting people with Alzheimer's and mild cognitive impairment (MCI), as well as healthy volunteers to be controls.

Find out more about participating in a clinical study through the Alzheimer's Association TrialMatch service [http://www.alz.org/research/clinical_trials/find_clinical_trials_trialmatch.asp], a free tool for people with Alzheimer's, caregivers, families, and physicians to locate clinical trials based on personal criteria (diagnosis, stage of disease) and location.

Chapter 28

Participating in AD Clinical Trials and Studies

When Margaret was diagnosed with early-stage Alzheimer disease at age 68, she wanted to do everything possible to combat the disease. She talked with her doctor about experimental treatments and clinical trials she had heard about in the news and worked with the doctor to find a trial that was right for her. Margaret appreciated being able to talk to experts about Alzheimer disease and felt she was doing something that might also help her children and grandchildren avoid the disease.

This is an exciting time for Alzheimer disease clinical research. Thanks to advances in our understanding of this disease and powerful new tools for "seeing" and diagnosing it in people, scientists are making great strides in identifying potential new interventions to help diagnose, slow, treat, and someday prevent the disease entirely.

But Alzheimer research can move forward only if people are willing to volunteer for clinical trials and studies. Before any drug or therapy can be used in clinical practice, it must be rigorously tested to find out whether it is safe and effective in humans. Today, at least 50,000 volunteers, both with and without Alzheimer disease, are urgently needed to participate in more than 175 actively enrolling clinical trials and studies in the United States. To reach that goal, researchers will need to screen at least half a million potential volunteers.

Excerpted from "Participating in Alzheimer's Disease Clinical Trials and Studies," by the National Institute on Aging (NIA, www.nia.nih.gov), part of the National Institutes of Health, September 2009.

This text describes Alzheimer disease clinical trials and studies, explains their scientific design, and offers key facts and questions to consider about volunteering for clinical research.

Comparing Alzheimer Disease Clinical Trials and Studies

Clinical research is medical research involving people. It includes clinical studies, which use long-term observation and analysis in large groups to determine how a disease or condition may occur and progress, and clinical trials, which test possible interventions to diagnose, prevent, treat, and someday cure a disease.

Clinical studies observe people in normal settings, with less direct intervention than in clinical trials. Researchers gather baseline information, group volunteers according to broad characteristics, and compare changes over time. Studies of Alzheimer disease may help identify new possibilities for clinical trials. The National Institute on Aging (NIA), part of the National Institutes of Health (NIH), sponsors several major ongoing studies, such as the following:

- Alzheimer's Disease Neuroimaging Initiative investigators study brain images and biomarkers in people with normal cognitive aging, mild cognitive impairment (MCI)—a disorder that may precede Alzheimer disease, and early-stage Alzheimer disease to develop better indicators of the disease and its progression. For example, they have found that certain changes in biomarkers, like proteins or enzymes in blood or cerebrospinal fluid, may signal early Alzheimer disease and have established a method and standard for testing these biomarkers.

- Alzheimer's Disease Genetics Studies researchers analyze DNA [deoxyribonucleic acid] from persons with and without the disease to identify genes that may be Alzheimer disease risk factors.

Clinical trials test interventions such as drugs or devices, as well as prevention methods and changes in diet or lifestyle. Drug testing is the focus of many clinical trials. Currently, more than 90 drugs are in clinical trials for Alzheimer disease, and more are in the pipeline awaiting Food and Drug Administration (FDA) approval to enter human testing. FDA-approved clinical trials are always preceded by laboratory analyses in test tubes and in tissue culture, followed by studies in laboratory animals to test for safety and efficacy. If these show favorable results, the FDA gives approval for the treatment or intervention to be tested in humans. Clinical trials advance through four well-defined phases to test the treatment, find appropriate dosage, and monitor side effects in increasing numbers of people. If investigators find an intervention safe and effective after undergoing the first three phases, the FDA decides whether to approve it for clinical use. In Phase IV, the FDA continues to monitor the effects of a new drug after its approval for marketing and clinical use. If problems occur, approval may be withdrawn and the drug recalled. After the efficacy of a drug for one health condition is established, Phase IV studies can evaluate the activity of the drug in other conditions.

Clinical Trials Seek Answers through Rigorous Testing

Scientists conducting Alzheimer disease research test a theory by using the classic scientific method. They first identify a valid question related to Alzheimer disease. The question is posed as a hypothesis that is either proven or disproven by the clinical trial.

For example, research has linked high blood cholesterol with Alzheimer disease. Scientists asked: Will medications that lower cholesterol also have an effect on Alzheimer disease? They formed a hypothesis: IF reducing blood cholesterol has a beneficial effect on Alzheimer disease, THEN: Statins (drugs to reduce cholesterol) will slow the progression of Alzheimer disease. To test that hypothesis, NIA has funded a number of clinical trials, which are ongoing.

Why Placebos Are Important

The "gold standard" for testing interventions in people is the randomized, placebo-controlled clinical trial, because it is designed to reduce error or bias. Volunteers are randomly assigned—that is, selected by chance—to either a test group receiving the experimental intervention or a control group receiving a placebo, an inactive substance resembling the drug tested.

Comparing results indicates whether changes in the test group result from the treatment. In many trials, no one—not even the research team—knows who gets the treatment, the placebo, or another intervention. When the participant, family members, and staff all are "blind" to the treatment, the study is called a double-blind, placebo-controlled clinical trial.

Placebo and test groups are equally important, as shown in the results of numerous clinical trials. For example, early research suggested that ginkgo biloba, an herbal supplement, might be effective in delaying dementia. To find out, NIA sponsored a 6-year, Phase III clinical trial with more than 3,000 participants age 75 and older. In 2008, scientists reported no significant differences in effect on dementia in adults who received ginkgo biloba or placebo.

This result was disappointing, but scientists gained a wealth of information to inform future research. For example, researchers learned more about subgroups of participants who may be at greater risk for developing dementia, and ginkgo's possible effects on cardiovascular disease, cancer, depression, and other age-related conditions. They also gained insights on issues related to the design and conduct of large dementia prevention trials in older adults, such as the number of participants needed to provide clinically significant measures on outcomes like occurrence of dementia.

Participating in a Trial or Study

Where to Find Alzheimer Disease Trials and Studies

Information about Alzheimer disease clinical trials and studies is available through a number of sources. First, talk to your doctor, who may know about local or specific research studies that may be right for you. NIA-supported Alzheimer's Disease Centers or specialized memory or neurological clinics in your community may also be conducting trials. You might also learn of clinical trials through newspapers or other media. To search more widely for trials or studies, you can also visit websites like ClinicalTrials.gov or the NIA Alzheimer's Disease Education and Referral (ADEAR) Center clinical trials database.

What Happens When a Person Joins a Clinical Trial?

First, it is important to learn as much as you can about the trial. Staff members at the research center are trained to explain the trial in detail and describe possible risks and benefits. They clarify participants' rights. Participants and their families can have this information repeated until they are sure they understand it.

After questions are answered, participants sign an informed consent form, which contains key facts about the trial. Next, they are screened by clinical staff to see whether they meet criteria to participate in the trial. Screening examines the characteristics people must have to participate in a particular trial, as well as characteristics that may exclude them. The screening may involve cognitive and physical tests that provide baseline information to compare with future changes. If participants meet all criteria, they are enrolled in the trial.

Informed Consent

Each participant must sign an informed consent agreement, affirming that he or she understands the trial and is willing to participate. Laws and regulations regarding informed consent differ across states and institutions, but they are all meant to ensure participant safety and protection, and to prevent unethical experimentation on vulnerable populations.

Researchers conducting clinical Alzheimer research must consider the declining memory and cognitive abilities of people with this disease or another dementia and must evaluate their ability to understand and consent to participate in research. If the person with Alzheimer disease is deemed unable to provide informed consent because of problems with memory and confusion, an authorized legal representative, or proxy (usually a family member), may be able to give permission for the person to participate, particularly if it is included in the patient's durable power of attorney. A durable power of attorney is a legal agreement designating who will handle the patient's affairs when he or she no longer can.

Inclusion and Exclusion Criteria

In the experimental protocol (written research plan), researchers define the inclusion criteria volunteers must meet to participate, such as age range, stage of dementia, racial and/or ethnic group, gender, genetic profile, and family history. The protocol also defines exclusion criteria, such as health conditions or medications that prevent volunteers from joining a trial. Many volunteers are needed for screening to find enough people for a study. Generally, volunteers can participate in only one trial or study at a time. It is important to realize that different trials have different inclusion and exclusion criteria, so being excluded from one trial does not necessarily mean exclusion from another.

What Happens during a Trial?

Usually, participants are randomly assigned to one of the trial groups. People in each group represent selected combinations of characteristics (such as age, sex, education, or cognitive ability). The test group receives the experimental drug or intervention. Other groups receive a different drug, a placebo, or another intervention.

Participants and family members follow strict instructions and keep detailed records. Every so often, they visit the research site to receive more physical and cognitive exams and talk with staff. Investigators collect

291

information on the effects of the test drug or treatment, evaluate disease progression, and see how the participant and caregiver are doing.

What Volunteers Need to Know

The following issues are some of the key concerns potential participants should consider before deciding whether joining a trial or study is right for them.

- **Expectations and motivations:** Single clinical trials and studies generally do not have miraculous results, and participants may not directly benefit.

- **Uncertainty:** Some people have problems because they are not permitted to know whether they are getting experimental treatment or a placebo, or may not know results. Can you live with these sorts of uncertainties?

- **Finding the right clinical trial or study:** Volunteers must meet the inclusion and exclusion criteria listed by researchers. Even if a participant is not eligible for one trial or study, another may be just right.

- **Time commitment and location:** Clinical trials and studies last days to years and may require multiple visits to study sites, such as private research facilities, teaching hospitals, Alzheimer disease research centers, or doctors' offices. How much time and travel are you willing and able to undertake?

- **Risk:** Researchers make every effort to ensure the safety of participants, but all clinical trials have some risk. What level of risk are you comfortable with?

Rights of Volunteers

Clinical trial volunteers have important rights, including the rights to receive clear, complete information and to withdraw from a trial anytime.

Right to Clear Information

Understanding what is involved in a clinical trial or study can relieve anxiety. Potential volunteers have the right to a thorough explanation and answers to all of their questions. Participants and family members can have information repeated and explained until they understand it.

Right to Withdraw

Volunteers can withdraw from a trial or study anytime they or their physician feels it is in their best interests. For example, a new health condition in a volunteer may require medications that are risky if combined with experimental treatments.

Questions to Ask about Clinical Trials and Studies

- What is the purpose?
- What tests and treatments will be given?
- What are the risks?
- What side effects might occur?
- What may happen with/without this research?
- Can I continue with treatments for Alzheimer disease and other conditions as prescribed by my regular doctor?
- How will you keep my doctor informed about my participation in the trial?
- Does the study compare standard and experimental treatments?
- How long will it last? How much time will it take?
- Where and when will the testing occur?
- How much flexibility will I have?
- How will it affect my activities?
- If I withdraw, will this affect my normal care?
- Will I learn the results?
- Could I receive a placebo?
- What steps ensure my confidentiality?
- Are expenses reimbursed?
- Will I be paid?

Clinical Trials and Studies Need All Kinds of People

Clinical trials and studies are a partnership between researchers and volunteer participants, who work together to answer questions about humans we can answer in no other way. Ensuring that those answers are correct requires including volunteers of all kinds—men and women, African Americans, Latinos, Native Americans, Asian Americans, whites, people with Alzheimer disease or a family history of the disease, people with conditions that may lead to Alzheimer disease, and those without the disease (controls).

An intervention may work differently in one group than in another. Without adequate representation of a particular group, questions about safety and effectiveness of a treatment in that group may remain unanswered. In addition to diversity, the number of people included in research can affect results. Changes or effects seen in smaller groups may or may not show up significantly in larger groups.

For More Information

To find out more, talk with your healthcare provider or contact NIA's ADEAR Center at 800-438-4380. Or, visit the ADEAR Center clinical trials database at www.nia.nih.gov/Alzheimers/ResearchInformation/ ClinicalTrials. You can sign up for e-mail alerts that identify new clinical trials added to the database. More information about clinical trials is available at www.ClinicalTrials.gov.

Alzheimer's Disease Education and Referral (ADEAR) Center
P.O. Box 8250
Silver Spring, MD 20907-8250
Toll-Free: 800-438-4380
Website: www.nia.nih.gov/Alzheimers

Chapter 29

Can AD Be Prevented?

Newspapers, magazines, the internet, and TV seem to be full of stories about ways to stay healthy, eat right, and keep fit. Many people are concerned about staying healthy as they get older. Along with keeping their bodies healthy, they want to keep their minds sharp. They also want to avoid brain diseases, such as Alzheimer disease (AD), that occur more often in older people than in younger people.

Currently, AD has no known cure, but the results of recent research are raising hopes that someday it might be possible to delay the onset of AD, slow its progress, or even prevent it altogether. Delaying by even 5 years the time when AD symptoms begin could greatly reduce the number of people who have this devastating disease.

Can We Prevent Complex Diseases Like AD?

Many diseases, such as diabetes, heart disease, and arthritis, are complex. They develop when genetic, environmental, and lifestyle factors interact to cause disease and/or make it worse. The importance of these factors may be different for different people.

AD is one of these complex diseases. It develops over many years and appears to be affected by a number of factors that may increase or decrease a person's chances of developing the disease. These factors

Excerpted from "Can Alzheimer's Disease Be Prevented?" by the National Institute on Aging (NIA, www.nia.nih.gov), part of the National Institutes of Health, April 2009.

include genetic makeup, environment, life history, and current life-style. We can't control some of these risk factors, but we can control others.

AD Risk Factors We Can't Control

Age

Age is the most important known risk factor for AD. The risk of developing the disease doubles every 5 years after age 65. Several studies estimate that up to half of all people older than 85 have AD. These facts are significant because of the growing number of people 65 and older. A 2005 Census report estimates that the number of Americans 65 and older will more than double to about 72 million by 2030. Even more significant, the group with the highest risk of AD—those older than 85—is the fastest growing age group in the United States.

Genetics

Genetic risk is another factor that a person can't control. Scientists have found genetic links to the two forms of AD—early-onset and late-onset.

Early-onset AD is a rare form of the disease, affecting only about 5 percent of all people who have AD. It develops in people ages 30 to 60. In the 1980s and early 1990s, researchers found that mutations (permanent abnormal changes) in certain genes cause most cases of early-onset AD. If a parent has any of these genetic mutations, his or her child has a 50-50 chance of inheriting the mutated gene and developing early-onset AD.

Late-onset AD, the much more common form of the disease, develops after age 60. In 1992, researchers found that three forms, or alleles (e), of a gene called apolipoprotein E (APOE) can influence the risk of late-onset AD:

- APOE e2, a rarely occurring form, may provide some protection against AD.

- APOE e3, the most common form, plays a neutral role, neither increasing nor decreasing risk.

- APOE e4, which occurs in about 40 percent of all people who develop late-onset AD and is present in about 25 to 30 percent of the population, increases risk by lowering the age of onset. Having this allele does not mean that a person will definitely develop AD; it only increases risk. Many people who develop AD do not have an APOE e4 allele.

Researchers think that at least half a dozen other risk-factor genes exist for late-onset AD and are intensively searching for them. In 2007, they found another likely risk-factor gene called SORL1. When this gene is active at low levels or in an abnormal form, levels of harmful beta-amyloid increase in the brain. Beta-amyloid is a component of amyloid plaques, one of the hallmarks of AD. Interestingly, the SORL1 gene also was identified as a risk-factor gene for certain aspects of cognitive decline, suggesting that cognitive decline and AD may share at least one predisposing genetic factor.

Finding AD risk-factor genes is essential for understanding the very early biological steps that lead to the vast majority of AD cases and for developing drugs and other prevention and treatment strategies. Finding these genes also will help scientists develop better ways to identify people at risk of AD and determine how the genes may interact with other genes or with lifestyle or environmental factors to affect an individual's AD risk.

The Search for AD Prevention Strategies

We can't do much about our age or genetic profile, but scientists are working hard to understand a variety of other factors that may be involved in the disease. Some scientists are examining the biological bases for AD. This research might lead to the development of drugs that could protect against or block biological processes leading to cognitive decline and AD.

Other scientists are studying health, lifestyle, and environmental factors—such as exercise and diet or the control of chronic diseases like diabetes—that may play a role in preventing or slowing AD or cognitive decline. Recent research suggests that maintaining good overall health habits may help lower our chances of developing several serious diseases, including brain diseases such as AD. This area is of particular interest because it appears that there may be things that individuals can do themselves to hold off AD.

Several of these potential factors have been identified in animal studies and in epidemiologic studies (studies that compare the lifestyles, behaviors, and characteristics of groups of people). At present, these factors are only associated with changes in AD risk. Further research, especially clinical trials, will be needed to determine cause and effect—whether these factors really do help prevent cognitive decline or AD directly.

Assessing Physical Activity

Accumulating evidence suggests that physical activity may be good for our brains as well as our hearts, waistlines, and ability to carry out activities of daily living. Epidemiologic studies have found associations between physical activity and improved cognitive skills or reduced AD risk. For example, investigators looked at the relationship of physical activity and AD risk in about 1,700 adults aged 65 years and older over a 6-year period. They found that the risk of AD was 35 to 40 percent lower in those who exercised for at least 15 minutes three or more times a week than in those who exercised fewer than three times a week.

Scientists have sought to confirm these associations in animal studies, hoping to clarify why physical activity might be related to reduced risk of cognitive decline and AD. For example, studies in older rats and mice have found that exercise increases the number of small blood vessels that supply blood to the brain and increases the number of connections between nerve cells. Other research has shown exercise to raise the level of specific brain-growth factors in an area of the brain that is particularly important to memory and learning.

Both epidemiologic and animal studies point to associations and help to explain them. However, epidemiologic studies can't tell us whether a true cause-and-effect relationship exists between a particular factor and AD risk. For example, people who exercise tend to be healthier in other ways, such as having decreased rates of heart disease or diabetes. They may also have healthier lifestyles, such as eating a nutritious diet. This means that even if people who exercise are less likely to develop AD, we don't know whether this is due to the exercise or the more healthful eating or other lifestyle differences that distinguish them from inactive people.

Likewise, animal studies can't tell us whether an intervention will definitely work in humans. That's why investigators conduct clinical trials—controlled studies involving humans. Clinical trials are the most reliable method for showing whether intervention strategies really can work to prevent or treat AD in people. This is because clinical trial participants are randomly assigned to receive or not receive a treatment (for example, exercise). Therefore, any differences between the groups should be due to the exercise program rather than other differences between the groups.

NIA supports clinical trials related to exercise and cognitive function. One completed trial used functional magnetic resonance imaging (MRI) tests to measure changes in brain activity in older adults before and after a 6-month program of brisk walking. Results showed that brain activity increased in specific brain regions as the participants' cardiovascular fitness increased. A similar study showed that brain volume increased as a result of a walking program.

These findings strongly suggest a biological basis for the role of aerobic fitness in helping to maintain the health and cognitive functioning of adults as they age, at least in the short term. Currently, a trial is underway to look at the effects of a 1-year aerobic fitness training program on cognition and brain activity and structure in older adults. Other NIA-supported research is examining whether exercise can delay the development of AD in people with mild cognitive impairment (MCI).

Exploring Dietary Factors

A number of studies suggest that how we eat may be linked to our risk of developing—or not developing—AD. This is another important area of current AD research. A nutritious diet—a diet that includes lots of fruits, vegetables, and whole grains and is low in fat and added sugar—can reduce the risk of many chronic diseases, including heart disease, type 2 diabetes, and obesity. Animal studies, epidemiologic studies, and clinical trials are looking at whether a healthy diet also can help preserve cognitive function or even reduce AD risk.

Studies have examined foods that are rich in antioxidants and anti-inflammatory components to find out whether those foods affect age-related changes in the brain. One study found that curcumin, the main ingredient of turmeric (a spice used in curry), can suppress the build-up of harmful beta-amyloid in the brains of rodents. Another study, in AD transgenic mice (those that are specially bred to have features of AD), found that DHA (docosahexaenoic acid, a type of omega-3 fatty acid found in some fish) reduced the presence of beta-amyloid and plaques. Other research has shown that older dogs perform better on learning tasks when they eat a diet rich in antioxidants and live in an enriched environment with many opportunities to play and interact with others.

In addition, studies in rats and mice have shown that dietary supplementation with blueberries, strawberries, and cranberries can improve cognitive function, both during normal aging and in animals that have been bred to develop AD. Scientists are beginning to identify some of the chemicals responsible for these berries' beneficial effects and think that the chemicals may act by neutralizing free radicals. This may reduce inflammation or stimulate neurons to protect themselves better against some of the adversities of aging and AD.

Several epidemiologic studies have shown an association between eating a diet rich in vegetables (especially green leafy vegetables and cruciferous vegetables like broccoli) and a reduced rate of cognitive decline. Researchers speculate that the beneficial effect may come from the antioxidant and folate content of the vegetables.

These results are interesting, but in their normal daily lives, people typically consume many different foods and nutrients. With this in mind, some investigators have conducted epidemiologic studies to examine a group's entire dietary pattern. One of these studies showed a reduced risk of AD in those who ate the Mediterranean diet—a diet that includes many fruits, vegetables, and beans; moderate amounts of fish; low-to-moderate amounts of dairy foods; small amounts of meat and poultry; regular but moderate amounts of wine; and olive oil.

These kinds of findings are exciting and suggestive, but they are not definitive. To confirm them, NIA is supporting several clinical trials to examine the relationship between specific dietary components and cognitive decline and AD.

Investigating Chronic Diseases

For some years now, scientists have been finding clues that damage to the vascular system (the body's vast system of large and small blood vessels) may contribute to the development of AD or affect its severity. Several common chronic diseases that affect older people, including heart disease, stroke, and type 2 diabetes, also affect the body's vascular system and have been tied to declines in cognitive function or increased AD risk. In addition, heart disease, high blood pressure, and diabetes to a large extent can be modified by diet, exercise, and other lifestyle changes. Therefore, scientists are keenly interested in learning whether reducing the risks of or controlling these conditions through lifestyle changes also may reduce the risks of cognitive decline or AD.

Much of the evidence so far about possible relationships between vascular diseases and cognitive decline or AD risk comes from epidemiologic studies. To clarify and build on these findings, scientists have conducted a variety of studies, including test tube, animal, and additional epidemiologic studies. NIA is supporting several clinical trials, including a trial to test the effect of lowering blood pressure and blood cholesterol levels on cognition in people with diabetes. Several other trials are examining whether intensive diabetes treatment can reduce cognitive decline. Researchers are also looking at increased stiffness of blood vessels with age as another potential treatment target.

Examining Social Engagement and Intellectually Stimulating Activities

Observations of nursing home residents and older people living in the community have suggested a link between social engagement and cognitive abilities. Having many friends and acquaintances and participating in many social activities also is associated with reduced cognitive decline and decreased risk of dementia in older adults. For example, the NIA-funded Chicago Health and Aging Project showed that more social networks and a higher level of social engagement were associated with a higher level of cognitive function at the beginning of the study. These factors also were related to a reduced rate of cognitive decline over time.

Studies have also shown that keeping the brain active is associated with reduced AD risk. In the Religious Orders Study, for example, investigators periodically asked more than 700 participants—older nuns, priests, and religious brothers—to describe the amount of time they spent in seven information-processing activities. These activities included listening to the radio, reading newspapers, playing puzzle games, and going to museums. After following the participants for 4 years, the investigators found that the risk of developing AD was 47 percent lower, on average, for those who did the activities most often than for those who did them least frequently.

Other studies have shown similar results. In addition, a growing body of research suggests that, even in the presence of AD plaques, the more formal education a person has, the better his or her memory and learning abilities.

Another NIA-funded study supports the value of lifelong learning and mentally stimulating activity. It showed that during early and middle adulthood, cognitively healthy older people had engaged in more mentally stimulating activities and spent more hours doing them than did those who ultimately developed AD. Other studies have shown that people who are bilingual or multilingual seem to develop AD at a later age than do people who only speak one language.

The reasons for this apparent link between social engagement or intellectual stimulation and AD risk aren't entirely clear, but scientists suggest four possibilities:

- Such activities may protect the brain in some way, perhaps by establishing cognitive reserve. (Cognitive reserve is the brain's ability to operate effectively even when some function is disrupted or the amount of damage that the brain can sustain before changes in cognition are evident.)

- These activities may help the brain become more adaptable and flexible in some areas of mental function so that it can compensate for declines in other areas.

- People who engage in these activities may have other lifestyle factors that protect them against developing AD.

- Less engagement with other people or in intellectually stimulating activities could be the result of very early effects of the disease rather than its cause.

The only way to really evaluate some of these possibilities is to test them in a controlled way in clinical trials. Several clinical trials have examined whether memory training and similar types of mental skills training can actually improve the cognitive abilities of healthy older adults and people with mild AD. In the Advanced Cognitive Training for Independent and Vital Elderly (ACTIVE) trial, for example, certified trainers provided 10 sessions of memory training, reasoning training, or processing-speed training to healthy adults 65 years old and older. The sessions improved participants' mental skills in the area in which they were trained. Even better, these improvements persisted for up to 5 years after the training was completed.

Other Clues to AD Prevention

NIA's program of AD research continues to add to what we know about AD and yield clues about possible ways to prevent the disease. The following sections briefly describe a few other areas that scientists are exploring.

Nonsteroidal Anti-Inflammatory Drugs (NSAIDs)

Inflammation in the brain is a common feature of AD, but it is unclear whether this is a cause or an effect of the disease. Some epidemiologic studies suggest an association between a reduced risk of AD and commonly used nonsteroidal anti-inflammatory drugs (NSAIDs), such as ibuprofen, naproxen, and indomethacin. So far, clinical trials have not demonstrated a benefit for AD from these drugs or from the newer cyclooxygenase-2 (COX-2) inhibitors, such as rofecoxib and celecoxib. However, scientists continue to look for ways to test how other anti-inflammatory drugs might affect the development or progression of AD.

Antioxidants

Damage during aging from highly active molecules called free radicals can build up in nerve cells and result in a loss of cell function, which could contribute to AD. Some population and laboratory studies suggest that antioxidants from dietary supplements or food may provide some protection against this damage (called oxidative damage), but other studies show no effect.

Clinical trials may provide some answers. Several current trials are investigating whether antioxidants, such as vitamins E and C, alpha-lipoic acid, and coenzyme Q, can slow cognitive decline and development of AD.

NIA-sponsored sub-studies to ongoing trials have looked at whether two treatments provide any protection against cognitive decline in women. One sub-study tested low-dose aspirin and antioxidant supplementation in healthy women, and the other tested antioxidant and folate supplements in women who already had heart disease. Initial results indicate that aspirin may provide some benefits for maintaining executive function but has no impact on other cognitive domains. For vitamin E, there was no overall benefit. Analysis of these studies is ongoing.

Another study added to a prostate cancer prevention trial is examining whether taking vitamin E and/or selenium supplements over a period of 7 to 12 years can help prevent memory loss and dementia. Although the primary trial was stopped because the supplements were shown not to prevent prostate cancer, researchers are continuing to follow participants to analyze longer term effects of the supplements.

The Memory Impairment Study compared the use of donepezil (Aricept®), vitamin E supplements, or placebo (an inactive substance) in participants with mild cognitive impairment (MCI) to see whether the drugs might delay or prevent progression to AD. People with MCI have more memory problems than normal for people their age, but their symptoms are not as severe as those with AD. More people with MCI, compared with those without MCI, go on to develop AD. The study found that taking vitamin E had no effect on progression to AD. It may be that this antioxidant did not help after memory declines had already started. Donepezil seemed to delay progression to AD during the first year of treatment; however, by the end of the 3-year study there was no benefit from the drug. The U.S. Food and Drug Administration (FDA) has not approved donepezil for treatment of MCI.

Estrogen

The hormone estrogen is produced by a woman's ovaries during her childbearing years, and its production declines dramatically after menopause. Over the past 25 years, some laboratory and animal research, as well as observational studies in women, have suggested that estrogen may protect the brain. Experts have wondered whether taking estrogen supplements could reduce the risk of AD or slow disease progression.

A number of clinical trials have shown that estrogen does not slow the progression of already-diagnosed AD and is not effective in treating or preventing AD if treatment is begun in later life. For example, a large trial found that women older than 65 who took estrogen (Premarin®) alone or estrogen with a synthetic progestin (Prempro®) were actually at increased risk of developing dementia, including AD. However, some questions, such as whether other forms of estrogen or starting treatment nearer menopause might be more effective, remain unanswered. These questions are now being investigated in clinical trials.

Researchers also are probing estrogen's possible beneficial effects on the brain. For example, scientists have developed estrogen-like molecules called SERMs (selective estrogen-receptor modulators) that protect against bone loss and other consequences of estrogen loss after menopause. These molecules may retain estrogen's neuron-protecting ability but may not have some of its other harmful effects on the body, such as increasing the risk of uterine cancer. One large clinical trial showed that raloxifene, a SERM used to prevent and treat osteoporosis and to reduce the incidence of breast cancer in women at high risk for the disease, lowered the risk of MCI in a group of postmenopausal women with osteoporosis. Another clinical trial is testing whether raloxifene can slow the rate of AD progression.

Immunization

Could a vaccine someday prevent AD? Early vaccine studies in mice were so successful in reducing deposits of beta-amyloid and improving brain performance on memory tests that investigators conducted preliminary clinical trials in humans with AD. These studies had to be stopped because life-threatening brain inflammation occurred in some participants. However, scientists are continuing to refine this strategy in animal models of AD, hoping to find ways of maintaining the vaccine's beneficial effects while reducing the unwanted side effects. Several pharmaceutical companies have obtained permission from the FDA to test several of these new vaccine strategies for safety in early-stage clinical trials.

So, What Can You Do?

Our knowledge about AD is growing rapidly as scientists expand their understanding of the many factors involved in this devastating disease. Although no treatments or drugs have yet been proven to prevent or delay AD, people can take some actions that are beneficial for healthy aging and that also might reduce the effect of possible risk factors for AD. For example, you can do the following:

- Exercise regularly.

- Eat a healthy diet that is rich in fruits and vegetables.

- Engage in social and intellectually stimulating activities.

- Control type 2 diabetes.

- Lower high blood pressure levels.

- Lower high blood cholesterol levels.

- Maintain a healthy weight.

These actions lower the risk of other diseases and help maintain and improve overall health and well-being. However, it is important to remember that they will not necessarily prevent or delay AD in any one person. Even if these actions were eventually proven effective, they might not offset a person's individual genetic and other risk factors enough to prevent the development of AD.

Whether you have memory problems or not, you can take one more important action—volunteer to participate in research. Participating in clinical trials is an effective way to help in the fight against AD. People who participate in these studies say that the biggest benefit is having regular contact with experts on AD who have lots of practical experience and a broad perspective on the disease. They also feel they are making a valuable contribution to future knowledge that will help scientists, people with AD, and their families.

Chapter 30

Recent AD Research

Chapter Contents

307

Section 30.1

Amyloid Deposits May Predict Risk for AD

From "Amyloid Deposits in Cognitively Normal People May Predict Risk
for Alzheimer's Disease," by the National Institute on Aging (NIA, www
.nia.nih.gov), part of the National Institutes of Health, December 14, 2009.

For people free of dementia, abnormal deposits of a protein associated
with Alzheimer disease are associated with increased risk of developing
the symptoms of the progressive brain disorder, according to two studies from researchers at Washington University in St. Louis. The studies,
primarily funded by the National Institute on Aging (NIA), part of the National Institutes of Health, linked higher amounts of the protein deposits
in dementia-free people with greater risk for developing the disease, and
with loss of brain volume and subtle declines in cognitive abilities.

The two studies are reported in the Dec. 14, 2009, online issue of
Archives of Neurology. The scientists used brain scans and other tests
to explore the relationship between levels of beta-amyloid, a sticky
protein that forms the hallmark plaques of Alzheimer disease, and
dementia risk in cognitively normal people. John C. Morris, MD, who
directs the NIA-supported Alzheimer's Disease Research Center at
Washington University in St. Louis, and his team conducted the research. Martha Storandt, PhD, also of Washington University in St.
Louis, directed one of the studies.

"Previous studies of brain pathology, cognitive testing, and brain
imaging have for some time suggested that Alzheimer pathology causes
changes to the brain many years before memory loss, confusion, and
other symptoms of the disease are apparent. But it remains difficult
to accurately predict whether a cognitively normal person will—or will
not—develop the disease," said NIA Director Richard J. Hodes, MD.
"These new studies suggest that beta-amyloid measured in the brains
of cognitively normal individuals may be a preclinical sign of disease."

Morris' team used a variety of measures to look for changes in the
brain in the two studies, including positron emission tomography (PET)
imaging using a radioactive form of Pittsburgh Compound B (PiB), an
agent specially developed to detect levels of beta-amyloid protein in
the living brain; magnetic resonance imaging (MRI) to measure brain

volume; and standardized clinical tests of memory and thinking abilities to determine cognitive health. Previously, the link between beta-amyloid load and Alzheimer disease could only be confirmed at autopsy.

The studies indicated that beta-amyloid might be present in the brain even in symptom-free people:

- Between 2004 and 2008, researchers used PiB scans to track 159 volunteers ages 51 to 88, who started the study with no signs of cognitive impairment, to see if there was a correlation between beta-amyloid levels and cognitive health. Over time, 23 participants developed mild impairments, and nine were eventually diagnosed with clinical Alzheimer disease. Compared with participants who remained cognitively normal, the nine who were eventually diagnosed clinically with Alzheimer's disease had high levels of PiB binding in the brain and experienced cognitive decline as well as volume loss in the parahippocampal gyrus, a part of the brain that controls memory. However, not every person who had beta-amyloid deposition in the brain developed cognitive impairment. Beta-amyloid deposition may be a risk factor for developing Alzheimer disease but its presence does not constitute a diagnostic finding.

- In 135 cognitively normal older adults aged 65 to 88, the level of beta-amyloid as measured by PiB binding correlated with atrophy, or shrinkage, in many parts of the brain and to declines on memory and thinking tests over many years.

"More study is needed in larger groups for longer periods, but these studies confirm the value of detecting and measuring amyloid load in the brains of living people as soon as possible," said Morris.

"These imaging tools are an important part of ongoing effort to create a profile of Alzheimer's in its earliest stages, even before symptoms appear, by linking imaging results with other biomarkers and clinical evaluations."

References

Morris JC, Roe CM, Grant EA, Head D, Storandt M, Goate AM, Fagan AM, Holtzman DM, Mintun MA. Pittsburgh Compound B imaging and prediction of progression from cognitive normality to symptomatic Alzheimer's disease. *Archives of Neurology,* Dec. 14, 2009.

Storandt M, Mintun MA, Head D, Morris JC. Cognitive decline and brain volume loss are signatures of cerebral amyloid beta deposition identified with PiB. *Archives of Neurology,* Dec. 14, 2009.

Section 30.2

Ovary Removal May Increase Risk of Dementia

From "Ovary Removal Linked to Cognitive Problems, Dementia" by the National Cancer Institute (NCI, www.cancer.gov), part of the National Institutes of Health. Adapted from the *NCI Cancer Bulletin,* vol. 4/no. 25, September 11, 2007.

Women who had one or both ovaries removed before menopause for noncancer reasons faced an increased risk of developing cognitive problems or dementia later in life, according to a study. But women who underwent estrogen replacement therapy until at least age 50 after having their ovaries removed were not at increased risk.

The study supports the hypothesis that there may be a "critical age window for the protective effects of estrogen on the brain," the researchers write in the September 11, 2007, issue of *Neurology.*

The study included nearly 3,000 women, who were followed for more than 25 years. Dr. Walter Rocca of the Mayo Clinic and his colleagues studied 813 women who had one ovary removed, 676 women who had both ovaries removed, and a comparison group of women who did not have their ovaries removed when the study began. About half the women had their ovaries removed because of a benign condition, such as cysts or inflammation; the others had their ovaries removed prophylactically to prevent ovarian cancer. Women who had the procedure for ovarian cancer or another estrogen-related cancer (usually breast cancer) were excluded because of their high risk of death shortly after surgery.

The researchers suggest three possible mechanisms to explain the association they observed. First, ovary removal may cause an estrogen deficiency that initiates biological changes leading to the elevated risk. Second, the association may involve a deficit of progesterone or testosterone rather than estrogen secreted by the ovaries. Third, the association may be caused by susceptibility genes that independently increase both the risk of ovary removal and cognitive impairment or dementia.

The study's strengths include the long follow-up and the fact that the women were representative of the general population. Its limitations include the use of telephone interviews to assess cognitive abilities and an overall interview participation rate of 62 percent. In addition, the surgeries were done between 1950 and 1987, when surgical practices and estrogen use may have differed from today.

Nevertheless, the findings should lead to a reassessment of prophylactic removal of the ovaries in premenopausal women and of the use of estrogen treatment following ovary removal, the researchers say. "The results of this study are important for the majority of women who do not have an increased risk of ovarian cancer," says Dr. Rocca. "Women should consult with their physicians when considering the risks and benefits of prophylactic removal of the ovaries, and when considering treatment afterwards."

Section 30.3

Changes Occur in High-Risk Seniors before AD Symptoms Appear

Reprinted by permission of the Society of Nuclear Medicine from "Alzheimer's Disease and Molecular Imaging," http://www.snm.org/docs/PET_PROS/Alzheimers.pdf. *PET PROS: PET Professional Resources and Outreach Source,* SNM PET Center of Excellence, June 2009. © Society of Nuclear Medicine (www.snm.org).

About Alzheimer's Disease

Alzheimer's disease is the most common form of dementia—a general term that describes memory loss or other mental impairments serious enough to interfere with daily life. More than 5 million people are currently living with Alzheimer's—and experts predict this number could triple by 2050. Alzheimer's usually sets in after age 60 and involves a progression of symptoms, beginning with impairments in learning and memory and later extending to every aspect of thinking, judgment, and behavior. New developments in molecular imaging technologies are contributing to our understanding of Alzheimer's disease and improving the ways in which Alzheimer's disease (AD) is diagnosed. Early detection of AD through molecular imaging techniques will assist the development and evaluation of medications to slow the progression of the disease and optimize patient care.

What are molecular imaging procedures, and how can they help Alzheimer's patients?

Molecular imaging (MI) procedures are highly effective, safe, and painless diagnostic imaging and treatment tools that present physicians with a detailed view of what's going on inside an individual's body at the cellular level. Most nuclear medicine procedures are molecular imaging procedures using radioactive substances.

The most commonly used molecular imaging procedure for diagnosing or guiding treatment of Alzheimer's disease is positron emission tomography (PET) scanning. Conventionally, the confirmation of Alzheimer's is a long process of elimination that may take 2 to 3 years of diagnostic and cognitive testing. However, MI technologies are now available that help physicians safely and painlessly identify abnormalities in the brain that indicate the presence of Alzheimer's disease. [For more information on PET/ CT scanning, please read SNM's fact sheet "PET/CT Scans: Get the Facts" on SNM's website at http://interactive .snm.org/index.cfm?PageID=7988.]

What MI technologies currently are available for Alzheimer's patients?

The MI technology most commonly used in diagnosing and guiding treatment of Alzheimer's patients is PET scanning. [See also "PET/CT scanning: Get The Facts."]

PET Scanning

How can PET scanning help Alzheimer's patients?

Specifically, PET scanning is a powerful tool for:

- diagnosing Alzheimer's earlier;

- differentiating Alzheimer's disease from other types of dementia; and

- monitoring the progression of the disease and the effectiveness of new therapies in clinical trials.

312

How does PET scanning work?

PET scanning is a molecular imaging procedure that allows physicians to obtain three-dimensional images of what is happening in a patient's body at the molecular and cellular level. For a PET scan, a patient is injected with a very small amount of a radiotracer such as fluorodeoxyglucose (FDG), which contains a sugar with a radioactive tag attached. The radiotracer is absorbed by the brain and will show the amount of sugar consumption in different regions of the brain. The brains of people with dementia consume less energy and therefore less sugar, and in patterns specific to the different types of dementia. In addition, radiotracers for amyloid plaques have been developed recently that show the presence and extent of plaques in the brain. This allows for early detection of Alzheimer's disease. Though still in clinical trial, new PET tracers for amyloid plaque are expected to be available for patient care within a few years. After the radiotracer is injected, the patient lies down on a table, and his or her head is moved to the center of a PET or PET/CT scanner. The PET scanner is composed of an array of detectors that receive signals emitted by the radiotracer. Using these signals, the PET scanner detects the amount of metabolic activity while a computer reassembles the signals into images. [For more information on PET/CT scans and how they work, visit "PET/CT Scanning: Get the Facts."]

How accurate are PET scans in detecting Alzheimer's disease?

Studies indicate that PET is very accurate at diagnosing Alzheimer's disease and differentiating it from other types of dementia. In one recent study that included seven centers in the United States and Europe, investigators at the New York University (NYU) School of Medicine used optimized FDG-PET analysis techniques to measure glucose metabolism in different regions of the brain.[1] More than 90 percent of the time, researchers were successfully able to distinguish patients with Alzheimer's disease from healthy subjects and patients with other dementias such as frontotemporal dementia—an umbrella term for a diverse group of rare disorders that primarily affect the frontal and temporal lobes of the brain—the areas generally associated with personality and behavior.

How can PET scanning help in the long-term management of Alzheimer's disease?

PET scanning can help physicians gain a clear understanding of the existence, progression, and aggressiveness of the disease. Researchers are experimenting with several new treatments for Alzheimer's disease. Molecular imaging tools such as PET can help determine whether treatments are working as intended. Molecular imaging may also help researchers learn more about the causes of Alzheimer's and how the disease progresses.

How long does it take to get PET scan results?

A trained radiologist or nuclear medicine physician will interpret the results and write a report for the physician who ordered the tests. A verbal report is available the day of the PET scan, and the written report is usually delivered to the physician within 2 or 3 days.

Will insurance reimburse for PET scans?

Insurance companies will cover the cost of most FDG PET scans. Because of the mounting evidence of the effectiveness of FDG PET/CT [computed tomography] scanning for the diagnosis and treatment of a wide range of cancers, coverage levels continue to expand. Coverage for PET scans that measure brain amyloid plaques is not yet available. For the most updated figures, check with your insurance carrier or physician, as the levels at which Medicare reimburses for PET are under review with CMS [Centers for Medicaid and Medicare Services] and subject to change.

Does PET show promise for identifying those at risk for developing Alzheimer's disease?

Postmortem studies suggest that the amyloid plaques of Alzheimer's are present for as long as a decade before dementia sets in. The results of several clinical trials indicate that PET imaging of amyloid plaques can identify patients destined to develop Alzheimer's disease several years before the development of dementia. For example, researchers at the University of Pittsburgh conducted a study of PET scanning with a radiotracer for amyloid plaques known as Pittsburgh Compound-B (PiB) in patients who had mild cognitive impairment, a condition that often—but not always—precedes Alzheimer's disease. Using PET with PiB, the researchers tracked patients with mild cognitive impairment for 4 years and found that only patients with brain plaques developed Alzheimer's. Other tracers are also being tested for this purpose.

Where can I get more information about Alzheimer's disease and molecular imaging?

To learn more about Alzheimer's disease, visit www.snm.org/facts. To learn more about PET/CT scanning or other nuclear medicine procedures, visit the SNM Molecular Imaging Center of Excellence (www.molecularimagingcenter.org).

Endnotes

1. *Journal of Nuclear Medicine,* "Multicenter Standardized 18F-FDG PET Diagnosis of Mild Cognitive Impairment, Alzheimer's Disease, and Other Dementias," Vol. 49, No. 3, 390–398, http://jnm.snmjournals.org/cgi/content/abstract/49/3/390.

Section 30.4

Family with AD May Carry Clues to Treatment

From "Family with Alzheimer's Disease May Carry Clues to Treatment," by the National Institute of Neurological Disorders and Stroke (NINDS, www.ninds.nih.gov), part of the National Institutes of Health, June 17, 2009.

In the brains of people with Alzheimer disease (AD), a toxic protein fragment called beta-amyloid accumulates in clumps that leave a path of damaged brain tissue. Although age is the most powerful risk factor for AD, a small fraction of people develop the disease because of genetic mutations that trigger beta-amyloid accumulation. In a 2009 study published in *Science,* researchers described a family with a mutation that causes beta-amyloid accumulation and AD in some individuals, but could protect against the disease in others.

This mutant beta-amyloid could serve as a template for small, artificial proteins designed to inhibit beta-amyloid accumulation and stave off AD in the roughly 400,000 people diagnosed with it each year.

The study was led by Fabrizio Tagliavini, MD, of the Istituto Nazionale Neurologico Carlo Besta in Milan, Italy; Mario Salmona, PhD, of the Istituto di Ricerche Farmacologiche Mario Negri in Milan; and

Efrat Levy, PhD, of New York University School of Medicine in Orangeburg, New York. It was funded in part by the National Institute of Neurological Disorders and Stroke (NINDS).

The study began when an Italian man with early-onset dementia visited Dr. Tagliavini's clinic in Milan. The man had begun to develop memory problems at age 36, and became completely dependent on caregivers by age 44. The man's younger sister also reported mild memory problems consistent with the first stages of AD. This unusually early, rapid course of the disease hinted at a genetic origin, the researchers say. Most people with AD have a sporadic form of the disease that is caused by a combination of genetic and environmental factors, and emerges sometime after age 60.

The researchers tested the patients' DNA for mutations in the few genes that have been linked to early-onset AD, including three genes called APP, presenilin-1 and presenilin-2. In both patients, the APP gene turned out to harbor a mutation, A673V, whose effects are unlike any other AD-linked mutation known.

Until now, all of the known genetic forms of AD were autosomal dominant, meaning that a mutation in just one copy of the APP gene or the presenilins is sufficient to cause the disease. (With the exception of genes on the Y chromosome, people normally have two copies of every gene.) In this study, the new APP mutation followed an autosomal recessive pattern. Each of the patients had the A673V mutation in both copies of the APP gene while several of their relatives, including an 88-year-old aunt, had the mutation in just one copy of the gene and remained disease free.

The APP gene encodes the amyloid precursor protein, which is the source of the beta-amyloid fragment. Even in the healthy brain, this protein is sliced apart by enzymes to produce the beta-amyloid fragment, but in the brains of people with AD, beta-amyloid changes its shape to form large amyloid deposits in the brain. The researchers found that the A673V mutation resides within the small piece of APP that becomes beta-amyloid, and that it has unusual effects on the formation of beta-amyloid clumps.

When the researchers made a synthetic version of the mutant beta-amyloid and let it incubate in a test tube, they found that it formed clumps—or aggregates—faster than normal beta-amyloid, the kind that accumulates in the brains of individuals with sporadic AD. However, when the mutant beta-amyloid was combined with normal beta-amyloid, the mixture formed aggregates more slowly than normal beta-amyloid did by itself. Finally, when the researchers exposed a neuronal cell line to the mutant beta-amyloid, normal beta-amyloid or a mixture, the mutant protein alone was most toxic to the cells and the mixture was least toxic.

Those findings show that when the mutant beta-amyloid encounters normal amyloid, it interferes with the formation of aggregates. The findings raise the surprising possibility that while having two copies of the A673V mutation is clearly detrimental, having just one copy of it might protect against AD, perhaps even the sporadic version of the disease. The researchers plan to test whether the A673V mutation can protect against AD in mice carrying the autosomal dominant mutations that are known to trigger the disease.

The researchers say it might be possible to design small, therapeutic proteins that mimic the effects of beta-amyloid containing the A673V mutation. The location of A673V within beta-amyloid might also have therapeutic implications, they say. It sits within the N-terminus, a region at one end of beta-amyloid that most experts did not consider important for the formation of aggregates. The study suggests that the beta-amyloid N-terminus could make an effective target not only for synthetic proteins, but for other kinds of drugs as well.

Di Fede G et al. "A Recessive Mutation in the APP Gene with Dominant-Negative Effect on Amyloidogenesis." *Science,* March 13, 2009, Vol. 323, pp. 1473–1477.

Section 30.5

Insulin May Improve Memory in People with AD

"Insulin is a Possible New Treatment for Alzheimer's,"
February 2, 2009, Northwestern University NewsCenter.
© 2009 Northwestern University. Reprinted with permission.

A Northwestern University-led research team reports that insulin, by shielding memory-forming synapses from harm, may slow or prevent the damage and memory loss caused by toxic proteins in Alzheimer's disease.

The findings, which provide additional new evidence that Alzheimer's could be due to a novel third form of diabetes, will be published online the week of Feb. 2 [2009] by the Proceedings of the National Academy of Sciences (PNAS).

In a study of neurons taken from the hippocampus, one of the brain's crucial memory centers, the scientists treated cells with insulin and the insulin-sensitizing drug rosiglitazone, which has been used to treat type 2 diabetes. (Isolated hippocampal cells are used by scientists to study memory chemistry; the cells are susceptible to damage caused by ADDLs, toxic proteins that build up in persons with Alzheimer's disease.)

The researchers discovered that damage to neurons exposed to ADDLs was blocked by insulin, which kept ADDLs from attaching to the cells. They also found that protection by low levels of insulin was enhanced by rosiglitazone.

ADDLs (short for "amyloid beta-derived diffusible ligands") were discovered at Northwestern and are known to attack memory-forming synapses. After ADDL binding, synapses lose their capacity to respond to incoming information, resulting in memory loss.

The protective mechanism of insulin works through a series of steps by ultimately reducing the actual number of ADDL binding sites, which in turn results in a marked reduction of ADDL attachment to synapses, the researchers report.

"Therapeutics designed to increase insulin sensitivity in the brain could provide new avenues for treating Alzheimer's disease," said senior author William L. Klein, a professor of neurobiology and physiology in the Weinberg College of Arts and Sciences and a researcher in North-western's Cognitive Neurology and Alzheimer's Disease Center. "Sensitivity to insulin can decline with aging, which presents a novel risk factor for Alzheimer's disease. Our results demonstrate that bolstering insulin signaling can protect neurons from harm."

The amyloid beta oligomers, or ADDLs, form when snippets of a protein clump together in the brain. In Alzheimer's disease, when ADDLs bind to nearby neurons, they cause damage from free radicals and a loss of neuronal structures crucial to brain function, including insulin receptors. This damage ultimately results in memory loss and other Alzheimer's disease symptoms. The Alzheimer's drug Namenda has been shown to partially protect neurons against the effects of ADDLs.

"The discovery that anti-diabetic drugs shield synapses against ADDLs offers new hope for fighting memory loss in Alzheimer's disease," said lead author Fernanda G. De Felice, a former visiting scientist in Klein's lab and an associate professor at the Federal University of Rio de Janeiro, Brazil.

"Recognizing that Alzheimer's disease is a type of brain diabetes points the way to novel discoveries that may finally result in disease-modifying treatments for this devastating disease," adds Sergio T. Ferreira, another member of the research team and a professor of biochemistry in Rio de Janeiro.

In other recent and related work, Klein, De Felice, and their colleagues showed that ADDLs bound to synapses remove insulin receptors from nerve cells, rendering those neurons insulin resistant.

The outcome of the molecular-level battle between ADDLs and insulin, which in the current *PNAS* study was found to remove ADDL receptors, may determine whether a person develops Alzheimer's disease.

In addition to Klein, De Felice, and Ferreira, other authors of the *PNAS* paper, titled "Protection of Synapses Against Alzheimer's-linked Toxins: Insulin Signaling Prevents the Pathogenic Binding of Alpha Beta Oligomers," are Wei-Qin Zhao, a former visiting scientist at Northwestern, now with Merck & Co., Inc.; Pauline T. Velasco, Mary P. Lambert, and Kirsten L. Viola, from Northwestern; and Marcelo N. N. Vieira, Theresa R. Bomfim, and Helena Decker, from the Federal University of Rio de Janeiro, Brazil.

This work was supported by the Alzheimer's Association, the American Health Assistance Foundation, the National Institute on Aging, the Howard Hughes Medical Institute, the Conselho Nacional de Desenvolvimento Cientifico e Tecnologico (Brazil), Fundacao de Amparo à Pesquisa do Estado do Rio de Janeiro (Brazil), and the Human Frontier Science Program.

Part Five

Living with AD
and Dementias

Chapter 31

Talking about Your Diagnosis

Chapter Contents

Section 31.1

Telling Others about an AD Diagnosis

When you learn that someone you care about has Alzheimer's, you may hesitate to tell the person that he or she has the disease. You may also have a hard time deciding whether to tell family and friends. Once you are emotionally ready to discuss the diagnosis, how will you break the news? Here are some suggestions for talking about the disease with others.

Respect the Person's Right to Know

- You may want to protect the person by withholding information. But your loved one is an adult with the right to know the truth. It can be a relief to hear the diagnosis, especially if the person had suspected he or she had Alzheimer's disease.

- In many cases, people who are diagnosed early are able to participate in important decisions about their healthcare and legal and financial planning.

- While there is no current cure for Alzheimer's, life will not stop with the diagnosis. There are treatments and services that can make life better for everyone.

Plan How to Tell the Person

- Talk with doctors, social workers, and others who work with people who have Alzheimer's to plan an approach for discussing the diagnosis.

- Consider a "family conference" to tell the person about the diagnosis. He or she may not remember the discussion, but may remember that people cared enough to come together. You may need to have more than one meeting to cover the details.

- Shape the discussion to fit the person's emotional state, medical condition, and ability to remember and make decisions.

- Pick the best time to talk about the diagnosis. People with Alzheimer's may be more receptive to new information at different times of the day.

- Don't provide too much information at once. Listen carefully to the person. They often signal the amount of information they can deal with through their questions and reactions. Later, you can explain the symptoms of Alzheimer's and talk about planning for the future and getting support.

Help the Person Accept the Diagnosis

- The person may not understand the meaning of the diagnosis or may deny it. Accept such reactions and avoid further explanations.

- If they respond well, try providing additional information.

- The person with Alzheimer's may forget the initial discussion but not the emotion involved. If telling them upsets them, hearing additional details may trigger the same reaction later.

- Reassure your loved one. Express your commitment to help and give support. Let the person know that you will do all you can to keep your lives fulfilling.

- Be open to the person's need to talk about the diagnosis and his or her emotions.

- Look for nonverbal signs of sadness, anger, or anxiety. Respond with love and reassurance.

- Encourage the person to join a support group for individuals with memory loss. Your local Alzheimer's Association can help you locate a group. To find an Association near you, please call 800-272-3900 or go to www.alz.org.

Telling Family and Friends

An Alzheimer diagnosis doesn't only affect the person receiving it. The lives of family members and friends may also drastically change.

- Be honest with family and friends about the person's diagnosis. Explain that Alzheimer's is a brain disease, not a psychological or emotional disorder.

- Share educational materials from the Alzheimer's Association. The more that people learn about the disease, the more comfortable they may feel around the person.

- Invite family to support groups sponsored by your local Alzheimer's Association.

- Realize that some people may drift out of your life, as they may feel uncomfortable around the person or may not want to help provide care.

- Alzheimer's disease can also impact children and teens. Just as with any family member, be honest about the person's diagnosis with the young people in your life. Encourage them to ask questions.

Section 31.2

Talking to Children about AD

"Helping Children Understand Alzheimer Disease," © 2007 Alzheimer Society of Canada (www.alzheimer.ca). Reprinted with permission.

You may have someone in your family who has Alzheimer's disease. Alzheimer's disease affects the person's brain. When people have this disease, they forget, they get confused, they have trouble speaking and taking care of themselves.

Scientists don't know why people get Alzheimer's disease, but they are working hard to find a cause so they can stop it from happening.

You can't get Alzheimer's disease from another person, like the cold or the flu. Just because someone in your family has the disease, it doesn't mean you will get it.

Alzheimer's disease is not a normal part of growing old. Most people who have the disease are over 65 but sometimes (not very often) people in their 40s and 50s get it too. As people get older, their chances of developing the disease increase.

People with Alzheimer's disease may forget your name, see or hear things that are not there, get lost, have trouble sleeping, or say the same things over and over. This can cause them to become frustrated or nervous and they may get angry with you for no reason. It is important to know that they do not mean to treat you badly. It is not your fault if the person gets upset. Alzheimer's disease makes the person act in this way.

Taking care of someone with Alzheimer's disease is a hard job. If your mom, dad or grandparent is taking care of someone with the disease, they are probably very busy.

You may find that they do not have as much time to spend with you or when they do, they are too tired to do anything. You may feel sad or angry about this. It is important to remember that they still love you. Talk to your family, a teacher, or a trusted adult about your feelings.

People with Alzheimer's disease need to know you care. When you hold their hand or give them a hug, they will always feel your love.

You may have questions about what is happening to the person with Alzheimer's disease. You can learn more about the disease and how to help the person.

Here Is a List of Things You Can Do

Remember Past Events

People with Alzheimer's disease like to remember things from long ago. You can help them remember by sitting with them and looking at old pictures or photo albums.

Make a Memory Box

You probably have many special memories about spending time with the person who has Alzheimer's disease. Fill a box with five special things that will help you to remember those times. Examples could be: fishing hook, a gold coin, a letter or card, a piece of jewelry (pin or brooch), a watch, a medal, a baseball, a theatre ticket stub.

Help around the House

People with Alzheimer's disease like to keep busy. You can help them make their bed, fold their laundry, help make lunch, go for walks or rake leaves in the yard.

To Learn More

Contact your local Alzheimer Society.

Book List

Here are a few suggestions to get you started. Check your public library, school library, or book stores for more resources.

- *The Memory Box* (Mary Bahr, 1992, Ages 6–11, ISBN 0807550531): Zach could hardly wait to spend his 3-week vacation with gram and gramps at the lake, fishing and listening to gramps tell his stories. But when gramps wants to start a memory box and forgets his way around the forest path, Zach begins to worry. Together the three fill the memory box with pictures, souvenirs, written memories—old and new—and prepare themselves for the changes in gramps and the summers ahead.

- *What's Happening to Grandpa?* (Maria Shriver, 2004, Ages 4–8, ISBN 0-316-00101-5): Grandpa has always been the best storyteller Kate has ever known, but lately, he seems different. He repeats himself, becomes easily frustrated, and then one day, he even forgets Kate's name. When her mother explains Grandpa's disease, Kate is overwhelmed. But with remarkable strength, Kate resolves to cherish her grandpa's life and memories.

- *If I Forget, You Remember* (Carol Lynch Williams, 1999, Ages 9–12, ISBN 0440414202): Elyse has just graduated from grade 6 and is looking forward to a busy summer. Then Elyse finds out that her grandmother is moving in for the summer. She has Alzheimer's disease and Elyse has to care for her while her mother works. Elyse thinks her grandmother will get better if Elyse is patient. But Elyse finds out it is not that easy and she learns to watch over her grandmother who was always there for her.

- *Mr. Knowsit™ Learns About Alzheimer's Disease* (Doug Stowe, 2000, Ages 4–6, Foresight Consultants, (905-268-5639): Why was Timothy's grandpa acting as if he didn't know him? Was it a practical joke? With some coaxing, a little affection and care, Mr. Knowsit helps Timothy learn the truth about his grandpa and something called "Alzheimer's disease." A candid and creative format to help children, and their families, understand this disease.

Chapter 32

Getting Support for AD and Dementia

The Basics of Alzheimer's Support Groups

Nearly every professional involved with Alzheimer's or other forms of dementia recommends support groups for caregivers and loved ones of people with the disease, simply because it can be so challenging— emotionally, mentally, and physically. As the disease progresses and alters a person you know, you're bound to experience a range of reactions and face ever-changing problems.

Being with other people in similar situations can be a source of practical help as you learn about new ideas and resources. But most of all, it's helpful to talk to or listen to others wrestling with similar problems and the complicated feelings they bring.

What are support groups?

Support groups come in different shapes and sizes:

- They may meet weekly, biweekly, monthly, or bimonthly.

- Some have fixed start and end dates, just like a series of classes.

- Others meet on a regular basis for anyone who drops in.

- Most are free.

"Alzheimer's Disease Support Groups," © 2010 Caring, Inc. (www.caring.com). Reprinted with permission.

- The individual meetings typically last about 2 hours each, and many are scheduled during evenings or weekends, to fit around working hours.

- Groups vary in size, usually being open to between six and 20 people per session. Ideally, they're small enough for everyone to contribute and feel comfortable with one another.

Who attends?

It depends on the group. Some are specifically organized to help a particular subgroup of caregivers—adult children, for example, or male caregivers. Some are set up for those whose family member is in a certain stage of the disease. Groups for early-stage Alzheimer's groups are increasingly available. Some gatherings have a faith-based or spiritual component.

Who leads support groups?

It's helpful to know about the group leader's background. Groups are generally led by medical professionals, social workers, experienced caregivers, or volunteers who've been trained to lead support groups (and who usually have had firsthand experience with the disease). If the facilitator isn't a professional, ideally she should be sponsored, supported, or trained by a trustworthy organization such as the Alzheimer's Association or the Alzheimer's Disease Research Center.

Facilitators should be able to wear several hats: They may lead discussions by introducing specific topics, may balance group members' opinions and advice with other perspectives, may teach or share useful information, and may offer reassurance and encouragement.

Typical Alzheimer's Support Group Meetings

What happens at meetings?

Groups vary in their purpose, organization, and "feel." Some support groups are formal, with guest lecturers scheduled to talk about common topics of interest to caregivers, like managing problematic behaviors or financial planning. Others are informal, inviting members to share stories about their experiences and give one another moral support. Many groups use a combination of these approaches, alternating candid conversations among members with lectures from special guests.

Despite the differences among support groups, they have one thing in common: All have the potential to become an essential component of a caregiver's well-being and success. By blending psychological support and practical knowledge, an Alzheimer's support group is a resource that can't be replicated just by reading up on the disease or by leaning on friends or a partner for moral support.

Support groups offer caregivers and family members the opportunity to ask questions, share stories, give and receive comfort and advice, and learn more about Alzheimer's disease (including its different stages, caregiving strategies, relevant legal advice, housing and other care options, local care contacts and resources, and more).

For many caregivers, a support group is a place to exhale. You may hesitate to confide certain information or experiences with family or friends who also know the person with Alzheimer's. You may fear that you'll be judged or criticized, or worry that what's said can affect family dynamics. It's often easier for any of us to talk with strangers who aren't involved in our particular situations.

And because the other group members have "been there," they may be more likely to listen compassionately to your expressions of guilt, frustration, or anxiety, or to stories about mistakes you feel you've made or challenging situations you've faced. A confidential, positive setting for sharing your experiences—and releasing your emotions—is known to be a tremendously important factor in how well one copes with caregiver stress.

Where can I find a group?

Groups are sponsored and organized by local Alzheimer's Association chapters, hospitals, churches, or other social-service or community organizations. Ask any of these institutions or the patient's doctor if they can suggest programs to investigate. These days they're easier to find than ever, as the disease affects ever-larger numbers and continues to lose its stigma and mystery.

Good sources of information on support groups, in addition to your local Alzheimer's Association chapter, include your local Area Agency on Aging, other social-service agencies, local hospitals, the patient's physician(s) and other health care professionals, a geriatric care consultant/coordinator/manager, adult day centers, and other caregivers. You can also find online support at http://www.caring.com/forums/alzheimers-forum.

How do I find one right that's for me?

The trick to getting the most out of a support group is to find a good fit. Consider whether a group is convenient to your schedule and location, addresses your specific needs, and feels comfortable to you.

It's important that you feel at ease and can open up about your experiences and ask questions—if not on your very first visit, then after you've sat in on a session or two. You may need to try out a few groups before settling on the right one. Don't be discouraged if one (or several) doesn't feel right to you—investigate another.

Some people benefit from joining more than one group. In addition to an Alzheimer's support group, you may want to consider a group for caregivers of people with dementia of all forms, or a group for caregivers in general.

If your schedule is tight or you can't find an appropriate group locally, try looking online. Numerous online support groups are available through reputable websites and organizations. One example: Alzheimer's List, a group organized by the Alzheimer's Disease Research Center at Washington University in St. Louis.

Chapter 33

Preventing Cognitive Decline If You Have AD or Dementia

Dementia is a loss of cognitive abilities in multiple domains that results in impairment in normal activities of daily living and loss of independence. Alzheimer disease (AD) is the most common cause of dementia, responsible for 60 to 80 percent of all dementia. AD causes severe suffering for patients, including progressive functional impairment, loss of independence, emotional distress, and behavioral symptoms. Families and caregivers often experience emotional and financial stress.

The major risk factor for AD is age, with the prevalence doubling every 5 years after the age of 65. Most estimates of the prevalence of AD in the United States are about 2.3 million for individuals over age 70, but some estimates are as high as 5.3 million individuals over the age of 65. The number of individuals with mild cognitive impairment exceeds the number with AD.

These individuals have mild impairment in cognition or daily functions that does not meet the threshold for a diagnosis of dementia, but they are at increased risk for development of AD, which makes them a prime target for intervention protocols.

Studies of selected risk or protective factors for cognitive decline and AD have been published, but it is not clear whether the results of these previous studies are of sufficient strength to warrant specific recommendations for behavioral, lifestyle, or pharmaceutical interventions/modifications targeted to these endpoints.

Excerpted from "Preventing Alzheimer's Disease and Cognitive Decline," by the Agency for Healthcare Research and Quality (AHRQ, www.ahrq.gov), April 26, 2010.

Methods

We searched MEDLINE® using Medical Subject Heading (MeSH) search terms, supplemented by keyword searches. In addition to MEDLINE®, we manually searched reference lists and searched the *Cochrane Database of Systematic Reviews* to identify relevant systematic reviews. For topics with a recent good-quality systematic review, we updated the search by identifying relevant primary literature published from 1 year prior to the search date of the review through October 27, 2009. When we did not identify a relevant good-quality review, we searched the primary literature for studies from 1984 through October 27, 2009. Because of the large volume of literature and the availability of specialized registries for genetic studies, we developed a separate search strategy for this topic and limited our review to select genes of special interest.

We restricted our review to human studies conducted in economically developed countries and published in English. We considered studies with participants greater than or equal to 50 years old, of both sexes, all racial and ethnic populations, and drawn from general populations. We limited the sample size to greater than or equal to 50 for randomized controlled trials (RCTs) and greater than or equal to 300 for observational studies. We required at least 1 year between exposure and outcomes assessment for studies of cognitive decline, and 2 years for studies of AD. For Key Questions 1 and 2, we evaluated studies using observational designs; for Key Questions 3 and 4, we evaluated RCTs. Two reviewers independently assessed study eligibility and study quality and abstracted data. For Key Questions 1 through 5, we considered factors identified by the OMAR (Office of Medical Applications of Research) planning committee in five major categories: (1) nutritional factors; (2) medical factors (including medical conditions and prescription and nonprescription medications); (3) social/economic/behavioral factors; (4) toxic and environmental factors; and (5) genetics. Data were synthesized qualitatively and, when appropriate, using quantitative methods. We rated the overall level of evidence for each factor as high, moderate, or low using principles developed by the Grading of Recommendations Assessment, Development and Evaluation (GRADE) working group. The level of evidence is considered "high" when further research is very unlikely to change our confidence in the estimate of effect, and "low" when further research is very likely to have an important impact on our confidence in the estimate of effect and is likely to change the estimate.

Results

A total of 25 systematic reviews and 250 primary studies met our inclusion criteria. The number of included studies differed markedly across the factors considered. Results are summarized immediately below by key question. We focus in this summary on the factors that showed an association with AD or cognitive decline. Among the many factors investigated, only a few have sufficient evidence to indicate a potential association with late-life cognitive outcomes.

Key Question 1—Factors Associated with Risk of Developing AD

The results reported here are based on observational studies of AD, but to fully understand the associations between factors and cognitive outcomes, it is important to consider the results from both observational studies and RCTs when the latter are available.

In the nutrition category, both higher levels of folic acid and higher adherence to a Mediterranean diet were associated with a small to moderate decrease in risk of AD. The level of evidence was low for both of these factors.

For medical conditions, diabetes (summary odds ratio [OR] 1.39; 95 percent confidence interval [CI] 1.17 to 1.66), hyperlipidemia in mid-life, depression (summary OR 1.90; 1.55 to 2.33), and traumatic brain injury in males (summary OR 2.29; 1.47 to 3.58) were all associated with increased risk of AD. The level of evidence was low for each of these factors. No other factors showed a consistent relation to AD.

In the medication category, use of statins (summary hazard ratio [HR] 0.73; 95 percent CI 0.57 to 0.94) showed an association with decreased risk of AD. The observational studies for estrogen (summary relative risk [RR] 0.50; 95 percent CI 0.30 to 0.80) and antihypertensives showed a likely protective association with AD. The level of the evidence was low for these factors.

In the social, economic, and behavioral category, current smoking (summary RR 1.79; 95 percent CI 1.43 to 2.23) was associated with increased risk of AD. Moderate use of alcohol (summary RR 0.72; 0.61 to 0.86), more years of education, and higher levels of cognitive engagement showed an association with a moderately decreased risk of AD. Participation in physical leisure activity (summary HR 0.72; 95 percent CI 0.53 to 0.98) was generally associated with decreased risk of AD. Limited data on marriage and social support suggest that never being married and having less social support are associated with a moderately increased risk of AD. The level of evidence for all of these factors was low.

For the environmental exposure category, case-control studies were included for the subtopics reviewed (solvents, pesticides, lead, and aluminum) because there were few cohort studies that met inclusion criteria. Only pesticides showed a consistent and large association with higher risk of AD, but the level of the evidence was low.

For the review of genes, we identified 10 genes with the strongest and best quality evidence of an association with AD based on a systematic review and quality ratings conducted by ALZGene, an online database of genetic association studies performed on AD phenotypes. Based on the selection criteria, it is not surprising that all genes showed a significant association with AD. It is noteworthy that the epsilon 4 allele of the apolipoprotein E gene (APOE e4) allele showed the highest and most consistent risk for AD (summary OR 3.68; 95 percent CI 3.3 to 4.1). The level of evidence was moderate for the APOE e4 allele.

Key Question 2—Factors Associated with Risk of Cognitive Decline

The results reported for this question are based on observational studies for cognitive decline. Effect sizes in all cases were small to moderate. In the nutrition category, low plasma selenium showed an association with higher risk of cognitive decline. Higher amounts of vegetable intake, adherence to a Mediterranean diet, and higher levels of omega-3 fatty acids showed a likely association with decreased risk of cognitive decline, but evidence was limited for some of these factors. The level of evidence was low for all of these factors.

For the medical category, diabetes, metabolic syndrome, and depression showed fairly consistent associations with a small increased risk of cognitive decline. There were no studies that met inclusion criteria on cognitive decline and traumatic brain injury, sleep apnea, resiliency, or anxiety.

For the medication category, two types of medication (non-steroidal anti-inflammatory drugs [NSAIDs] and estrogen) showed possibly decreased risk for cognitive decline in select subgroups, but the other medications evaluated (statins, antihypertensives, and cholinesterase inhibitors) showed no association or no consistent association with cognitive decline.

Among the social, economic, and behavioral factors, smoking showed an increased risk of cognitive decline. Participation in non-physical/ non-cognitive leisure activities, cognitive engagement, and physical activity all showed a fairly consistent protective association against cognitive decline. For observational studies, the level of evidence was low for these factors.

There were no eligible studies identified for the environmental exposure category. In the genetic category, only APOE has been assessed in relation to cognitive decline. The studies fairly consistently report that APOE e4 is associated with greater cognitive decline on selected cognitive measures that were not consistent across studies. The level of evidence was rated as low for this factor.

Key Question 3—Interventions to Delay the Onset of AD

There were relatively few RCTs assessing the association between the factors examined and AD. This is at least partially attributable to the fact that many of the factors are not amenable to testing in an RCT. There were also sparse, if any, data on differences in outcomes among subgroups because the few RCTs conducted have generally not been designed to assess such differences.

For the nutrition category, there was one RCT on vitamin E and one on gingko biloba that showed no association with AD. There were no other RCTs for nutritional factors, including folic acid and Mediterranean diet, factors suggested to decrease risk by observational studies.

The factors in the medical conditions category are not appropriate for randomization. For the medications category, the three RCTs using antihypertensive medication showed no association with AD, but findings were limited by low power to detect a clinically important effect and assessment for all-cause dementia rather than AD. The eight RCTs using cholinesterase inhibitors showed no association with AD (moderate level of evidence). The two RCTs assessing NSAIDs showed increased risk of AD with rofecoxib, a medication that was subsequently withdrawn from the market for safety reasons, and increased risk for non-specific dementia with naproxen (HR 3.57; 95 percent CI 1.09 to 11.7) but the study was stopped early and findings were based on few cases. In intervention trials, estrogen alone showed no association, but estrogen combined with progesterone showed an increased risk of AD (HR 2.05; 95 percent CI 1.21 to 3.48). The level of evidence was rated as moderate for estrogen combined with progesterone and low for NSAIDs.

For the social, economic, and behavioral factors, there were no intervention trials for any factors, including physical activity and cognitive engagement, interventions suggested to be beneficial by observational studies.

Key Question 4—Interventions to Improve or Maintain Cognitive Ability or Function

There were few RCTs assessing the effect of the various factors on cognitive decline. Additionally there was no information on differential outcomes by subgroups.

For the nutrition category, intervention trials of vitamin B6 and B12, vitamin E, and folic acid showed either no effect on cognitive decline or no consistent effect across trials. The level of evidence was judged to be high for vitamin E and moderate for the other supplements. We did not identify any trials that evaluated the Mediterranean diet or diets high in vegetables, practices that have been associated with lower risk of cognitive decline in observational studies.

The medical conditions were not appropriate for RCTs. For the medication category, there was no effect of statins (level of evidence = high), antihypertensive medications (low), cholinesterase inhibitors (moderate), or estrogen (high).

Some of the types of NSAIDs showed no effect, but one (naproxen) showed increased risk of cognitive decline. The level of evidence for NSAIDs was rated as low. Observational studies had suggested lower risk for both NSAIDs and estrogen.

For the social, economic, and behavioral categories, physical activity and cognitive training interventions showed a small protective association against cognitive decline. The level of the evidence for cognitive training was rated high, but that for physical activity was rated low.

Key Question 5—Relationships between Factors Affecting AD and Cognitive Decline

To address this question, we used the results from Key Questions 1 through 4 to compare the evidence for the effects of each exposure on risk of AD and cognitive decline. For factors with both RCT and observational evidence, we first compared the consistency of findings across study designs for each outcome. RCTs were preferred when of high quality. When studies showed a consistent effect on risk that was in the same direction for both AD and cognitive decline, we judged the results concordant. For many factors, the available data are quite limited, and concordant evidence across outcomes should not necessarily be interpreted as a robust finding.

For other factors, not only were data limited but there was also marked heterogeneity in exposure or outcome measures across studies, so it was not possible to draw a conclusion about concordance.

It is important to note that risk modification was generally small to moderate when factors were associated with AD (i.e., odds ratios and relative risk ratios were often substantially less than 2.0). For cognitive decline, it is more difficult to determine the threshold for a meaningful change due to the numerous cognitive measures used to assess cognitive decline. But generally the differences in annual rate of decline between the exposed and unexposed groups were quite small.

Factors showing an association for both AD and cognitive decline were the following:

Increased Risk

- Diabetes
- APOE e4
- Smoking
- Depression

Decreased Risk

- Mediterranean diet (limited data)
- Cognitive engagement
- Physical activities

Chapter 34

Nutrition, Exercise, and Therapeutic Recommendations

Chapter Contents

Section 34.1

Questions and Answers about AD, Diet, and Exercise

Excerpted from "Alzheimer's Diet, Exercise, and Complementary Health,"
© 2010 Fisher Center for Alzheimer's Research Foundation. Reprinted
with permission. For additional information, visit www.alzinfo.com.

How can overall health and well-being be maintained in a person suffering from Alzheimer's disease?

It's important for the person with Alzheimer's to be under the continual supervision of a qualified medical doctor in order to stay in the best overall health possible. Poor overall health is associated with greater symptoms of Alzheimer's, so maintaining healthy habits may reduce symptoms. Attention must be paid to proper exercise, diet, and to any new or long-standing health problems. Hearing and vision should also be evaluated regularly and treated appropriately if faltering. Ongoing consultation with a primary care physician may be supplemented with visits to specialists or other health professionals as necessary to address specific needs.

Co-existing medical conditions should be identified and properly managed, as they may negatively impact Alzheimer's behaviors. For example, frequent urinary tract infections may increase wandering, and depression disrupts sleep and deepens social withdrawal.

Do people with Alzheimer's need to follow a special diet?

People with Alzheimer's should eat well-balanced, nutrient-rich meals, but a special diet is usually not necessary. However, even healthy older people experience changes in eating habits as they age: Food may not smell or taste the same; it may become more difficult to chew and digest food, and our cells may not be able to utilize the energy from food as efficiently. These problems may be more pronounced in people with Alzheimer's and may be compounded by other challenges posed by the disease. In addition, Alzheimer's may cause appetite control systems in the brain to malfunction as nerve cells in those areas deteriorate, resulting in extreme eating behaviors (overeating or not eating at all).

In early stages of the disease, people with Alzheimer's may have difficulty preparing meals. They may forget they have food in the oven or cook something and forget to eat it. Step-by-step written or verbal instructions clearly delineating what to do to prepare and eat meals may be beneficial in such cases.

Food preparation problems may progress to difficulty eating. Nerve cell death eventually steals the ability to recognize thirst or hunger. At the same time, depth perception may be compromised due to changes in the visual and "mapping" areas of the brain, making the process of eating more frustrating. The person may no longer know how to use a knife or fork and may lose interest in food altogether.

Severe eating problems put the person with Alzheimer's at risk for weight loss, dehydration, and malnutrition. See your doctor if you notice significant weight loss or changes in eating behavior. Ask about ways to increase your loved one's food intake and find out if nutritional supplementation might be warranted. Keep in mind that supplements should be used with caution and only under a doctor's supervision, as they may interact with prescription medications.

Is it important for a person who has Alzheimer's to exercise?

Maintaining a reasonable level of exercise is important for many reasons, both for overall health and to address issues specific to Alzheimer's. Exercise can improve mobility and help one maintain independence. In normal people, moderately strenuous exercise has been shown to improve cognitive functioning.

In people with Alzheimer's, studies show that light exercise and walking appear to reduce wandering, aggression, and agitation. Incorporating exercise into daily routines and scheduled activities can also be beneficial in alleviating problem behaviors. The type of exercise should be individualized to the person's abilities. Talk with your doctor about what is right.

Section 34.2

Physical Activity Benefits Nursing-Home Residents with AD

A couple hours a week of moderate activity allowed seniors with Alzheimer's who were living in a nursing home to boost stamina and better carry out everyday activities than those who did not receive a structured exercise program. Those with Alzheimer's who participated in the fitness program showed slower physical deterioration than their more sedentary peers and performed better on tests that measure walking, strength, balance, and flexibility.

The findings, from French scientists at Hospital La Grave-Casselardit in Toulouse, France, add to a growing body of evidence that exercise is good not just for the body but for the brain as well. A rigorous study from 2003, published in the *Journal of the American Medical Association,* found that a home exercise program eased depression and boosted physical vitality of those suffering from Alzheimer's. [See the article, "Exercise Boosts Mood, Performance of Alzheimer's Patients" (http://www.alzinfo.org/?p=1360)] People with Alzheimer's who got regular physical activity showed greater stamina and better general functioning and mood, even 2 years later.

In the current study, scientists studied 110 elderly men and women with Alzheimer's living in nursing homes. Their average age was 83. Some were assigned to the exercise program, which focused on an hour of walking, strength, balance, and flexibility training twice a week. Others continued to receive routine care. By the end of the study, 1 year later, those who had completed the training were able to walk faster and did better on strength and balance tests. The results were published in the *Journal of the American Geriatrics Society.*

Exercise Good for Everyone

Another study published in that journal found that exercise benefits healthy older seniors as well, and not just those with Alzheimer's.

Researchers at the Rush Alzheimer's Disease Center in Chicago found that for healthy seniors with intact memory (average age 80), the risk of becoming disabled fell 7 percent for every hour spent each week being physically active. Regular physical activity also greatly cut the risk of dying.

Exercise also allowed older adults to better carry out everyday activities like walking short distances, eating meals, getting dressed, preparing meals, shopping, and housekeeping.

Regular physical activity boosts blood flow to organs throughout the body, including the brain, and may provide an extra boost for those with or without Alzheimer's, the research suggests.

And it's never too early to get off the couch. Numerous studies show that walking and other moderate exercise benefits men and women regardless of age. For more information, visit www.ALZinfo.org.

By www.ALZinfo.org, The Alzheimer's Information Site. Reviewed by William J. Netzer, PhD, Fisher Center for Alzheimer's Research Foundation at The Rockefeller University.

Source: *Journal of the American Geriatrics Society,* February 2007.

Section 34.3

Alternative Medicine Therapies for AD and Dementia

Excerpted from "Alzheimer's Diet, Exercise, and Complementary Health," © 2010 Fisher Center for Alzheimer's Research Foundation. Reprinted with permission. For additional information, visit www.alzinfo.com.

Health treatments for people with Alzheimer's disease can also employ so-called complementary health approaches. These may include herbal remedies, acupuncture, and massage. This area of treatment is presently the subject of a great deal of research, with far more proposed. It's important to understand that complementary or alternative health approaches, including vitamins and herbal supplements, are not subject to the same kind of critical government review for safety and efficacy that new drugs are, so one must be cautious when considering such approaches. While there are a growing number of legitimate researchers investigating these approaches, there is also a great deal of misinformation in the public domain, and unsubstantiated claims are rampant. Ask your doctor to help you understand the benefits and risks of such approaches, and do not take herbal or vitamin supplements without first discussing it with your doctor, since many of these pills can interact negatively with prescription or nonprescription medications.

Gingko biloba, an herbal supplement with antioxidant properties, has been the subject of much hype regarding its supposed effects on cognition and memory. Some studies have shown that some people with dementia (of unspecified types) may benefit from gingko biloba supplements, but rigorous evidence of the herb's effectiveness is so far lacking. More studies are ongoing, including ones that are investigating whether gingko biloba can help improve symptoms of Mild Cognitive Impairment. Like other herbal supplements, gingko biloba can have side effects and may interact with prescription medications, so it should only be taken under a doctor's supervision.

Acupuncture, a core component of traditional Chinese medicine that has been used for thousands of years to treat all manner of health complaints, has recently been investigated for its use in Alzheimer's disease. Scientists at two medical institutions, the Wellesley College Center for Research on Women in Wellesley, Massachusetts, and the University of Hong Kong, reported the promising findings of two small studies at a recent medical meeting for Alzheimer's researchers.

In the Wellesley study, 11 people with dementia (10 with Alzheimer's, one with vascular dementia, a related condition) were treated with acupuncture twice a week for 3 months. Tests completed before and after the study measured cognitive function and mood in the study subjects, and an analysis showed that the treatments significantly reduced depression and anxiety. The Hong Kong study, in which eight patients with Alzheimer's were treated for a total of 30 days each, demonstrated significant improvements in cognition, verbal skills, motor coordination, and in an overall measure of the severity of Alzheimer's symptoms. Additional studies are ongoing to repeat the results and further explore the effectiveness of acupuncture for treating mood and behavioral disturbances associated with Alzheimer's disease.

Massage can be therapeutic for a number of health conditions, and a great deal of research has documented its benefits in general health. Fewer studies have investigated its usefulness in Alzheimer's, but there is some evidence that massage therapy may reduce behaviors such as wandering, aggression, and agitation.

Chapter 35

Dental Care and the Dementia Patient

Dementia is the permanent loss of multiple intellectual functions resulting from neuronal death. Dementia afflicts 10% of individuals over the age of 65 and these patients survive approximately 7 years with their cognitive impairment. Most (60%) nursing home residents have cognitive impairment. Although Alzheimer's disease is the most common cause of dementia (65%), other causes include vascular (15%), alcoholic (5%–15%), as well as multiple rare diseases. These dementias have similar clinical features. Patients with dementia have ongoing needs for oral care. Oral pathology can result in poor nutrition, pain, distress, and agitation. Dementia patients need special consideration for management by the dentist.

The basic symptoms of dementia include: (1) amnesia, i.e., memory loss, (2) aphasia, i.e., communication difficulties, (3) apraxia, i.e., inability to perform complicated motor tasks, and (4) agnosia, i.e., inability to recognize previously learned sensory input—e.g., faces. Some dementia patients also manifest psychiatric symptoms that include hallucinations, delusions, depression, personality changes, and aggressive behavior. This combination of cognitive and psychiatric symptoms makes dementia patients a challenge for oral care. Most dementia patients deny or hide their cognitive disability.

Patients with dementia and other types of structural brain injury are predisposed to delirium (i.e., abrupt onset, temporary confusion

"Dental Care and the Dementia Patient," © 2008 Richard E. Powers, MD. For additional information, visit www.alzbrain.org, an educational website sponsored by the Dementia Education & Training Program, or call 800-457-5679.

caused by medical problems or psychotropic medications). Medications prescribed by dentists such as narcotics and benzodiazepines may cause dementia patients to become more confused and unsteady. Approximately 15% of patients over age 65 admitted to the hospital and 3% of nursing home patients suffer from delirium.

The cognitive symptoms of Alzheimer's disease can complicate the dental management in patients. Amnestic patients will forget symptoms and instructions. Since the 5-minute recall of Alzheimer's patients is quite limited, patients may need frequent reminders during the dental procedure as to your identity and instruction on how to cooperate. Aphasic patients may fail to understand spoken word (receptive aphasia) or may have difficulty communicating (expressive aphasia). These patients may require a little extra time to elicit clinical symptoms and may not understand all the questions about their dental care. The family caregiver should be present during the clinical assessment to assure accurate history. Amnestic patients may forget allergies to medication and a clinical history from a dementia patient should always involve a knowledgeable family caregiver. Non-verbal communication with significantly aphasic patients is helpful. A frequent smile, a calm, gentle voice and touch, as well as pointing and mimicking can assist with communication in the patient with receptive aphasia.

Apraxic patients frequently forget how to perform complex motor tasks such as brushing teeth, or insertion of dentures. Forgetful patients can place dentures in different parts of the home or nursing home and frequently lose them. Patients in the dental chair may be unable to perform complicated movement with their mouth. The practitioner should aid oral care by talking with family. More profoundly demented patients may resist attempts to brush their teeth or insert dentures. The family and dentist may need to develop creative approaches toward assuring minimal oral care to instructions on insertion of dentures, bridges, etc. Visual agnosia is common in the elderly and many forget the faces of familiar people. Your long-term dental patient who develops Alzheimer's disease may forget who you are. They may identify you as someone else and fail to recognize the dental office as a scene of medical care. Gentle reminders and frequent reassurances are helpful in lowering the anxiety of the patient. It is better to distract the patient than dispute their false beliefs.

Many Alzheimer patients develop psychiatric symptoms during the course of their illness. Hallucinations (25%), delusions (30%), hostility (25%), and depression (30%) are some of the many behavioral symptoms present in Alzheimer patients and other dementias. Few Alzheimer patients are a threat to dental office staff; however, precaution can be taken with at-risk patients. The family should contact the local physician to assess level of risk and an appropriate PRN [pro re nata, or as-needed] medication can be used to sedate potentially aggressive patients. For example, a one-time dose of Ativan (0.25–1 mgm) may produce sufficient sedation for the oral procedure. Adequate use of topical anesthetics will lessen the risk of impulsive activity on the part of the patients. Gas or other major sedatives may worsen confusion rather than improve patient management. A constant, steady, compassionate management style is most effective in reassuring the patient and obtaining maximum patient compliance.

Creutzfeldt-Jakob disease is a prion mediated (infectious particle smaller than virus) that accounts for less than 1% of all dementia. Creutzfeldt's patients progress rapidly and most die within 18 months in contrast to Alzheimer patients who survive for prolonged periods of time. There is no recorded transmission of Creutzfeldt's disease through human bites or blood products. Transmission requires inoculation with central nervous system tissue. The Creutzfeldt's prion is not destroyed by standard autoclave or aseptic technique and requires specialized procedures to assure inactivation. Creutzfeldt's disease is a difficult clinical diagnosis that requires a neurologist with expertise in the dementias.

Good oral care is essential in the management of Alzheimer patients. Most dementia victims survive approximately 7 years with a range from 3–18 years. Alzheimer's disease can be divided into multiple phases; however, dentists should recognize three stages of illness— early, middle, and late. Early stages (first 3 years) are characterized by mild forgetfulness and most patients should be able to maintain reasonable oral care. Patients may forget appointments, lose dentures, and usually hide their cognitive deficits. Middle stages (3–6 years) include all the cognitive symptoms and many psychiatric symptoms. Families may have difficulty providing oral care for mid-stage patients who may be slightly resistive to examination and dental procedures. Late stage patients usually have overwhelming brain injury and forget how to eat, walk, talk, or tend to their bodily needs. These patients require passive oral care to prevent oral infection. Many require syringe feedings, feeding tubes, or may have PEG [percutaneous endoscopic gastrostomy] tube placement. Alzheimer's patients lose weight for a variety of reasons. Dentists should assure that oral disease is not limiting oral intake. Unrecognized dental pain may be a cause of agitation in the midphase patient who is unable to explain his oral symptoms. Painful, broken teeth or abscesses may provoke agitation that is unresponsive to Haldol or Ativan.

The relationship between dental disease and weight loss is unclear. Dentate patients with dementia lose more weight than the edentulous (Hand 1994). Psychotropic medications may promote dental disease, (e.g., xerostomia) and induce buco-oral movement disorders (e.g., teeth grinding) with tardive dyskinesia.

Dementia is often undiagnosed or misdiagnosed in the elderly. Approximately 20% of confused elders have some other disease that is improved with appropriate treatment. Dentists should encourage families to seek accurate diagnosis of dementia. The local mental health center, neurologist, or psychiatrist can perform a mental status examination to screen for dementia. The local physician can perform basic exclusionary studies such as thyroid screen, CAT [computerized axial tomography] scan, etc., to exclude treatable causes. Assistance for rural or suburban residents includes home health care, support groups, caregiver education, and specialty referral clinics for the dementia patient. Dentists should encourage families to seek appropriate assessment and utilize support services that will assure maximum quality of life for both the patient and the family caregiver.

Chapter 36

Hearing Loss, AD, and Dementia

There is a correlation between hearing loss and certain medical ailments such as diabetes and cardiovascular diseases, among others. But there is also compelling evidence to suggest a link between hearing loss, dementia, and Alzheimer's, both of which are degenerative diseases that lead to progressive memory loss in the elderly.

In fact, multiple research studies have shown that hearing loss not only exacerbates the symptoms of Alzheimer's and dementia, but may also be an important risk factor.

Many symptoms of hearing loss—especially those related to difficulty in understanding and communicating—are similar to some of those found in Alzheimer's. For example, both Alzheimer's and hearing loss are known to affect speech and language skills. Depression is also a common feature of both conditions.

Hearing Loss and Memory: A Proven Link

A number of studies have demonstrated a correlation between Alzheimer's, dementia, and hearing loss.

One study conducted at the University of Washington with Alzheimer's patients who also had hearing loss demonstrated a strong correlation between the severity of cognitive decline and the degree of hearing loss.

Another study carried out in the 1980s found that 83 percent of the 30 patients diagnosed with senile dementia also suffered from a significant hearing loss, higher than normally expected for that age group. However, there was some promising news that came out of that research: 33 percent of those with memory and hearing loss were re-classified to a less severe category of dementia once the hearing loss was treated with hearing aids.

That was also demonstrated in yet another study conducted a decade ago, which showed a significant drop in communication problems in Alzheimer's patients whose hearing loss had been tested and corrected with the use of hearing aids.

The message here is clear: Hearing aids can be extremely beneficial for the Alzheimer's and dementia patients, as they are for anyone with hearing loss. It is possible, however, that health care providers who do not routinely deal with elderly people the way audiologists or geriatricians do, may not be aware of the importance of screening these patients for hearing loss. As a matter of fact, there is plenty of evidence to suggest that many seniors diagnosed with dementia or Alzheimer's don't undergo tests to rule out hearing loss.

So if anyone you know is suffering from memory loss, or displaying any symptoms of Alzheimer's or dementia, encourage them to be screened for hearing loss as well. If a hearing loss is found, assistive technology such as hearing aids can, as demonstrated above, make a big difference in improving all the essential cognitive functions.

Once appropriate treatment is implemented, these people can benefit from other measures that improve the failing memory—such as music therapy.

Music to Your Brain

The common denominator in both functions—auditory and memory—is the brain, so naturally, anything we can do to boost its ability to properly process hearing, language, and memory, will be beneficial. In other words, treating hearing loss will allow the brain to continue to be stimulated and active, allowing the patient to stay alert.

And this is where the beneficial effects of music for people with cognitive deficiencies can be seen. Studies conducted at University of California, Davis, found that Alzheimer's patients who have difficulty with their memory still respond to music.

Other research has indicated that music stimulates the motor region of our brain and listening to familiar songs may restore a certain degree of cognitive functions in people with memory loss.

For example, Dr. Concetta Tomaino of the Institute for Music and Neurologic Function in the Bronx, NY, found that music stimulates areas of the brain that have become dormant due to degenerative diseases such as Alzheimer's. She reported that 45 patients with mid- to late-stage dementia, who had 1-hour personalized music therapy sessions three times a week, were able to boost their cognitive functions by an average of 50 percent within less than a year.

Again, this is where the importance of assistive hearing technology comes in, since it makes it possible for people to hear and respond to music, thus boosting their diminishing cognitive functions.

Look at it this way: Good hearing is essential to stimulating parts of our brain required for memory and is also the foundation of so many other therapies that are crucial to our health and well-being.

Take this message to heart and pass it on to those you know suffering from dementia or Alzheimer's.

Chapter 37

Pain and Dementia

Dementia is a condition of declining mental abilities. A diagnosis of dementia means that the patient may have difficulty reasoning over time. The patient may have problems remembering things and even people they love. Your loved one may not be able to communicate his or her thoughts, feelings, needs, or physical problems. In fact, he or she may not even fully understand physical problems, such as pain.

Sadly, persistent pain is common among older persons, because they are more likely to suffer from problems such as arthritis and other chronic medical conditions. Many people think that pain is to be expected with aging and that nothing can be done. Older persons commonly have multiple medical problems which, when combined with dementia, can make diagnosis difficult. If your loved one has dementia, determining if he or she is experiencing pain may be up to you. Often, older persons deny that they have pain. Instead, asking your loved one whether he/she experiences discomfort, aching, or hurting may result in a more truthful answer.

Even if dementia makes it impossible for your loved one to respond, your careful observation can reveal important clues to let you know that he or she is experiencing pain.

Used with permission from the American Geriatrics Society. "Pain in Dementia: A Family and Caregivers Guide to Assessment and Treatment" http://www.healthin aging org/public_education/pain/pain_dementia.pdf from the American Geriatrics Society. For more information visit the AGS online at www.americangeriatrics.org. Reviewed by David A. Cooke, MD, FACP, February 17, 2011.

What Are the Clues?

- **Facial expressions:** Does your loved one frown, look frightened, grimace, wrinkle his or her brow, keep eyes closed tightly, blink rapidly, or exhibit any distorted expression?

- **Verbalizations/vocalizations:** Does he or she moan, groan, sigh, grunt/chant/call out, breathe noisily, ask for help, or become verbally abusive?

- **Body movements:** Is your loved one's body posture rigid and/or tense? Does he or she fidget, pace or rock back and forth, have restricted movement, gait or mobility changes?

- **Behavioral changes:** Does he or she refuse food or have an appetite change? Is there any change in sleep/rest periods? Has he or she suddenly stopped common routines or begun wandering?

- **Mental status changes:** Does he or she cry, become more confused, irritable, or distressed?

When Does the Pain Occur?

- **During movement?** Does your loved one grimace or groan during personal care (such as bathing), walking, or transferring (from bed to chair, for example)?

- **When there is no movement involved?** Does your loved one appear agitated or have other behavioral changes, such as trouble sleeping, loss of appetite, or reclusiveness?

The Pain Assessment

If you see any of these clues, talk to your health care provider right away. If your loved one has mild-to-moderate dementia and is able to communicate adequately, your health care provider will question him or her directly and should use pain evaluation tools and scales. The health care provider may ask the patient to give pain a number from 1 to 10, or use pictures of faces or a pain thermometer to help measure the pain.

If your loved one is not able to communicate adequately, you must describe your loved one's signs of pain with as much detail as possible. Tell the health care provider what you have noticed and give examples. Focus on when the pain occurs. You can describe how it seems to be experienced (for example, comes and goes or is constant; and whether the pain occurs with or without movement). Tell what—if anything—

358

relieves the pain; the health care provider will be able to make a diagnosis and offer a plan to help relieve the pain.

An important part of the pain assessment is a history of all prescription and over-the-counter medicines your loved one now takes and has taken in the past. Write down all medications and dosages the patient has taken and give it to the health care provider.

The health care provider should also perform a physical examination that will focus on the site(s) of pain, often the muscle/bone and nervous systems. The health care provider will evaluate the patient's physical function (walking, range of motion of joints, etc). Laboratory tests and/or x-rays may be performed, as well.

Treatments

Medication is the most common way of controlling pain in older persons. Around-the-clock doses of acetaminophen (Tylenol) are effective for most patients with mild-to-moderate muscle/bone pain, like arthritis. Non-steroidal anti-inflammatory drugs, such as aspirin and ibuprofen, can be effective but may have more side effects in older persons. Because they have to be taken every day over a long period of time they may cause such problems as bleeding ulcers. There is another type of nonsteroidal anti-inflammatory drug, Cox-2 Inhibitors (Celecoxib), that may be useful if bleeding is a potential problem. This new class of drugs has some distinct advantages, but also risks—especially for long-term use—that should be considered in selecting the best medication.

For more serious pain, there are the opioid drugs, such as Vicodin or Roxicet to name just a couple of the many different products that are now available for moderate to severe pain. These drugs can be very effective in some cases.

For pain that is due to damage to nerves, a wide variety of drugs used for control of depression and even epilepsy have been found to be helpful. If movement causes pain, the health care provider can prescribe medication to be taken before the movement. He or she may suggest ways to alter the movement or activity that causes pain. If the pain is caused by something other than movement, the health care provider will investigate other causes and ask questions like: Are the patient's basic needs being met? Is there an infection? Is the patient constipated? Treatment needs to be prescribed based on each patient's specific situation.

Pain is a serious problem for many older persons. Alleviating pain in patients with dementia often depends on the observations of the family/caregiver. You and your health care provider can work together to relieve the patient's pain and achieve a better quality of life for your loved one in his/her later years.

Where Can I Get More Information?

For more tools of persistent pain management visit The Foundation for Health in Aging (www.healthinaging.org).

Chapter 38

Sexuality and AD

The physicians who diagnose Alzheimer's disease discuss the cognitive and behavioral changes a patient will experience during the course of the disease, and how these changes will affect their partner. But how will the diagnosis affect the intimate relationship between patients and their partners? Many couples are too embarrassed to ask the questions they really need answered.

Sex is important; to some people it is a non-negotiable need. Many couples find it beneficial to have a discussion soon after diagnosis about their individual expectations. Navigating the territory of sexuality and dementia can be murky. Ideally, decisions should be based on what works for both people individually and as a couple.

Most Alzheimer's patients are diagnosed in their mid-seventies. Although the aging body is no stranger to erectile dysfunction, vaginal dryness, or changes in frequency, intensity, or even ability to orgasm or ejaculate, these issues can often be accommodated with products, pharmaceuticals, or good old-fashioned innovation. A dementia diagnosis not only introduces other sexual issues, it can also exacerbate existing problems. As a person's cognition changes, so do the ways in which they relate to their partner.

The ebb and flow of dementia symptoms can create tension in and out of the bedroom. A person with dementia may not always recognize his or her partner, and may respond inappropriately to verbal or physical cues. Personality changes can mean a person who was once meek may be more aggressive or vice versa. Dementia patients may make sexual advances toward strangers or forget their marriage vows, which they formerly treated as serious and binding oaths. Mistaking a relationship with one's partner is not uncommon. For example, a woman could think her husband is her father, deem his advances inappropriate, and react accordingly. Proper sequencing, something that is primary to both sex and intimacy, deteriorates with Alzheimer's. The unspoken language of a couple becomes disjointed. Partners often express a desire for sex in nonverbal ways, but these subtle cues may not be picked up or understood by someone with Alzheimer's. It's not just the couple's sex life that may suffer as a result, but any sustained form of intimacy.

In couples who have been together for decades, these changes can be disconcerting or even shocking for the partner without dementia. During the sex act, dementia-related symptoms such as limited attention span and lack of focus can make the partner without dementia feel unsatisfied, poorly treated, or "used." The idea of being used is also fed by common situations such as a person with dementia not recalling their partner's name, yet continually making sexual advances. Conversely, some partners wonder if the person with dementia can give informed consent for the sex act—even questioning whether their behavior could be classified as rape.

A partner without dementia can sometimes misunderstand what is occurring; some actions aren't unequivocally sexual in the context of dementia. For example, a person with dementia might undress because his or her clothing feels uncomfortable, but will not explain the behavior, which may make it seem like a sexual overture. Hypersexuality in dementia patients, usually associated with men, is a myth based on accounts of disinhibition that can result in behaviors such as public undressing. According to the Alzheimer's Association, about 50 percent of men with Alzheimer's experience erectile dysfunction.

Most sex-related issues only are present in the early to moderate stages of dementia. In late stages, intercourse usually isn't possible due to physical constraints. However, the agitation often experienced by late-stage Alzheimer's patients can sometimes be alleviated by gentle touching and soothing words. The sexual parameters of this part of the disease course primarily encompass a softer form of physical comfort rather than more intense sexual encounters.

Many late-stage Alzheimer's patients live in nursing homes where workers generally aren't trained to see residents as sexual beings. Hence, even innocent interactions such as snuggling fully clothed with one's partner can be met with anything from dubious stares to outright chastisement. There are some notable exceptions throughout the country where residents and their partners are accommodated by the facility. Several videos are available online to train staffers how to graciously allow nursing home residents their intimate moments.

What makes sexuality and dementia a particularly thorny issue is that many couples view sex as the ultimate expression of the love they feel for their partner. To these couples, it is yet another form of communication that dementia has robbed them of. Communication is further complicated when the person without dementia acts as both a caregiver and a partner. The duality of roles can be difficult, troubling and, for some, seemingly impossible. Support groups are essential for most couples dealing with a dementia diagnosis—and critical for partners without dementia. The Alzheimer's Association is a good place to start searching for resources in your community.

Chapter 39

Sleep Problems and Dementia

Chapter Contents

Section 39.1

Treatment for Dementia-Related Sleep Changes

This section contains text from "A Good Night's Sleep," by the National Institute on Aging (NIA, www.nia.nih.gov), part of the National Institutes of Health, March 2009, and text excerpted from "Side Effects of Sleep Drugs," by the U.S. Food and Drug Administration (FDA, www.fda.gov), July 31, 2007.

A Good Night's Sleep

Ever since he retired, Edward dreads going to bed at night. He's afraid that when he turns off his light, he will just lie there with his eyes open and his mind racing. "How can I break this cycle?" he asks. "I'm so tired—I need to get some sleep."

Just like Edward, you want a good night's rest. Getting enough sleep helps you stay healthy and alert. But many older people don't sleep well. If you're always sleepy, it may be time to see a doctor. You shouldn't wake up every day feeling tired.

Sleep and Aging

Older adults need about the same amount of sleep as young adults—7 to 9 hours each night. But seniors tend to go to sleep earlier and get up earlier than when they were younger. Older people may nap more during the day, which can sometimes make it hard to fall asleep at night.

There are two kinds of sleep—REM (rapid eye movement) sleep and non-REM sleep. We dream mostly during REM sleep and have the deepest sleep during non-REM sleep. As people get older, they spend less time in deep sleep, which may be why older people are often light sleepers.

Sleep Problems

There are many reasons why older people may not get enough sleep at night. Feeling sick or being in pain can make it hard to sleep. Napping during the day can disrupt sleep at night. Some medicines can keep you awake. No matter the reason, if you don't get a good night's sleep, the next day you may experience the following:

- Be irritable
- Have memory problems or be forgetful
- Feel depressed
- Have more falls or accidents
- Feel very sleepy during the day

Insomnia

Insomnia is the most common sleep problem in adults age 60 and older. People with insomnia have trouble falling and staying asleep. Insomnia can last for days, months, or even years. If you're having trouble sleeping, you may experience the following:

- Take a long time to fall asleep
- Wake up many times in the night
- Wake up early and be unable to get back to sleep
- Wake up tired
- Feel very sleepy during the day

There are many causes of insomnia. Some of them you can control, but others you can't. For example, if you are excited about a new activity or worrying over your bills, you may have trouble sleeping. Sometimes insomnia may be a sign of other problems. Or, it could be a side effect of a medication or an illness.

Often, being unable to sleep becomes a habit. Some people worry about not sleeping even before they get into bed. This may even make insomnia worse.

Older adults who have trouble sleeping may use more over-the-counter sleep aids. Using prescription medicines for a short time might help. But remember, medicines aren't a cure for insomnia. Developing healthy habits at bedtime may help you get a good night's sleep.

Sleep Apnea

Sleep apnea is another serious sleep disorder. A person with sleep apnea has short pauses in breathing while sleeping. These pauses may happen many times during the night. If not treated, sleep apnea can lead to other problems such as high blood pressure, stroke, or memory loss.

You can have sleep apnea and not even know it. But your loud snoring and gasping for air can keep other people awake. Feeling sleepy during the day and being told you are snoring loudly at night could be signs that you have sleep apnea.

If you think you have sleep apnea, see a doctor who knows about this sleep problem. You may need to learn to sleep in a position that keeps your airways open. Sometimes a medical device called Continuous Positive Air Pressure (CPAP), a dental device, or surgery can help.

Movement Disorders

Restless legs syndrome, periodic limb movement disorder, and rapid eye movement sleep behavior disorder are common in older adults. These movement disorders can rob you of needed sleep.

People with restless legs syndrome, or RLS, feel like there is tingling, crawling, or pins and needles in one or both legs. It's worse at night. Moving the legs brings some relief, at least for a short time. RLS tends to run in families. See your doctor for more information about medicines to treat RLS.

Periodic limb movement disorder, or PLMD, causes people to jerk and kick their legs every 20 to 40 seconds during sleep. Some people have hundreds of these movements each night, which may result in loss of sleep and feeling tired and sleepy the next day. Medication, warm baths, exercise, and learning ways to relax can help.

Rapid eye movement sleep behavior disorder, also known as REM sleep behavior disorder, is another condition that may make it harder to get a good night's sleep. REM sleep, or rapid eye movement sleep, is the most active stage of sleep when dreaming often occurs. During normal REM sleep, your muscles cannot move, so your body stays still. But if you have REM sleep behavior disorder, your muscles can move, and your sleep is disrupted.

Alzheimer's Disease and Sleep—A Special Problem

Alzheimer's disease often changes a person's sleeping habits. For example, some people with Alzheimer's disease sleep too much; others don't sleep enough. Some people wake up many times during the night; others wander or yell at night. The person with Alzheimer's disease isn't the only one who loses sleep. Caregivers may have sleepless nights, leaving them tired for the challenges they face.

If you're caring for someone with Alzheimer's disease, there are steps you can take for his or her safety and that might help you sleep better at night. Try the following:

- Make sure the floor is clear of objects.

- Lock up any medicines.

- Attach grab bars in the bathroom.

- Place a gate across the stairs.

Getting a Good Night's Sleep

Being older doesn't mean you have to feel tired all the time. There are many things you can do to help you get a good night's sleep. Here are some ideas:

- Follow a regular sleep schedule. Go to sleep and get up at the same time each day, even on weekends. Try to avoid napping in the late afternoon or evening, as it may keep you awake at night.

- Develop a bedtime routine. Take time to relax before bedtime each night. Some people watch television, read a book, listen to soothing music, or soak in a warm bath.

- Keep your bedroom dark, not too hot or too cold, and as quiet as possible.

- Have a comfortable mattress, a pillow you like, and enough blankets for the season.

- Exercise at regular times each day but not within 3 hours of your bedtime.

- Make an effort to get outside in the sunlight each day.

- Be careful about when and how much you eat. Large meals close to bedtime may keep you awake, but a light snack in the evening can help you get a good night's sleep.

- Stay away from caffeine late in the day. Caffeine (found in coffee, tea, soda, and hot chocolate) can keep you awake.

- Drink fewer beverages in the evening. Waking up to go to the bathroom and turning on a bright light break up your sleep.

- Remember that alcohol won't help you sleep. Even small amounts make it harder to stay asleep.

- Use your bedroom only for sleeping. After turning off the light, give yourself about 20 minutes to fall asleep. If you're still awake and not drowsy, get out of bed. When you feel sleepy, go back to bed.

Safe Sleeping

Try to set up a safe and restful place to sleep. Make sure you have smoke alarms on each floor of your house or apartment. Lock the outside doors before going to bed. Other ideas for a safe night's sleep are the following:

- Keep a telephone with emergency phone numbers by your bed.

- Have a good lamp within reach that turns on easily.

- Put a glass of water next to the bed in case you wake up thirsty.

- Use nightlights in the bathroom and hall.

- Don't smoke, especially in bed.

- Remove area rugs so you won't trip if you get out of bed in the middle of the night.

- Don't fall asleep with a heating pad on; it may burn.

Sweet Dreams

There are some tricks to help you fall asleep. You don't really have to count sheep—but you could try counting slowly to 100. Some people find that playing mental games makes them sleepy. For example, tell yourself it's 5 minutes before you have to get up, and you're just trying to get a few extra winks. Other people find that relaxing their body puts them to sleep. You might start by telling yourself that your toes feel light as feathers and then work your way up the rest of the body saying the same words. You may drift off to sleep before getting to the top of your head.

If you feel tired and unable to do your activities for more than 2 or 3 weeks, you may have a sleep problem. Talk to your doctor about changes you can make to get a better night's sleep.

Side Effects of Sleep Drugs

Eating a little bit of chocolate was a treat that Teresa Wood looked forward to after work. The Fairfax Station, Virginia, resident allowed herself two small pieces of chocolate candy a day.

But after taking a drug to help her sleep at night, Wood awoke in the morning to find an empty box on the table in place of a pound of chocolates that had been there the night before.

"I couldn't believe it," says Wood. "I started looking all around the house—I even looked under the bed. I thought for sure someone came into the house during the night and ate them." But she was alone.

A few weeks later, Wood awoke to find a near-full box of chocolates gone again. "I just don't remember eating all that candy," she says.

Complex Sleep-Related Behaviors

Wood and her doctor determined that she had been getting up during the night and "sleep eating," an occurrence known as a complex sleep-related behavior. Other behaviors include making phone calls, having sex, and getting into the car and driving while not fully awake. Most people do not remember these events later.

Complex behaviors are a potential side effect of sedative-hypnotic products—a class of drugs used to help a person fall asleep and stay asleep.

"Complex behaviors, such as sleep-driving, could be potentially dangerous to both the patients and to others," says Russell Katz, MD, director of the Food and Drug Administration's Division of Neurology Products.

Allergic Reactions

Other rare but potential side effects of sedative-hypnotic drugs are a severe allergic reaction (anaphylaxis) and severe facial swelling (angioedema), which can occur as early as the first time the product is taken.

"Severe allergic reactions can affect a patient's ability to breathe and can affect other body systems as well, and can even be fatal at times," says Katz. "Although these allergic reactions are probably very rare, people should be aware that they can occur, because these reactions may be difficult to notice as people are falling asleep."

Stronger Warnings

To make known the risks of these products, FDA requested in early 2007 that all manufacturers of sedative-hypnotic drug products strengthen their product labeling to include warnings about complex sleep-related behaviors and anaphylaxis and angioedema.

"There are a number of prescription sleep aids available that are well-tolerated and effective for many people," says Steven Galson, MD, MPH, director of FDA's Center for Drug Evaluation and Research. However, after reviewing the available information on adverse events that occurred after the sedative-hypnotic drugs were on the market, FDA concluded that labeling changes were necessary to inform health care providers and consumers about risks, says Galson.

In addition to the labeling changes, FDA has requested that manufacturers of sedative-hypnotic products do the following:

- Send letters to health care providers to notify them about the new warnings (Manufacturers sent these letters beginning in March 2007.)

- Develop Patient Medication Guides for the products to inform consumers about risks and advise them of precautions that can be taken (Patient Medication Guides are handouts given to patients, families, and caregivers when a medicine is dispensed. The guides will contain FDA-approved information, such as proper use and the recommendation to avoid ingesting alcohol or other central nervous system depressants.)

- Conduct clinical studies to investigate the frequency with which sleep-driving and other complex behaviors occur in association with individual drug products

The revised labeling and other actions to make risks known affect these sedative-hypnotic products:

- Ambien, Ambien CR (zolpidem tartrate)

- Butisol sodium

- Carbrital (pentobarbital and carbromal)

- Dalmane (flurazepam hydrochloride)

- Doral (quazepam)

- Halcion (triazolam)

- Lunesta (eszopiclone)

- Placidyl (ethchlorvynol)

- ProSom (estazolam)

- Restoril (temazepam)

- Rozerem (ramelteon)

- Seconal (secobarbital sodium)

- Sonata (zaleplon)

Precautions

FDA advises people who are treated with any of these products to take the following precautions:

- Talk to your health care provider before you start these medications and if you have any questions or concerns.

- Read the Medication Guide, when available, before taking the product.

- Do not increase the dose prescribed by your health care provider. Complex sleep-related behaviors are more likely to occur with higher than appropriate doses.

- Do not drink alcohol or take other drugs that depress the nervous system.

- Do not discontinue the use of these medications without first talking to your health care provider.

Over-the-Counter Sleep Aids

Not all sleep medications are prescription. FDA has approved over-the-counter (OTC) medications for use up to 2 weeks to help relieve occasional sleepiness in people ages 12 and older. "If you continue to have sleeping problems beyond 2 weeks, you should see a doctor," says Marina Chang, RPh, pharmacist and team leader in FDA's Division of Nonprescription Regulation Development.

OTC sleep aids are non-habit-forming and do not present the risk of allergic reactions and complex sleep-related behaviors that are known to occur with sedative-hypnotic drugs.

But just because they're available over the counter doesn't mean they don't have side effects, says Chang. "They don't have the same level of precision as the prescription drugs. They don't completely stop working after 8 hours—many people feel drowsy for longer than 8 hours after taking them."

Chang advises reading the product label and exercising caution when taking OTC sleep aids until you learn how they will affect you. "They affect people differently," she says. "They are not for everybody."

Section 39.2

Light Therapy

"Does Light Therapy Help Alzheimer's Patients Sleep?,"
© 2009 Remedy Health Media. Reprinted with permission.

Many people with Alzheimer's have trouble sleeping, which can leave them exhausted during the day. Fatigue takes a toll on both patients and their caregivers. Indeed, irregular sleeping is a major reason why families move relatives with Alzheimer's into long-term care. Light therapy is a promising treatment under investigation for people with Alzheimer's who struggle with sleep.

Alzheimer's patients who have trouble sleeping should first be evaluated for underlying sleep disorders and medical conditions that cause sleep trouble. Also, stopping medications that affect sleep or switching to more tolerable drugs may help.

No studies have found that conventional sleep aids, like Ambien (zolpidem) and Sonata (zaleplon), or sedative antidepressant medications like trazodone (Desyrel) effectively treat disturbed sleep in Alzheimer's patients. And supplements that boost levels of melatonin (a hormone that makes people feel tired) have limited effect, perhaps because Alzheimer's patients have fewer melatonin receptors in the brain than people without dementia.

Light therapy—regular exposure to sunlight or special bright lamps that mimic natural light—is another option. Exposure to bright light signals to the brain that it is daytime and helps set the body's circadian rhythms—regular mental and biological changes that occur over a 24-hour cycle and regulate important functions, like preparing the body for sleep at night.

How well does light therapy work for Alzheimer's patients? In a 3-week study from the University of North Carolina at Chapel Hill, 66 adults with dementia living in long-term care facilities were exposed for varying amounts of time to bright ceiling lights installed in common areas.

Compared with participants who did not spend time under the lights, those who were exposed to light therapy for 2 and a half hours in the morning slept 16 minutes longer; those who were exposed for about 8 and a half hours off and on throughout the day slept 14 minutes longer. The morning group was also able to fall asleep 29 minutes earlier, which is important since Alzheimer's patients often can't fall asleep until late at night.

But not all studies have produced positive results, and there are questions about the appropriate dosage. The amount of light prescribed for other conditions may not be sufficient for older patients with Alzheimer's; eyes transmit less light with age, and visual problems are particularly common in patients with Alzheimer's disease.

While researchers have yet to determine the ultimate benefits of light therapy or how much is needed to have an effect, "It's still reasonable to encourage people with Alzheimer's to stay in well-lit areas during the day," says Peter Rabins, MD, Director of Geriatric Psychiatry and Neuropsychiatry at Johns Hopkins.

This may be more practical than purchasing specialized equipment, he notes. "The light-therapy boxes used by people with disorders like depression require sitting still in front of a bright lamp, and this can be a challenge for those with Alzheimer's." Spending time outside in the morning may be a convenient way to produce similar effects.

More Tips for Caregivers

The Alzheimer's Association offers these tips for better sleep:

- Maintain regular meal times and sleep schedules.

- Discourage alcohol, caffeine, and nicotine use.

- Encourage daily exercise (but no later than 4 hours before bedtime).

- Don't give Alzheimer's drugs before bedtime.

- Discourage watching TV or staying in bed during wakeful periods.

Chapter 40

Driving and Dementia

Safe Driving and Mild Cognitive Impairment

Changes in the brain that affect memory, thinking skills, and the control of body actions eventually affect driving ability. Early brain cell changes may lead to a very small amount of decline in short-term memory, some minor difficulty in keeping up with managing complex events such as overseeing a business or organizing a class or family reunion. Occasionally the person may experience some delay when trying to recall an exact name or word. Despite these mild difficulties, driving skills may remain strong. Driver skills are most likely strong if there are no changes in driver ability, no recent accidents, no difficulties parking the car, no problems handling surprise moves by other drivers, and no near misses, scrapes, or fender benders.

However, some early brain cell changes that lead to a decline in body movement, such as coordinated hand movements (for example, using a tool to do a home repair such as fixing a door knob, using a knife and fork when eating, or buttoning a jacket), may affect driving skills. The decline in hand skills may result in less ability to manage driving a motor vehicle, whether it is a car, truck, motor boat, or simple lawn

Excerpted from "Driving and Progressive Dementia," by Leilani Doty, PhD, Director, University of Florida Cognitive & Memory Disorder Clinics. Reprinted with permission from Alzheimer's Caregiver Support Online (http://alzonline .phhp.ufl.edu), a project sponsored by the State of Florida Department of Elder Affairs and the University of Florida Center for Telehealth and Healthcare Communications. © 2007.

mower. Driving may be less safe, not only for the passengers with the struggling driver but also for people in other cars on the road. Anyone who has difficulty moving one or both hands or arms should undergo a medical exam. If this difficulty is the beginning of a progressive disorder, a regular medical check-up is essential to make sure that driving safety is not reduced.

Warning Signs

Are you a safe driver? A "yes" to any of the following questions should lead to a talk with your family and your doctor to see if a health change may mean you are at a higher risk as a driver.

1. Have you noticed any change in your driving skills in the past few months or within the past year?

2. In the past 6 months has anyone commented about your unsafe driving?

3. Are you less sure of your overall driving skill?

4. This past year did you, while driving, ever forget where you were going?

5. In the past year have you become lost while driving?

6. Do other drivers honk at you or show signs of being angry at you?

7. This past year, has anyone riding in the car with you suddenly said, "Watch out!" or "Be careful of that driver . . ." or "Don't hit that . . ."?

8. In the past year has anyone refused to ride with you as the driver?

9. In the past year has anyone asked you to stop driving?

10. In the past year have you had any car accidents?

11. In the past year have you almost had a car accident (any close calls)?

12. In the past 6 months, have you had any slight scrapes or fender benders with other cars in parking lots?

13. In the past 6 months while driving, have you scraped other objects in the garage or bushes, fence, trees along your driveway? How about the mailbox?

14. In the past year, have you received any traffic warnings or tickets for speeding, going too slow, turning improperly, not stopping, etc.?

15. Have you missed seeing a traffic sign or red light?

16. Are you having problems with parking: scraping curbs, bumping other cars, not able to fit in between the lines or into the space?

17. In the past year have you confused the gas pedal and brake pedal?

18. In the past year have you been more unsure about where to turn or exit?

19. Do you need a "copilot" to drive?

The Driver with Mild Cognitive Impairment

People who have only a short-term memory loss are often diagnosed as having a Mild Cognitive Impairment. Sometimes people with Mild Cognitive Impairment, often called MCI, will also have very mild, occasional difficulty recalling specific names during conversations. They may have other occasional mild thinking difficulties such as keeping up with many topics that come up when many people talk at a meeting. Or, they may have trouble managing complicated projects, such as leading the annual fund raiser for their religious community. Generally speaking, however, they manage their paid job, home duties, and relationships just fine.

With a healthy lifestyle many of these people will not experience any further brain cell decline and will continue to be skilled, safe drivers. Others, despite their best and healthiest efforts, seem to convert over time to slow, progressive declines in memory and other thinking functions.

Short-Term Memory and Driving

Short-term memory and thinking functions are important for safe driving:

- **If there is a mild decline in short-term memory:** A person must be able to remember information that was just heard or seen to be a safe driver. For example, remembering a sign or lit message board by the roadside about upcoming road repair or road hazards from weather changes is important in order to drive more cautiously before approaching the hazardous area. For example, road surfaces on a bridge become icy and increase the hazards of skidding before the temperature drops to freezing; 37 degrees Fahrenheit is considered as the point of such danger.

- **Mild decline in naming:** A person must be able to read quickly and to understand language such as names of places and signs with directions while driving along at the speed limit.

Early Medical Exam Is Important

Often an early medical evaluation when the symptoms such as problems with memory first appear will lead to help. Recommendations may improve function and slow the rate of decline that is occurring. At the point of beginning decline, the person with Mild Cognitive Impairment probably still is fully safe as a driver of motor vehicles.

To determine if decline is ongoing in the person with Mild Cognitive Impairment, a medical check-up every 3 to 6 months with the physician offers a way to monitor changes. If medical findings suggest a decline in driver skills, then the physician may recommend limits on driving. In some cases the physician may decide that a comprehensive driver evaluation should occur before the person continues to drive.

If there are any reports from the person or the family (or significant other) that any of the risks in the preceding list of questions have occurred, then a comprehensive driver evaluation should occur before the person continues driving. Sometimes as a result of such testing, a driver refresher course or training with a driver safety specialist may update the driver's skills. A driver safety specialist may suggest adding features such as a wider rear-view mirror or larger side-view mirrors to the vehicle to increase the visual field of the driver.

A comprehensive (full) driver evaluation is more extensive than the regular driver test of the Department of Motor Vehicles and Highway Safety. The comprehensive driver evaluation test involves different vision tests, tests of memory and cognitive functions, as well as an on-the-road test (some places use a virtual test, an indoor set-up that was designed to imitate on-the-road driving situations).

A driver safety specialist who is certified in comprehensive driver evaluation is trained in assessment and may offer some driver rehab. Some of these specialists are occupational therapists; others have different training.

Chapter 41

Living Alone with AD or Dementia

Background

An increasing number of older people live alone. If they also have Alzheimer's disease or a related dementia, they are more likely to be diagnosed later in the disease because their symptoms often go unrecognized.

Our society values independence and the ability to live alone. Moving people away from home to live, for example, with a son or daughter, or in a long-term care setting, is often viewed as a loss of independence. This is not necessarily so, as a move may offer people not just better support and safety but also an environment that supports independence.

The Issues

For people with Alzheimer's disease:

- **Loss of independence:** Some people with Alzheimer's disease can tell when living alone is no longer safe or desirable. Others may want to stay in their own home for as long as possible, even if there are some safety issues. They may be concerned that a move away from home would mean a loss of self-reliance and control in their daily lives.

"Living Alone," © 2007 Alzheimer Society of Canada (www.alzheimer.ca). Reprinted with permission.

- **Premature move from home:** The person with the disease may have a higher tolerance for risk than family members and caregivers and may feel pressured into moving out of the home earlier than necessary.

For family members, caregivers, and health-care professionals:

- **Determining when living alone is no longer safe or desirable:** When people with Alzheimer's disease no longer have an understanding of their own safety and ability to look after themselves, family members and health-care professionals often have to determine if it is still suitable for the person to live alone. This includes weighing the risks of living alone against the benefits of providing support that enables the person to live at home.

- **Barriers within the health-care, community care, and legal systems:** Family members and health-care professionals often face barriers when trying to determine if a move from home is needed or if additional support can be provided in the home. These barriers include the difficulty of sharing information under privacy and confidentiality regulations; the limited availability of services to support independent living; and the complexities of competency legislation (the laws that determine when a person is no longer able to make a certain decision).

Preferred Choice

Living Environments That Provide Safety, Quality of Life, and Support

People with Alzheimer's disease need to live in environments that best support their safety and quality of life. For some, this may mean living at home with support services, even if there is some risk. If risks have been identified, it is important that family members and health-care professionals try to lessen them, wherever possible. For example, if a person frequently leaves the stove on, consider disconnecting the stove and finding other ways to provide hot food, for example, Meals on Wheels.

The amount and type of support available are important factors in determining if a person can live alone. For example, a person with a large family living in a community with many services may be better able to live alone than someone with no family living in a community with limited services.

Wherever possible, the person with the disease should take part in discussions concerning whether to continue living alone.

Some Factors to Consider

Overall well-being:

- Does the person have a good quality of life at home?
- Is there enough stimulation during the day?
- Could the person benefit from the level of care and support provided by another environment, such as a son or daughter's home, retirement home, or long-term care facility?

Health:

- Is the person able to take medication properly?
- If sick, would the person be able to understand and take appropriate action, such as calling for help?
- Is the person able to take care of personal hygiene, such as bathing and toileting?
- Are there current or past health problems that might put the person at risk of harm?

Nutrition:

- Is the person able to maintain a proper weight?
- Is the person able to eat nutritiously throughout the day?
- Is the person able to store foods properly?

Safety:

- Is the person at risk of harm? If yes, is the amount of risk acceptable to the person, to family members, to caregivers?
- Is it possible to find a level of risk with which everyone is comfortable? For example, the risk of falling on the stairs might be considered an acceptable risk if the person has no problems with balance or walking.
- Does the person pose a risk to others? For example, does the person live in an apartment and regularly cause fires with the stove or cigarettes?

- Is the person able to react and take action in an emergency, such as a fire?

- Is the person's home safe? For example, are stairs well lit?

- Are there handrails?

Finances:

- Can the person handle day-to-day financial transactions, such as keeping track of bills and paying bills promptly?

- Is the person at risk of exploitation or abuse regarding finances?

The day-to-day strategies in Table 41.1 may help provide support to a person with Alzheimer's disease who lives alone. The abilities of the person should be assessed before initiating any of these strategies.

In Closing

Living in a place that is safe, familiar, and comfortable is important to everyone, including people with Alzheimer's disease. A diagnosis of Alzheimer's disease does not automatically mean that a person is incapable of living alone. Some people may be capable of living on their own for some time after the diagnosis. Others may be at too much risk to continue living alone. It is often difficult to decide when a person living at home is at too much risk to continue living alone. However, a premature move from home should be avoided. Each person's living situation should be monitored and assessed carefully, as the disease progresses.

Some of the barriers to making informed decisions about a person's ability to live at home include privacy of information regulations, availability of community support programs and competency legislation. With growing numbers of people with Alzheimer's disease living on their own, there is a need for more public discussion of these issues.

Resources

"Freedom Fading: On Dementia, Best Interests, and Public Safety." Bruce Jennings, *Georgia Law Review* 2001;35(2): 593–619.

At Home with Alzheimer's Disease: Useful adaptations to the home environment. Canada Mortgage and Housing Corporation, 2001. Also available at: www.cmhc-schl.gc.ca or 800-668-2642.

Table 41.1. Strategies to Enhance Independent Living

Concern	Strategy	Benefits	Drawbacks
Safety	Leave a set of house keys with trusted neighbours.	Access to the home is available. Someone can enter if there is a problem.	Neighbours not always at home.
	Arrange for someone to call or visit once a day.	Regular checks can reassure person as well as family. May be able to monitor areas of concern.	Only once a day. Problems may arise at other times.
	Register with Alzheimer's Association's Safe Return program.	Provides peace of mind for the person and family should the person wander away from home and become confused.	
	Appliance safety measures: Automatic shut off kettle; Stove safety— remove fuses, put burners on timers, shut off gas; lower temperature of hot water heater.	Minimizes the chance of accident.	Some people may find the changes confusing or frustrating.
	Emergency call system	Person has 24-hour access to help should a problem arise.	Person may not be able to understand concept or use of call button.
Daily living	Get help with tasks, such as housekeeping and meal preparation.	Someone is in the home to supervise activity and provide companionship. Tasks get accomplished.	Person with disease may be reluctant or resistant to accepting help.
	Sort closets and dresser drawers to make only the necessary clothes available.	Makes decisions about what to wear easier.	Does not help if person has trouble knowing when or how to dress.

Continued on next page

Table 41.1. Strategies to Enhance Independent Living, *continued*

Concern	Strategy	Benefits	Drawbacks
Food	Meals on Wheels	Delivery of hot meal once a day	No way to monitor if food has been eaten or stored properly.
	Provide toaster oven or microwave for heating food.	Good alternatives to stove. Allows use of pre-prepared foods with little work.	Person may not know how to use or may not be able to read or follow in-structions. Concern about use of metal in microwave.
	Use prepared foods, non-perishable foods, and foods that do not need to be stored in a refrigerator.	Preparation is easier. Less concern about spoilage.	Preparation may still be too complex. The person may not like the food.
Medication	Simplify medica-tion routines. For example, use a pill dispenser. Have someone visit to give pills.	Allows only a small supply of pills at once. Helps person take the pills on the right day and time.	Possibility for confu-sion about day and time. May not prevent per-son from taking extra medication, if more than one day's sup-ply is available.
Finances	Bank-at-home services	Person does not have to leave home. Personalized service.	Person may not be able to deal with fi-nances.
	Make someone else, such as a substitute decision-maker, responsible for han-dling finances, such as writing cheques, paying bills, monitor-ing accounts.	Allows person to manage finances with some indepen-dence yet provides protection.	Does not protect from overpayment/ nonpayment of bills, or from scams. Person may not be willing to use new methods or have someone help with finances.
	Direct deposit of cheques and direct payment of bills	This hands-free ap-proach to banking offers fewer chances for problems.	

Chapter 42

Financial Concerns and AD

Putting financial plans in place is important for everyone, but understanding money matters is especially vital for the person with dementia.

Dementia is a general term for the loss of memory, decision-making, and other intellectual abilities serious enough to interfere with daily life. Alzheimer's disease is the most common form of dementia.

Once a person is diagnosed, family and friends should help the person make financial plans. The sooner plans can begin, the more the person with dementia may be able to participate.

Getting Started

Begin putting financial plans in place as soon as the diagnosis has been made. Careful planning can help you secure a healthy financial future.

In addition to planning for the cost of care, there are many ongoing financial duties, including:

- paying bills;
- arranging for benefit claims;
- making investment decisions;
- preparing tax returns.

Get started by putting in place all of the information, resources, and support you'll need.

Gather Financial and Legal Documents

Carefully go over all financial and legal documents, even if you're already familiar with them.

Legal documents include:

- living wills;
- medical and durable powers of attorney;
- wills.

Financial documents include:

- bank and brokerage account information;
- deeds, mortgage papers, or ownership statements;
- insurance policies;
- monthly or outstanding bills;
- pension and other retirement benefit summaries;
- rental income paperwork;
- Social Security payment information;
- stock and bond certificates.

At this point, it may also be helpful to identify which necessary documents are not in place. Professional financial and legal advisers can assist you with this task.

Discuss Financial Needs and Goals

After the diagnosis, determine financial needs and goals. Discussing these early on enables the person to still understand the issues and to talk about what his or her wishes are.

Involve all other people concerned as much as possible. Talk about putting financial and care plans in place. If others are available to help, encourage the sharing of caregiving duties. Discuss how finances might be pooled to provide necessary care.

Get Professional Assistance

Now is also a good time to find the professionals you will need. They will be valuable sources of information and assistance.

Start by contacting your local Alzheimer's Association office. Our staff can match you with the right professional services, including qualified attorneys, financial planners, and accountants.

Financial Advisers

Professional financial advisers, such as financial planners and estate planning attorneys, can help you:

- identify potential financial resources;
- identify tax deductions;
- avoid bad investment decisions that could deplete your finances.

When selecting a financial adviser, check qualifications such as:

- professional credentials;
- work experience;
- educational background;
- membership in professional associations;
- areas of specialty.

Also, ask the financial adviser if he or she is familiar with elder care or long-term care planning.

Legal Advisers

Seek an experienced elder law attorney to help:

- address estate planning issues;
- prepare legal documents.

If you cannot afford legal assistance, find out if pro bono (no cost) legal aid is available in your community.

Look at Factors That Affect Income

When making financial plans for the person with dementia, be sure to consider his or her:

- age;
- types of assets;
- types of insurance;

- tax issues;

- long-term health outlook.

Costs You May Face

Begin planning a long-term budget now. Consider all the costs you might face, now and in the future. Keep in mind that Alzheimer's is a progressive disease, and the person's needs will change over time.

Costs may include:

- ongoing medical treatment for Alzheimer's, including diagnosis and follow-up visits;

- treatment for other medical conditions;

- prescription drugs;

- personal care supplies;

- adult day care services;

- in-home care services;

- full-time residential care services.

These costs vary depending upon where you live.

To learn about care options in your area, contact your local Alzheimer's Association office or visit the Alzheimer's Association Care-Source™ at www.alz.org/caresource. There you'll find a set of online tools and services that will help you coordinate and plan to pay for care. A financial adviser can help design a plan that's unique to the person's financial needs—both immediate and long-term.

How to Cover the Costs

A number of financial resources may be available to help cover the costs throughout the course of the disease. Some may apply now, others in the future.

Insurance: Health-Care Coverage

If you are 65 or older, the primary source of health care coverage is usually Medicare.

However, private insurance, a group employee plan or retiree health coverage may also be in effect. No matter what the age of the person with dementia, it's vital to keep active any existing health care plans that meet his or her needs.

Medicare covers inpatient hospital care and some of the doctors' fees and other medical items for people with Alzheimer's who are age 65 or older. Medicare also covers outpatient prescription drugs.

If the person with dementia is younger than 65, Medicare can provide coverage if he or she has been on Social Security disability for at least 24 months.

Medicare provides some home health care, including skilled nursing care and rehabilitation therapy, under certain conditions.

Custodial long-term nursing home care is not covered by Medicare. Medicare will only pay for up to 100 days of skilled nursing home care under limited circumstances. Medicare will pay for home or inpatient hospice care for qualified people who are terminally ill.

You may be able to choose a "managed care" form of Medicare, such as:

- Medicare health maintenance organization (HMO);
- preferred provider organization (PPO);
- point of service (POS) plan.

These options may provide services not covered by traditional Medicare. But these forms of Medicare usually have limits on which hospitals, doctors, and other health care providers you can use.

To learn about the many Medicare options, and whether they are right for the person with dementia, read each plan carefully. You can also contact your State Health Insurance Assistance Program (SHIP) for free one-on-one help and publications. Call us at 800-272-3900, and ask for the SHIP location nearest you.

You also may be able to supplement the person's Medicare coverage with Medigap insurance, which fills gaps in Medicare coverage, such as paying for coinsurance. The more expensive Medigap policies may cover additional items.

Learn more about Medicare: Call 800-633-4227 or visit www.medicare .gov or find your state's SHIP at www.medicare.gov/contacts/static/ allStateContacts.asp.

If the person with dementia is younger than 65 years old (considered younger-onset Alzheimer's), he or she may have private insurance, a group employee health plan, or perhaps retiree medical coverage.

If he or she changes policies, check how soon expenses from Alzheimer's disease will be covered under the new policy.

Most policies do not cover "pre-existing conditions" for up to a year. However, these exclusion periods (when coverage is not provided) don't apply in all cases.

The exclusion period won't apply if the person:

- has been covered for the past 12 or 18 months, depending on the policy,

- has already met an exclusion period, and

- has not been without health coverage for more than 62 days.

COBRA may be another option for a person younger than age 65. COBRA stands for the Consolidated Omnibus Budget Reconciliation Act of 1985. COBRA applies to employers with 20 or more employees.

Under COBRA, an employee may continue group plan coverage for up to 18, 29, or 36 months, depending on the circumstances, if he or she:

- leaves the employer;

- has his or her hours reduced to the point that he or she no longer qualifies for the health plan.

The insured employee must pay the full cost of coverage, plus up to 2 percent more to cover administrative costs.

COBRA can be especially helpful until the person with dementia:

- gets new coverage through an employer, or

- becomes eligible for Medicare.

You must activate the COBRA option within 60 days of when the person with dementia leaves work or has work hours reduced.

Some private health care plans will extend coverage under a disability extension of benefits. In other words, even though the medical plan may lapse, an insured's disability (in this case, Alzheimer's disease) remains covered.

Disability Insurance

Disability insurance provides income for a worker who can no longer work due to illness or injury.

With an employer-paid disability policy, 60 to 70 percent of a person's gross (overall total) income is usually provided. Benefits paid out of an employer-paid plan are taxed as income.

If the person with dementia bought a personal disability policy, then the benefits paid will be the amount he or she chose. The benefits from a personal disability policy are not taxed as income.

Long-Term Care Insurance

If long-term care insurance is in place, carefully review the policy to find out:

- Is Alzheimer's disease covered? Most policies say they cover Alzheimer's disease, but take a closer look to be sure.

- When can the person with dementia begin to collect benefits? Most policies require a defined level of physical or cognitive impairment.

- What is the daily benefit, and is it adjusted annually for inflation?

- How long will benefits be paid?

- Is there a maximum lifetime payout?

- What kind of care will the policy cover? Examples include skilled nursing home, assisted living, custodial care, and licensed home care.

- How long after diagnosis will the policy begin to pay? This is often called the elimination period.

- Are there tax implications for getting this money?

Unfortunately, after symptoms of Alzheimer's disease appear, it is usually no longer possible to purchase many types of insurance, like disability and long-term care insurance.

Life Insurance

Life insurance can be a source of cash.

You may be able to borrow from a life insurance policy's cash value. Or the person with dementia may be able to receive a part of the policy's face value as a loan. This is called a viatical loan and is paid off upon the person's death.

Some life insurance policies may offer accelerated death benefits. This means that some of the insurance benefits can be paid if the insured person is not expected to live beyond the next 6 to 12 months because of a terminal illness.

The payout may run as high as 90 to 95 percent of the policy's face value and will not be taxed as income.

See if any policies contain a waiver of premium rider. That means that the insured, if disabled, does not have to pay premiums to continue coverage.

393

Work-Related and Personal Resources

Employment

In the early stages of dementia it's often possible that a person will continue working. This may mean adapting job duties to fit the current level of ability.

The Americans with Disabilities Act (ADA) offers limited protection to those with Alzheimer's.

The ADA requires that companies with at least 15 or more employees make "reasonable" accommodations for job applicants and employees with physical or mental disabilities. For example, an employer may switch the worker to a less demanding job or reduce work hours.

Be sure the employer is educated about Alzheimer's disease and its symptoms.

If you think the person with dementia has been treated unfairly at work, first try to resolve the issue with the employer. If that doesn't work, you can file a claim under the ADA through the federal Equal Employment Opportunity Commission or under your state's disability law.

Employee Benefits

If the person with dementia continues to work:

- Review the employer's benefits handbook.

- Ask the benefits specialist what benefits may be available. For example, the employer may provide paid sick leave or other short-term disability benefits (usually for 1 year or less).

- Keep written confirmation of all benefits. The employee may be able to convert an employer provided life insurance policy to an individual plan.

If the person with dementia is still working, he or she may have available a flexible spending account. This allows payment for out-of-pocket medical expenses with pretax dollars, for potential savings of about 20 to 30 percent.

Retirement Benefits

Retirement plans include:

- individual retirement accounts (IRAs);

- annuities.

Benefits from retirement plans can provide critical financial resources, even if the person with dementia hasn't reached retirement age.

Pension plans typically pay benefits before retirement age to a worker defined as disabled under the plan's guidelines.

The person with dementia may also be able to withdraw money from his or her IRA or employee-funded retirement plan before age 59 1/2 without paying the typical 10 percent early withdrawal penalty.

This money usually will be considered regular income, and taxes will have to be paid on the amount withdrawn.

In that case, if withdrawals can be delayed until after the person leaves work, income taxes due will likely be less because he or she will probably fall into a lower income-tax bracket.

Social Security benefits are also available before retirement age if Social Security disability requirements are met.

Personal Savings, Investments, and Personal Property

Investment assets like these can be sources of income:

- Stocks

- Bonds

- Savings accounts

- Real estate

- Personal property, such as jewelry or artwork

For example, the equity in a home could be converted into income, a process called a reverse mortgage. This is a type of home equity loan that allows a person age 62 or older to convert some of the equity in his or her home into cash while remaining the homeowner.

The amount the person is eligible to borrow is generally based on the:

- person's age;

- home's equity;

- lender's interest rate.

Reverse mortgages do not have an impact on Social Security or Medicare benefits, but they may affect qualifying for other government programs.

Government Assistance

In addition to Medicare, the person with dementia may qualify for a number of public programs. These programs provide income support or long-term care services to people who are eligible.

Social Security Disability Income (SSDI)

A worker who is younger than age 65 may qualify for Social Security disability payments.

To qualify for SSDI, the person must meet the Social Security Administration's definition of disability. Meeting the definition of disability generally means proving that:

- the person with dementia is unable to work in any occupation;

- the condition will last at least a year or is expected to result in death.

Family members also may be eligible to receive SSDI benefits. File for SSDI benefits as soon as possible:

- Benefits do not begin until the sixth full month of disability.

- The Social Security Administration often takes a long time to decide whether to approve a claim.

- It's not unusual for disability applicants to be rejected initially. Be prepared to appeal. Your professional advisers can assist in this process.

After receiving SSDI benefits for at least 24 months, the person with dementia will qualify for Medicare benefits.

Supplemental Security Income (SSI)

SSI guarantees a minimum monthly income for people who:

- are age 65 or older,

- are disabled or blind, and

- have very limited income and assets—these asset and income levels vary from state to state.

To qualify for SSI benefits, the person with dementia must meet the Social Security Administration's definition of disability.

If you think he or she qualifies for SSI benefits, begin the application process as quickly as possible after the diagnosis. SSI payments begin upon approval of the application.

Learn more about SSDI and SSI: Call 800-772-1213 or visit www .ssa.gov.

Medicaid

Medicaid is a program jointly funded by federal and state governments. It is administered by each state.

Medicaid pays for:

• medical care for people with very low income and asset levels;

• long-term care for people who have used up most of their own money, under most circumstances.

Most Medicaid dollars go toward nursing home care, but most states have home- and community-care options for some people who qualify for nursing home care. (Not all nursing homes accept Medicaid, so choices are limited.)

In most states, Medicaid will pay for hospice care. If the person with dementia is eligible for SSI, he or she usually is automatically eligible for Medicaid.

Those not on SSI must have minimal income and assets. The amount is determined by each state.

There are also specific guidelines about protecting spouses from impoverishment (the depleting of finances) in determining income and asset levels. The person with dementia should be very careful about giving away assets to family members to qualify for Medicaid. Strict laws govern this area.

Be sure you are fully aware of the legal and financial results of transferring property and wealth. Check with your legal adviser before you proceed.

Learn more about Medicaid:

• Your state's Medicaid telephone number may be listed in the blue (government) pages of the telephone directory.

• Call the general information telephone number for your state or county human services or social services department.

• Visit www.cms.hhs.gov/medicaid.

Veterans Benefits

Veterans may qualify for government benefits, including health and long-term care. These benefits often change, so call a Veterans Affairs benefits counselor or visit the VA website for the latest information.

Learn more about veterans benefits—Contact the Department of Veterans Affairs: Call 877-222-8387 for health care benefits; call 800-827-1000 for general benefits; or visit www.va.gov.

Other Public Programs

Many states have state-funded, long-term care, including:

- adult day care;
- respite care.

Learn more about other public programs:

- Local Alzheimer's Association office
- Local Area Agency on Aging or the Eldercare Locator: Call 800-677-1116 or visit www.eldercare.gov.

Tax Benefits

Some financial benefits are available for the caregiver from the Internal Revenue Service (IRS):

- Income tax deductions
- Income tax credits

The person with dementia is likely considered your dependent for tax purposes. If so, you may be allowed to itemize his or her medical costs. Keep careful records of all medical expenses. You may be entitled to the Household and Dependent Care Credit if you need to pay someone to care for the person so you can work. This credit can be subtracted directly from the tax shown on your return.

Learn more about tax issues:

- Alzheimer's Association publication, Taxes and Alzheimer's disease, available from your local chapter or at www.alz.org
- Your tax adviser
- Internal Revenue Service (IRS): Call 800-829-1040 or visit www.irs.gov

Financial Help That You Provide

You may choose to pay out of your own pocket for some or most of the care. Review your own resources, such as savings and insurance policies.

Flexible Spending Account

If the person with dementia is a dependent under the tax rules, you might be able to use your own workplace flexible spending account. This money can cover the person's out-of-pocket medical costs or dependent care expenses in some cases.

Family and Medical Leave Act

If you work for an employer with 50 or more employees, you may be able to use the federal Family and Medical Leave Act (FMLA) to help balance your caregiving responsibilities. FMLA allows you to take off up to 12 weeks of unpaid leave each year to provide caregiving. Most workers are guaranteed to keep their jobs.

Paid Time Off

Some employers provided limited paid time off. You may be able to adjust your schedule or work fewer hours.

In-Home Care

If you hire a professional to work in your home to help with caregiving, you may be responsible for paying his or her Social Security and unemployment taxes. Ask your financial adviser to be sure.

Support Services in Your Community

Many community organizations provide low-cost or even free services, including:

- respite care;
- support groups;
- transportation to social events;
- meals delivered to the home.

Learn more about support services:

- Your local Alzheimer's Association office

- Eldercare Locator: Call 800-677-1116 or visit www.eldercare.gov

- Your local religious organization

- Hospital social worker or discharge planner

Learn more about financial issues and planning by visiting your local Alzheimer's Association or one of the following resources:

Alzheimer's Association CareSource™

Website: www.alz.org/caresource

Benefits CheckUp

Website: www.benefitscheckup.org

Eldercare Locator

Toll-Free: 800-677-1116
Website: www.eldercare.gov

Financial Planning Association

Toll-Free: 800-322-4237
Website: www.fpanet.org

Internal Revenue Service

Toll-Free: 800-829-1040
Website: www.irs.gov

National Academy of Elder Law Attorneys

Website: www.naela.com

Ten Quick Tips: Money Matters

1. Don't put off talking about finances and future care wishes.

2. Organize and review important documents.

3. Get help from well qualified financial and legal advisers.

4. Estimate possible costs for the entire disease process.

5. Look at all of your insurance options.

6.   Work-related salary/benefits and personal property should be considered as potential income.

7.   Find out for which government programs you are eligible.

8.   Learn about income tax breaks for which you may qualify.

9.   Explore financial assistance you can personally provide.

10.   Take advantage of low-cost and free community services.

Chapter 43

Medicare and AD

Chapter Contents

Section 43.1

Understanding Medicare

"Medicare," © 2010 Fisher Center for Alzheimer's
Research Foundation. Reprinted with permission.
For additional information, visit www.alzinfo.com.

What is the difference between Medicaid and Medicare?

This is a very common question. Medicaid is a type of government program that offers health insurance to people with limited incomes. It is available to people of all ages, including children, and it can vary from state to state.

Medicare, on the other hand, is a government health insurance program only available to people 65 and over, people under 65 with certain disabilities, and people of all ages with end-stage renal disease.

What is the difference between Medicare Part A, Part B, Part C, and Part D?

- Part A is hospital insurance.

- Part B helps pay for general medical services that Part A doesn't cover.

- Part C is called Medicare Advantage. If you have Parts A and B, you can choose this option to receive all of your health care through a provider organization, like an HMO.

- Part D is prescription drug coverage. It helps pay for some medicines.

Medicare Part A, Hospital Insurance helps cover inpatient care in hospitals, including critical access hospitals, and skilled nursing facilities (not custodial or long-term care). It also helps cover hospice care and some home health care, but it does not usually cover dental, vision, and prescription drugs. Certain conditions must be met to get these benefits. Many people do not have to pay a monthly premium for Part A because they or a spouse paid Medicare taxes while working.

Most people are enrolled in Part A when they turn 65. To see if you are enrolled, look at your Medicare card and if you are covered, it will list Hospital Part A.

Medicare Part B, Medical Insurance helps cover doctors' services and outpatient care. It also covers some other medical services that Part A doesn't cover, such as some of the services of physical and occupational therapists, and some home health care. Part B helps pay for these covered services and supplies when they are medically necessary.

Medicare Part B is optional. You can sign up for Part B anytime during a 7-month period, which begins 3 months before you turn 65. Unlike Medicare Part A, Medicare Part B does have a premium, which is paid each month, and there is also a deductible. Part B is typically paid for out of your Social Security check or a civil retirement plan payment. There may be state funds available to help cover the costs of the monthly premium and the deductible, so if you are concerned about these costs, you should contact your local Medicare office. Use our Resource Locator [http://www.alzinfo.org/resource-locator] to find the office nearest you.

Medicare Advantage, Part C is a health insurance plan offered by a private company that is approved by Medicare. These plans offer you all the protection of Medicare Part A and Medicare Part B, plus extra coverage on things like vision, hearing, dental, and/or health and wellness programs. Most plans will also offer prescription drug coverage.

Medicare Part D is Medicare prescription drug coverage run by private companies approved by Medicare. There are two types of plans:

- Medicare Prescription Drug Plans: These plans (sometimes called "PDPs") add drug coverage to Original Medicare, some Medicare Cost Plans, some Medicare Private Fee-for-Service (PFFS) Plans, and Medicare Medical Savings Account (MSA) Plans. You must have Medicare Part A and/or Medicare Part B to be eligible for the PDPs.

- Medicare Advantage Plans (like an HMO or PPO) are other Medicare health plans that offer Medicare prescription drug coverage. You get all of your Part A and Part B coverage, and prescription drug coverage (Part D), through these plans. Medicare Advantage Plans with prescription drug coverage are sometimes called "MA-PDs." In order to be eligible for this plan, you must have Medicare Part A and Medicare Part B.

Does Medicare cover care for people with Alzheimer's?

Thanks to a recent, important policy change, Medicare beneficiaries can no longer be denied coverage for mental health services, hospice care, and home healthcare solely because they have Alzheimer's disease or any other preexisting condition. Prior to this policy change, people with Alzheimer's could be denied coverage for such services.

The services Medicare now covers include "reasonable and necessary" doctors' visits; physical, occupational, or speech therapy; psychotherapy or behavioral management therapy by a mental health professional; and skilled home-care services (such as skilled nursing, speech, or physical therapy).

Another policy change, which was officially in place as of late 2001 but only became public in March 2002, reflects recent scientific evidence indicating that people with Alzheimer's can often benefit from mental health services and specialized types of therapy. Alzheimer's experts say the new rules will enable people with the disease to stay at home longer by providing access to services that help improve activities of daily living and help people with the disease maintain a better quality of life.

Medicare still does not pay for prescription drugs for Alzheimer's (unless you enroll in Medicare Part C or D), adult day care, room and board at assisted-living facilities, or custodial care in a nursing home, though it will pay for medically necessary skilled-care services at assisted-living facilities or nursing homes.

I have questions about Medicare. Who do I contact?

Medicare can seem complicated, but do not worry, there is help available. Find your local Medicare office through our Resource Locator [http://www.alzinfo.org/resource-locator] or call the Medicare Help Line to get your questions answered at 800-MEDICARE. You can also read more online at Medicare.gov.

Sources

U.S. Department of Health and Human Services, Centers for Medicare and Medicaid Services: http://www.cms.gov

Medicare.gov: The Official US Government Site for Medicare: http://www.medicare.gov

MedlinePlus, National Institutes of Health: http://www.nlm.nih.gov/medlineplus/medicare.html

Section 43.2

Choosing a Medicare Drug Plan for People with AD

Prescription drug coverage is available to all Medicare beneficiaries. All plans made changes for 2011. If you (or a family member) enrolled in a drug plan in 2010, you should have received a letter explaining what changes it made in 2011. It is important to review the changes, especially the list of covered drugs (formulary) to make sure the plan is still best for you. If you (or a family member) have Alzheimer's disease, you should consider the following important factors before making a decision about which drug plan is right for you.

If you currently have drug coverage through an employer, union, government agency, or other organization that is "as good as" the Medicare benefit, you may not want to sign up for a Medicare drug plan at this time. In November, you should receive a letter or booklet from your current provider indicating if your coverage is "as good as" the new drug benefit. You will need to decide if you are happy with your current plan or whether you want to get your drug coverage through Medicare.

Important Change to Medicare Drug Coverage: Beginning January 1, 2011, for the first time, you will not have to pay all of the costs of your drugs while you are in the coverage gap. You will get a 50% discount on brand name prescription drugs on your plan's formulary while you are in the coverage gap. You will get this discount at the time you buy the drugs. You will get a 7% discount of the cost of generic drugs on the plan's formulary during the coverage gap. These changes do not apply if you already receive Extra Help.

Key Things to Consider

All plans are not the same. Here are important factors to consider when choosing a plan:

Will the drug plan pay for all or most of the drugs you take now?

Each plan has a list of drugs for which it will pay. This is called a formulary. Are your current drugs on the plan's formulary? Are your Alzheimer drugs on the formulary? At least two cholinesterase inhibiters and memantine must be on every plan formulary.

Does the plan cover the doses of the drugs that you take? Check the plan formulary to make sure it covers the actual doses that you take. For example, not all plans cover Aricept 23 mg on their formularies although you can file a formal request (called an exception) for the plan to cover it.

Do the plan's rules or policies limit coverage of your Alzheimer drugs and/or your more costly drugs by requiring prior approval or by requiring you to try a less expensive, similar drug (step therapy) before the plan will pay for your drug(s)? Are there limits on the number of pills that a prescription may cover (quantity limits) over a specific period of time?

What will the plan cost you?

Compare the monthly premiums for each plan, the annual deductible, and cost sharing for each drug you currently take that is covered by the plan. For an additional premium, some plans will provide some drug coverage in the coverage gap (donut hole). Remember, if one or more of your drugs is not on the plan's formulary, you may have to pay the entire cost of the drug(s) yourself. This is especially important this year because the cost-sharing for Medicare beneficiaries has increased significantly in many drug plans.

Be sure to compare all of the costs for each plan, including the deductible, copayments, or co-insurance, not just the amount of the monthly premiums.

Is my local pharmacy in the plan's pharmacy network?

For each plan, find out if your pharmacy is in the plan's network. If it is in the network, find out if it is a preferred pharmacy. For some plans, your co-payments may be less if you buy your drugs from a preferred pharmacy.

If you prefer to use mail order for your drugs, does the plan offer it as an option?

Review Your Current Plan, Compare It to Other Plans, and Make a Decision

Take your time and consider the information about the drug plans and evaluate your choices. Call the provider to confirm all the information you have about the plan before you make a decision. If you are staying with your current plan, you don't have to do anything. If you decide to change plans, you need to complete the enrollment form by phone, online, or mail.

Where to Get Plan Information

Get the information necessary to make your decision from several sources:

- Medicare's website at www.medicare.gov: It has information about which plans are available in each state and which drugs each plan will cover. It also has several tools to help individuals decide which plan is best for them.

- Medicare's toll-free number at 800-MEDICARE: Call for information about the plans available in each state.

- Each plan's website or customer service telephone number: You can get this information from www.medicare.gov or 800-MEDICARE.

- The Alzheimer's Association website has fact sheets on the Medicare drug benefit and Alzheimer's disease at www.alz.org.

- Medicare Access for Patients Rx (MAPRx): Access information and interactive tools to help evaluate Medicare drug plan options at www.maprx.info.

Questions and Answers

For the Medicare beneficiary who has Alzheimer's disease, there are some special considerations to think about before choosing a drug plan.

Will the Medicare drug plans cover Alzheimer drugs?

Yes. Through the Association's advocacy efforts, all Medicare drug plans are required to cover and have at least two cholinesterase

409

inhibitors and memantine on their formularies (list of drugs the plan covers). Each plan will decide what the co-payment amount is for each drug. Plans are allowed to charge different amounts for different drugs. Consumers will need to check with each plan to find out the specific amount of the co-payment for specific drugs.

Is it true that Medicare will not pay for Xanax, Valium, Ativan, and other benzodiazepines?

Yes. Standard or basic Medicare drug plans are forbidden by law from paying for benzodiazepines, such as Xanax, Valium, and Ativan. In addition, Medicare will not pay for barbiturates (such as Phenobarbital or Nembutal), which are often used for sedation or to control seizures. State Medicaid programs and state pharmacy assistance programs may still pay for them. In addition, Medicare drug plans can offer supplemental or additional benefits beyond the standard Medicare package for an additional premium. These enhanced plans can cover benzodiazepines, barbiturates, or other medications not covered by Medicare.

Will Medicare drug plans cover antidepressants and anti-anxiety drugs which are often prescribed to Alzheimer beneficiaries?

Yes. Medicare plans must cover "all or substantially all" antidepressants (such as Celexa and Zoloft), antipsychotics (such as Abilify, Zyprexa, Seroquel, and Risperdal), and anticonvulsants (such as Tegretol and Depakote), which many Medicare beneficiaries with Alzheimer's disease need.

Can a Medicare drug plan put restrictions on access to drugs even if the drugs are on the formulary?

Yes. The Medicare drug plans can require that individuals get prior approval from the plan for specific drugs before the plan will pay for it. This is called prior authorization.

In addition, plans can require that an individual try a different, less expensive drug before agreeing to pay for the one originally prescribed by the doctor. This is often called step therapy or fail first. However, an individual can request that step therapy or fail first not be required if the individual or the treating doctor can prove that there would be adverse effects or the prescribed drug would be more effective.

Some health plans have specific policies on how much of a drug is covered by limiting the number of pills or number of days a prescription may cover. This is called quantity limits. The Alzheimer's Association has developed a chart that provides information about which of the national plans require prior approval, step therapy, or quantity limits for the Alzheimer drugs. The chart is available on the website: www .alz.org.

If my mother has Alzheimer's and does not have the capacity to sign up for a plan, who can do it for her?

Medicare rules allow an individual who has legal authority under state law to act on behalf of the beneficiary (your mom) to enroll or disenroll her from a Medicare drug plan.

Depending on the state law where your mom lives, this may include attorneys-in-fact or agents who have authority under a durable power of attorney document, guardians appointed by the court, or individuals authorized to make healthcare decisions under state health care consent laws.

My father has Alzheimer's disease, takes several medications, and is stable. If one or more of his current drugs are not on his drug plan's formulary, is there anything he can do to get the drugs paid for by his plan?

Yes. Your father, his authorized representative, or his treating physician can ask the plan to cover the non-formulary drug for him. This request is called an "exception" and generally requires a physician's statement in support of the request. You can get specific information about the exceptions process from the drug plan organization.

Section 43.3

Medicare's Hospice Benefit for People with AD

What is hospice care?

Hospice is a special way of caring for people who are terminally ill, and for their family. This care includes physical care and counseling. Hospice provides palliative or comfort care for an individual at the end-of-life. The primary purpose of hospice care is to manage the pain and other symptoms of the terminal illness, rather than provide treatment for the illness.

How does my father become eligible to receive hospice under Medicare?

Medicare covers hospice care if:

- your father has Medicare Part A;

- his physician and a hospice medical director certifies that he is terminally ill, that is, his life expectancy is 6 months or less, if the illness runs its normal course; and,

- he chooses or elects to receive hospice care and gives up (waives) the right for Medicare to pay for any other services to treat the terminal illness. Instead, Medicare pays the hospice and any related physician expenses. Medicare will continue to pay for your father's care for any services not related to the terminal illness.

Are there guidelines to determine if someone with Alzheimer's disease is terminally ill?

The National Hospice and Palliative Care Organization has published guidelines to help identify which dementia patients are likely

412

to have a prognosis of 6 months or less, if the disease runs its normal course. Remember, these are only guidelines to assist doctors in determining whether a patient may be appropriate for hospice care. Some Medicare contractors, that are responsible for paying the hospice claims, have specific rules for payment of hospice for dementia patients.

What services can my wife receive from a hospice under Medicare?

Under the hospice benefit, Medicare will pay for your wife's:

- physician's services;
- nursing services;
- physical, occupational, and speech therapy;
- medical social services;
- home health aide and homemaker services;
- counseling services for your wife and your family;
- short-term inpatient care;
- respite care;
- prescription drugs;
- medical appliances and supplies;
- and bereavement counseling for your family.

Where can my mother receive these services?

Your mother can receive hospice care at home, in a free-standing hospice facility, or in a hospital or nursing facility. If your mother is a resident of a nursing facility, Medicare will only pay for the hospice services provided, not for her room and board.

What will hospice care cost my husband?

There will be no deductibles and only limited coinsurance payments for his hospice services. Your husband will have to pay 5 percent of the cost of a drug or biological, not to exceed $5. For respite care, there is a coinsurance payment of 5 percent of the Medicare payment for each respite care day.

413

How long can my wife receive hospice services?

Your wife may elect to receive benefits for two periods of 90 days each, and an unlimited number of periods of 60 days each. If at any time she changes her mind, she can decide to stop receiving hospice care and immediately begin to receive her other Medicare benefits.

For Additional Information

- Centers for Medicare and Medicaid Services (www.cms.hhs.gov)

- Medicare Website (www.medicare.gov)

- National Hospice and Palliative Care Organization (www.nhpco.org)

Chapter 44

Getting Your Affairs in Order

Chapter Contents

415

Section 44.1

Planning for the Future

From "Getting Your Affairs in Order," by the National Institute on Aging (NIA, www.nia.nih.gov), part of the National Institutes of Health, May 2010.

Ben has been married for 47 years. He always managed the family's money. But since his stroke, Ben can't walk or talk. His wife, Shirley, feels overwhelmed. Of course, she's worried about Ben's health. But on top of that, she has no idea what bills should be paid or when they are due.

Across town, 80-year-old Louise lives alone. One night, she fell in the kitchen and broke her hip. She spent a week in the hospital and 2 months in a rehabilitation nursing home. Even though her son lives across the country, he was able to pay her bills and handle her Medicare questions right away. That's because, several years ago, Louise and her son made a plan about what he should do in case Louise had a medical emergency.

Plan for the Future

No one ever plans to be sick or disabled. Yet, it's just this kind of planning that can make all the difference in an emergency. Long before she fell, Louise had put all her important papers in one place and told her son where to find them. She gave him the name of her lawyer as well as a list of people he could contact at her bank, doctor's office, insurance company, and investment firm. She made sure he had copies of her Medicare and other health insurance cards. She added her son's name to her checking account, allowing him to write checks from that account. His name is on her safe deposit box at the bank as well. Louise made sure Medicare and her doctor had written permission to talk with her son about her health or any insurance claims.

On the other hand, Ben always took care of family money matters, and he never talked about the details with Shirley. No one but Ben knew that his life insurance policy was in a box in the closet or that the car title and deed to the house were filed in his desk drawer. Ben never expected that his wife would have to take over. His lack of planning has made a tough job even tougher for Shirley.

Steps for Getting Your Affairs in Order

- Put your important papers and copies of legal documents in one place. You could set up a file, put everything in a desk or dresser drawer, or just list the information and location of papers in a notebook. If your papers are in a bank safe deposit box, keep copies in a file at home. Check each year to see if there's anything new to add.

- Tell a trusted family member or friend where you put all your important papers. You don't need to tell this friend or family member about your personal affairs, but someone should know where you keep your papers in case of emergency. If you don't have a relative or friend you trust, ask a lawyer to help.

- Give consent in advance for your doctor or lawyer to talk with your caregiver as needed. There may be questions about your care, a bill, or a health insurance claim. Without your consent, your caregiver may not be able to get needed information. You can give your okay in advance to Medicare, a credit card company, your bank, or your doctor. You may need to sign and return a form.

Legal Documents

There are many different types of legal documents that can help you plan how your affairs will be handled in the future. Many of these documents have names that sound alike, so make sure you are getting the documents you want. Also, state laws do vary, so find out about the rules, requirements, and forms used in your state.

- Wills and trusts let you name the person you want your money and property to go to after you die.

- Advance directives let you make arrangements for your care if you become sick. There are two ways to do this:

  - A living will gives you a say in your health care if you are too sick to make your wishes known. In a living will, you can state what kind of care you do or don't want. This can make it easier for family members to make tough health care decisions for you.

  - A durable power of attorney for health care lets you name the person you want to make medical decisions for you if you can't make them yourself. Make sure the person you name is willing to make those decisions for you.

417

For legal matters, there are two ways to give someone you trust the power to act in your place:

- A durable power of attorney allows you to name someone to act on your behalf for any legal task. It stays in place if you become unable to make your own decisions.

- A general power of attorney also lets you give someone else the authority to act on your behalf, but this power will end if you are unable to make your own decisions.

What Exactly Is an Important Paper?

The answer to this question may be different for every family. The following lists can help you decide what is important for you. Remember, this is a starting place. You may have other information to add. For example, if you have a pet, you will want to include the name and address of your vet.

Personal Records

- Full legal name
- Social Security number
- Legal residence
- Date and place of birth
- Names and addresses of spouse and children
- Location of birth and death certificates and certificates of marriage, divorce, citizenship, and adoption
- Employers and dates of employment
- Education and military records
- Names and phone numbers of religious contacts
- Memberships in groups and awards received
- Names and phone numbers of close friends, relatives, and lawyer or financial advisor
- Names and phone numbers of doctors
- Medications taken regularly
- Location of living will

Financial Records

- Sources of income and assets (retirement funds, IRAs, 401(k)s, interest, etc.)

- Social Security and Medicare information

- Insurance information (life, health, long-term care, home, car) with policy numbers and agents' names and phone numbers

- Names of your banks and account numbers (checking, savings, credit union)

- Investment income (stocks, bonds, property) and stockbrokers' names and phone numbers

- Copy of most recent income tax return

- Location of most up-to-date will with an original signature

- Liabilities, including property tax—what is owed, to whom, when payments are due

- Mortgages and debts—how and when paid

- Location of original deed of trust for home and car title and registration

- Credit and debit card names and numbers

- Location of safe deposit box and key

Resources

You may want to talk with a lawyer about setting up a general power of attorney, durable power of attorney, joint account, trust, or advance directive. Be sure to ask about the fees before you make an appointment.

You should be able to find a directory of local lawyers at your library or you can contact your local bar association for lawyers in your area. An informed family member may be able to help you manage some of these issues.

Section 44.2

Elder Law Attorneys

What is an elder law attorney?

Elder law attorneys focus on the special legal needs of older persons and persons with disability to protect their autonomy, quality of life, and financial security as they age.

Most elder law attorneys do not handle all legal issues affecting the elderly. It is important that you find out whether the attorney regularly handles matters in the area in which you need assistance.

What role does an elder law attorney play?

An elder law attorney must be knowledgeable about both identifying and addressing the problems facing the elderly or disabled client, and how those problems can be handled within the state laws. Issues that may be addressed include: (1) qualification for Medicare and Medicaid benefits or other public benefits; (2) effective estate planning, using durable powers of attorney, trusts, wills, and other legal/financial tools; (3) substitute decision making in the event of incapacity; and (4) planning for the possible need for long-term care for the disabled client. For example, a client who has a disabled spouse may wish to focus on issues that may arise in the event of the client's death.

An elder law attorney may also draft durable powers of attorney and health care proxy forms, as well as handle guardianship matters. The elder law attorney's job does not necessarily end with the preparation of required documentation. There may be a need to review your situation periodically to ensure that past solutions are suitable for today and in the future. Therefore, an ongoing relationship with an attorney may be appropriate.

When should an elder law attorney be contacted?

In the case of an elderly person whose health is declining or who has been diagnosed with a debilitating disorder, an elder law attorney should be contacted. If an elder law attorney is contacted at an early stage, there may be more options available.

Following is a list of questions compiled by the New York City Department for the Aging that can assist you in preparing for a visit with an attorney. The goal of the questions is to establish the needs of the family as well as the person who has Alzheimer's, the emotional environment of the family, and the availability of the family and others to assist in the future care of the person with Alzheimer's disease.

Most of the questions can be answered without the advice of an attorney. Do as many as you can and bring the results with you to your first attorney visit.

- Describe the current stage of the illness.

- What needs are being met?

- How well is the person with Alzheimer's able to care for him/herself?

- To what extent can he/she handle financial affairs?

- Can he/she live at home at present and how soon will assistance in daily living activities be needed?

- Does he/she have any disabilities?

- Do insurance or entitlements cover the disabilities?

- What are the overall financial needs of this family member?

- Will he/she qualify for any federal or state benefits? Which ones?

- What needs do you (as the well spouse/child/friend) have as a caregiver? Are you likely to become disabled?

- Who will look after the person with Alzheimer's in the event of your disability or death?

- Are there other family members who must or should be provided for, such as a child with a disability? What are their needs?

- How will others feel if the needs of the person with Alzheimer's deplete the available resources? How will they react toward him/her?

- Are there other family members or friends who are willing to help? On what basis? Do they have the time and necessary expertise? Can they be trained to handle the problems?

421

- When naming someone to hold power of attorney or healthcare proxy, can you trust the person to carry out wishes and/or act in the best interests of the person with Alzheimer's?

- If no family member or friend can or will help, you may need outside help. Who can help you? What will you have to pay for such help?

- What are your long-term goals for yourself and for the person with Alzheimer's?

- What are the person's assets and liabilities? Carefully inventory all assets, all sources of income, and all liabilities.

How do I find an elder law attorney?

An elder law attorney can be contacted either by referral from a trusted advisor or by a close review of the attorney's credentials. You should consider the attorney's activity in professional and community organizations as well as other credentials. Use the Resource Locator [http://www.alzinfo.org/resource-locator] to find an attorney near you.

How do I choose an elder law attorney?

Ask lots of questions before selecting and elder law attorney. You don't want to end up in the office of an attorney who can't help you. Start with the initial phone call. It is not unusual to speak only to a secretary, receptionist, or office manager during an initial call or before actually meeting with the attorney. If so, ask this person your questions.

- How long has the attorney been in practice?

- Does his/her practice emphasize a particular area of law?

- How long has he/she been in this field?

- What percentage of his/her practice is devoted to elder law?

- Is there a fee for the first consultation and if so, how much is it?

- Given the nature of your problem, what information should you bring with you to the initial consultation?

The answers to your questions will assist you in determining whether that particular attorney has those qualifications important to you for a successful attorney/client relationship. If you have a specific legal issue that requires immediate attention, be sure to inform the office of this during the initial telephone conversation.

How much does an elder law attorney cost?

There are many different ways of charging fees and each attorney will choose to work differently. Be aware of how your attorney charges. You will also want to know how often he/she bills. Some attorneys bill weekly, some bill monthly, some bill upon completion of work. Ask about these matters at the initial conference, so there will be no surprises! If you don't understand, ask again. If you need clarification, say so. It is very important that you feel comfortable in this area.

Some attorneys charge by the hour with different hourly rates for work performed by attorneys, paralegals, and secretaries. If this is the case, find out what the rates are. Other attorneys charge a flat fee for all or part of the services. This is not unusual, for example, if you are having documents prepared. Your attorney might use a combination of these billing methods.

In addition to fees, most attorneys will charge you out-of-pocket expenses. Out-of-pocket expenses typically include charges for copies, postage, messenger fees, court fees, disposition fees, long distance telephone calls, and other such costs. Find out if there will be any other incidental costs.

The attorney may ask for a retainer. This is money paid before the attorney starts working on your case. It is usually placed in a trust account and each time the attorney bills you, he/she pays himself or herself out of that account. Expenses may be paid directly from the trust account. The size of the retainer may range from a small percentage of the estimated cost to the full amount.

Sources: National Academy of Elder Law Attorneys, Inc., Questions and Answers When Looking for an Elder Law Attorney [http://www .naela.org]; "Caring: A Guide to Caring for Persons with Alzheimer's Disease," New York City Department for the Aging, Alzheimer's and Long-Term-Care Unit.

Section 44.3

Legal and Health Care Planning Documents

From "Legal and Financial Planning for People with Alzheimer's Disease
Fact Sheet," by the National Institute on Aging (NIA, www.nia.nih.gov),
part of the National Institutes of Health, August 2010.

Many people are unprepared to deal with the legal and financial consequences of a serious illness such as Alzheimer disease. Legal and medical experts encourage people recently diagnosed with a serious illness—particularly one that is expected to cause declining mental and physical health—to examine and update their financial and health care arrangements as soon as possible. Basic legal and financial instruments, such as a will, a living trust, and advance directives, are available to ensure that the person's late-stage or end-of-life health care and financial decisions are carried out.

A complication of diseases such as Alzheimer disease is that the person may lack or gradually lose the ability to think clearly. This change affects his or her ability to participate meaningfully in decision making and makes early legal and financial planning even more important. Although difficult questions often arise, advance planning can help people with Alzheimer disease and their families clarify their wishes and make well-informed decisions about health care and financial arrangements.

When possible, advance planning should take place soon after a diagnosis of early-stage Alzheimer disease while the person can participate in discussions. People with early-stage disease are often capable of understanding many aspects and consequences of legal decision making. However, legal and medical experts say that many forms of planning can help the person and his or her family even if the person is diagnosed with later-stage Alzheimer disease.

There are good reasons to retain the services of a lawyer when preparing advance planning documents. For example, a lawyer can help interpret different state laws and suggest ways to ensure that the patient's and family's wishes are carried out. It's important to understand that laws vary by state, and changes in situation—for instance, a divorce, relocation, or death in the family—can influence how documents are prepared and subsequently maintained.

Legal, Financial, and Health Care Planning Documents

When families begin the legal planning process, there are a number of strategies and legal documents they need to discuss. Depending on the family situation and the applicable state laws, some or all of the following terms and documents may be introduced by the lawyer hired to assist in this process. Broadly speaking, these documents can be divided into two groups:

- Documents that communicate the health care wishes of someone who may no longer be able to make health care decisions

- Documents that communicate the financial management and estate plan wishes of someone who may no longer be able to make financial decisions

See Table 44.1 for an overview of medical, legal, and financial planning documents.

Table 44.1. Overview of Medical, Legal, and Financial Planning Documents

Medical Document	How It Is Used
Living Will	Describes and instructs how the person wants end-of-life health care managed
Durable Power of Attorney for Health Care	Gives a designated person the authority to make health care decisions on behalf of the person with Alzheimer disease
Do Not Resuscitate Form	Instructs health care professionals not to perform CPR [cardiopulmonary resuscitation] in case of stopped heart or stopped breathing
Legal/Financial Document	**How It Is Used**
Will	Indicates how a person's assets and estate will be distributed among beneficiaries after his/her death
Durable Power of Attorney for Finances	Gives a designated person the authority to make legal/financial decisions on behalf of the person with Alzheimer disease
Living Trust	Gives a designated person (trustee) the authority to hold and distribute property and funds for the person with Alzheimer disease

Advance Directives for Health Care

Advance directives for health care are documents that communicate the health care wishes of a person with Alzheimer disease. These decisions are then carried out after the person no longer can make decisions. In most cases, these documents must be prepared while the person is legally able to execute them.

A living will records a person's wishes for medical treatment near the end of life. It may do the following:

- Specify the extent of life-sustaining treatment and major health care the person wants

- Help a terminal patient die with dignity

- Protect the physician or hospital from liability for carrying out the patient's instructions

- Specify how much discretion the person gives to his or her proxy about end-of-life decisions

A durable power of attorney for health care designates a person, sometimes called an agent or proxy, to make health care decisions when the person with Alzheimer disease no longer can do so. Depending on state laws and the person's preferences, the proxy might be authorized to do the following:

- Refuse or agree to treatments

- Change health care providers

- Remove the patient from an institution

- Decide about making organ donations

- Decide about starting or continuing life support (if not specified in a living will)

- Decide whether the person with Alzheimer disease will end life at home or in a facility

- Have access to medical records

A Do Not Resuscitate (DNR) order instructs health care professionals not to perform cardiopulmonary resuscitation if a person's heart stops or if he or she stops breathing. A DNR order is signed by a doctor and put in a person's medical chart.

Access to private medical information is closely regulated. The person with AD must state in writing who can see or use personal medical records.

Advance Directives for Financial and Estate Management

Advance directives for financial and estate management must be created while the person with Alzheimer disease still can make these decisions (sometimes referred to as "having legal capacity" to make decisions). These directives may include some or all of the following documents.

A will indicates how a person's assets and estate will be distributed upon death. It also can specify the following:

- Arrangements for care of minors

- Gifts

- Trusts to manage the estate

- Funeral and/or burial arrangements

Medical and legal experts say that the newly diagnosed person with Alzheimer disease and his or her family should move quickly to make or update a will and secure the estate.

A durable power of attorney for finances names someone to make financial decisions when the person with Alzheimer disease no longer can. It can help people with the disease and their families avoid court actions that may take away control of financial affairs.

A living trust provides instructions about the person's estate and appoints someone, often referred to as the trustee, to hold title to property and funds for the beneficiaries. The trustee follows these instructions after the person no longer can manage his or her affairs.

The person with Alzheimer disease also can name the trustee as the health care proxy through the durable power of attorney for health care.

A living trust can:

- include a wide range of property;

- provide a detailed plan for property disposition;

- avoid the expense and delay of probate (in which the courts establish the validity of a will);

- state how property should be distributed when the last beneficiary dies and whether the trust should continue to benefit others.

Who Can Help?

Health care providers: Health care providers cannot act as legal or financial advisors, but they can encourage planning discussions

427

between patients and their families. Qualified clinicians can also guide patients, families, the care team, attorneys, and judges regarding the patient's ability to make decisions.

Elder law attorneys (ELAs): An ELA helps older people and families do the following:

- Interpret state laws
- Plan how their wishes will be carried out
- Understand their financial options
- Learn how to preserve financial assets while caring for a loved one

The National Academy of Elder Law Attorneys and the American Bar Association can help families find qualified ELAs.

Geriatric care managers (GCMs): GCMs are trained social workers or nurses who can help people with Alzheimer disease and their families do the following:

- Discuss difficult topics and complex issues
- Address emotional concerns
- Make short- and long-term plans
- Evaluate in-home care needs
- Select care personnel
- Coordinate medical services
- Evaluate other living arrangements
- Provide caregiver stress relief

Steps for Getting Your Affairs in Order

- Gather everything you can about your income, property, investments, insurance, and savings.
- Put copies of legal documents and other important papers in one place. You could set up a file, put everything in a desk or dresser drawer, or just list the information and location of papers in a notebook. If your papers are in a bank safe deposit box, keep copies in a file at home. Check regularly to see if there's anything new to add.
- Tell a trusted family member or friend where you put your important papers. You don't need to tell this friend or family

member your personal business, but someone should know where you keep your papers in case of emergency. If you don't have a relative or friend you trust, ask a lawyer to help.

Other Advance Planning Advice

- Start discussions early. The rate of decline differs for each person with Alzheimer disease, and his or her ability to be involved in planning will decline over time. People in the early stages of the disease may be able to understand the issues, but they may also be defensive or emotionally unable to deal with difficult questions. Remember that not all people are diagnosed at an early stage. Decision making already may be difficult when Alzheimer disease is diagnosed.

- Review plans over time. Changes in personal situations—such as a divorce, relocation, or death in the family—and in state laws can affect how legal documents are prepared and maintained. Review plans regularly, and update documents as needed.

- Reduce anxiety about funeral and burial arrangements. Advance planning for the funeral and burial can provide a sense of peace and reduce anxiety for both the person with Alzheimer disease and the family.

Resources for Low-Income Families

Families who cannot afford a lawyer still can do advance planning. Samples of basic health planning documents can be downloaded from state government websites. Area Agency on Aging officials may provide legal advice or help.

Other possible sources of legal assistance and referral include state legal aid offices, the state bar association, local nonprofit agencies, foundations, and social service agencies.

Summary

Facing Alzheimer disease can be emotionally wrenching for all concerned. A legal expert and members of the health care team can help the person and family address end-of-life issues. Advance health care and financial planning can help people diagnosed with Alzheimer disease and their families confront tough questions about future treatment, caregiving, and legal arrangements.

Section 44.4

Making End-of-Life Choices

"End-of-Life Decision-Making," © 2008 Family Caregiver Alliance. Reprinted with permission. To view the complete text of this article including recommendations for further reading and related organizations and websites, visit www.caregiver.org.

Americans are a people who plan. We plan everything: Our schedules, our careers and work projects, our weddings and vacations, our retirements. Many of us plan for the disposition of our estates after we die. The one area that most of us avoid planning is the end of our life. Yet, if we don't plan, if we don't at least think about it and share our ideas with those we love, others take over at the very time when we are most vulnerable, most in need of understanding and comfort, and most longing for dignity.

Big issues confront us when we think about our own death or that of someone we love. Our attitudes and beliefs about religion, pain, suffering, loss of consciousness, and leaving behind those we love come into play. We can let things unfold as they may, and for some of us that's exactly right. For others of us, it is good to plan.

This text is not intended to provide a comprehensive planning tool. It outlines areas we need to think about and resources that can help, whether we are caring for someone who is already incapacitated, or making decisions for ourselves.

How to Begin

Begin simply with yourself. Try to confront and understand any fears you might have: Do they relate to the possibility of pain? Loss of dignity while undergoing treatment? Not being clearly understood by those around you? Being alone? Being overly sedated or in a lingering state of unconsciousness? Leaving loved ones or unfinished projects behind? Leaving your loved ones without adequate financial resources? Dying in a strange place?

Once you know that you want to explore these topics and make some plans, most experts suggest that you begin by talking. Talk openly to family and friends about your values and beliefs, your hopes and fears about the end stage of your life and theirs. Someone who is uncomfortable with the subject can be led to talk with indirect topics. Use "openings" in conversations, such as recalling a family event and talking about a future event where you might not be present. Talk about whom you wish to leave a possession to, whom you'd like to have near if you were seriously ill.

Ask your doctor for a time when you can go over your ideas and questions about end-of-life treatment and medical decisions. Tell him or her you want guidance in preparing advance directives. If you are already ill, ask your doctor what you might expect to happen when you begin to feel worse. Let him or her know how much information you wish to receive about your illness, prognosis, care options, and hospice programs.

Discuss with your lawyer and/or financial adviser whether your legal and financial affairs are in order. Talk to a religious adviser about spiritual concerns.

What Do You Need to Talk About?

Specific issues relate to the end of one's life. They include:

- Whom do you want to make decisions for you if you are not able to make your own, both on financial matters and health care decisions? The same person may not be right for both.

- What medical treatments and care are acceptable to you? Are there some that you fear?

- Do you wish to be resuscitated if you stop breathing and/or your heart stops?

- Do you want to be hospitalized or stay at home, or somewhere else, if you are seriously or terminally ill?

- How will your care be paid for? Do you have adequate insurance? What might you have overlooked that will be costly at a time when your loved ones are distracted by grieving over your condition or death?

- What actually happens when a person dies? Do you want to know more about what might happen? Will your loved ones be prepared for the decisions they may have to make?

Taking Control

Financial Decisions

Sometimes the easiest place to begin taking control of planning is in your estate and finances because the content is more concrete. Make sure you have a valid, up-to-date will, or trust documents if desired or needed. A durable power of attorney for financial affairs is a legally binding document that you prepare, or have prepared for you to sign, that designates a trusted person to act for you if you become incapacitated. A lawyer should help you complete these documents.

Keep all your insurance information—medical, long-term care, life, and special needs policies—in an accessible place. Tell a trusted person where these documents are located. You should also think about, and write out, instructions for your funeral, burial or cremation preferences, and how they will be paid for.

Keep a list of your documents in an accessible place, and either give a copy to a trusted relative or friend or let them know where they can find it when needed. (See Where to Find My Important Papers on the Family Caregiver Alliance's website, http://caregiver.org/caregiver/jsp/content_node.jsp?nodeid=851.)

Medical Decisions

Medical advances make it possible to keep a person alive who, in former times, would have died more quickly from the serious nature of their illness, injury, or infection. This has set the stage for ethical and legal controversy about the patient's rights, the family's rights, and the medical profession's proper role. To complicate matters further, the state also has an interest in protecting its citizens from harm.

Each American has the constitutional right, established by a Supreme Court decision, to request that medical treatment be withdrawn or withheld. The right remains valid even if you become incapacitated. Another aspect of end-of-life decision-making is the right to insist on receiving, rather than refusing, treatment. This issue relates to "medical futility," when medical personnel deem further treatment to be useless except if in the nature of comfort or palliative care.

To begin, understand that you have the right to make your own decisions about your care. You can also appoint an "agent" to be your proxy or surrogate should you become incapacitated. In the event you become legally incapacitated (which may require involvement of both medical experts and a court of law) very specific legal steps must be followed before decisions about your care are made.

All states have adopted laws that make it easier for you to plan for the care you wish to receive should you not be able to communicate these wishes in the future. These means are called "advance directives" and take different forms in different states. No one can force you to sign a directive, but they are a helpful tool for you and for those who must step in for you.

Care Options

Most people do not die traumatically. Instead, the last days of their lives are spent in a hospital, nursing home, or in their own home. In your advance directive, you can state your preferences about where you wish to be in the event of terminal illness or during the process of dying. If you choose to be at home, many home care options are available, including home health and custodial care.

Hospice care—a program designed to aid the person who has been given only a short time to live and his or her family—can be provided in the home or in a facility, depending on the program. Hospice is an interdisciplinary approach that can enhance the quality of life. Pain control and emotional support for family members as well as the person who is ill are key elements of hospice. Contact your local hospice program or national association for more information.

Advance Directives

Advance directives are written instructions which communicate your wishes about the care and treatment you want to receive if you reach the point where you can no longer speak for yourself. Medicare and Medicaid require that health care facilities that receive payments from them provide patients with written information concerning the right to accept or refuse treatment and to prepare advance directives. Every state now recognizes advance directives, but the laws governing directives vary from state to state.

Probably the most commonly used form of advance directive is the durable power of attorney for health care. A more limited type of advance directive is the living will. There are important differences between these two documents.

The durable power of attorney for health care (also called the "medical power of attorney") names someone—a relative or friend—to make medical decisions for you when you are not able. Depending on the state where you live, the person you designate is called an agent, attorney-in-fact, proxy, or surrogate. (California uses the first two terms.) A durable power of attorney deals with all medical decisions unless you decide to limit it. You can also give specific instructions about treatments you want or don't want, or about other issues that concern you. For example, your agent will have access to your medical records unless you limit this right.

Because a durable power of attorney is a legal document, special forms are available and the power of attorney must be signed to be valid. Some states require witnesses and have specific rules about who can witness. It is important to select a proxy who knows you well and whom you trust. You should also name a backup proxy in case the first person is unavailable. A relative or friend can be your proxy, but an attending physician or hospital staff person usually cannot be.

The agent will be able to make all decisions regarding your health care, from flu shots to the need for surgery. And your agent or proxy can decide whether to withdraw or withhold life-sustaining procedures. While you can be as specific as you wish in the guidelines you give in the document, remember that your agent must also have the flexibility to make decisions in changing circumstances. You do not need a lawyer to complete a DPA-HC, nor can a nursing home require you to sign one before admission.

The living will, in some states called "instructions," "directive to physicians," or "declaration," states your desires regarding life-sustaining or life-prolonging medical treatment. These instructions generally apply to specific circumstances that may arise near the end of your life, such as prolonged unconsciousness. They do not appoint a surrogate to make decisions for you. Most states include these types of instructions in their medical durable power of attorney forms. Not all states recognize separate living wills as legally binding; California does not.

California's Health Care Decisions law, effective July 1, 2000, combines the durable power of attorney for health care and the instructions for health care decisions into one form called the Advance Health Care Directives. New forms are available from several agencies and web sites. Older forms, executed before July 1, 2000, are still valid, however. Note that the durable power of attorney for health care does not authorize anyone to make legal or financial decisions for you. That is done through a separate financial durable power of attorney, as discussed in the preceding under "Taking Control—Financial Decisions."

Other forms or methods of instruction may also be available to you, including:

- a Do Not Resuscitate or DNR order, which instructs medical personnel, including emergency medical personnel, not to use resuscitative measures;

- a preferred intensity of care document, a form for your physician that outlines your preferences for care under special circumstances.

Check with the laws in your state regarding oral directives. Some allow you to designate a surrogate without a written directive, with some restrictions.

Why Would I Want to Prepare an Advance Directive?

It is wise to prepare an advance directive so that medical personnel and your loved ones will know what care and services you prefer and what treatment you would refuse, in the event that you are unable to communicate your wishes. You also can designate the person or more than one person who you would like to make decisions on your behalf. In a surprising number of families, there is disagreement over what a very ill relative would prefer. The advance directive makes your wishes clear.

What Are the Care or Treatments Covered by Advance Directives?

Most advance directives cover life-sustaining treatment such as artificial feeding, mechanical ventilators, resuscitation, defibrillation, antibiotics, dialysis, and other invasive procedures.

You can give broad or specific instructions for care providers for each type of circumstance or treatment. For example, you can state that you do not want life-prolonging treatments if you will never recover your physical and mental health to live without constant care and supervision. Or you can state that you want your life prolonged as long as possible. You can address what you wish to occur in the event of trauma, a prolonged state of unconsciousness, a diagnosis of dementia, and so on.

You can also state that you wish to receive only palliative or comfort care. Such care is designed to manage terminal symptoms, including pain. It is important to understand these terms before making decisions about your preferences. Your surrogate should also become informed about the difference between comfort care and life-sustaining treatments. Health professionals and family members may disagree on the nature of a particular treatment. For example, a relative may become alarmed to see that fluids are being administered and think that this will extend life against the patient's wishes. However, the physician might believe fluids are making the dying person more comfortable and are appropriate palliative care. Another example could be the temporary need for a ventilator (mechanical breathing apparatus) and antibiotics following routine surgery.

Pain alleviation or management is among the most controversial end-of-life topics. Because of ethical concerns and the confusion over laws regulating drug addiction, Congress is debating the role of habit-forming and potentially lethal drugs in the management of pain and discomfort at the end of life. Studies have found that addiction among seriously ill people is rarer than once thought. Some individuals, however, fear being over-sedated at the very time when they want and need to recognize and interact with others.

Before making decisions about these treatments they should be discussed with a well-informed health professional. You can also ask what to expect during the last days and hours of your life, and what your surrogate and other loved ones should expect.

What Other Decisions Can My Proxy Make?

Depending on where you live and your written instructions, your proxy or agent can be authorized to decide where you will die (at home or in a facility), and can arrange for autopsy, organ donation, disposition of remains, and funeral or memorial plans.

Whom Should I Select to Be My Proxy or Agent?

Choose a responsible person to be your surrogate who shares your values and beliefs about medical care and dying. You must also make sure that the person is willing to take on this responsibility before you name her or him in the directive. An alternate should also be selected (and informed of your choice). Some states do not allow certain people, such as health care providers or health facility operators, to serve as agents. Remember also that the person you select to be your surrogate does not have to be the same person who oversees your financial affairs.

Can Someone Take over Making Decisions before I'm Ready?

Though laws vary by state, most states ensure that you remain in charge of your care as long as you are able. Usually laws are in place that require at least two physicians to declare you to be incapacitated. Agents/proxies are not allowed to commit you to a mental institution or to consent for experimental mental health research, psychosurgery, or electroconvulsive treatment. Your proxy may not deny comfort measures for you.

Can a Medical Professional Refuse to Observe My Wishes?

A health care provider may refuse to observe your stated wishes or the decisions of your agent because of conscience or the institution's policies or standards. The provider must inform you or your surrogate immediately and transfer to another provider should be arranged.

Advance directives must be reviewed periodically and kept current. Keep the original and give copies of the signed documents to your proxy/agent (including alternates), your physician, and your hospital. Put a card or notation in your wallet or purse stating that you have an advance directive. You may also leave a copy with your lawyer. Some people take their directives with them when they travel. If you spend extended time in another state you should also complete advance directives there, using that state's forms and rules. Advance directives remain in effect until they are revoked. Any written change you make on a directive may invalidate it, so consult with a professional or hospital if you wish to make changes.

Where to Get Forms and Instructions

A local hospital, Long-Term Care Ombudsman program, senior legal service or senior information and referral program, a local or state medical society, or your physician usually have forms appropriate for your state. Some medical centers offer classes in preparing directives. Attorneys may also draft their own forms. Compassion & Choices (formerly Compassion In Dying) has forms and instructions that can be downloaded from its website (www.compassionindying.org).

What If I Don't Sign an Advance Directive?

Someone has to make decisions when an ill person cannot. Without directives in the person's medical or hospital files, and without the appointment of a surrogate through the durable power of attorney, your doctors, hospital staff, and loved ones will do the best they can. To your spouse or child or life-long friend, this might mean struggling with what they think you would want. To the medical staff, it means letting their training and professional experience guide them. Unfortunately, in a world of good intentions, that training has traditionally led health care professionals to do all they can to keep you alive. Recent laws are making it easier for these able professionals to find the best ways to make you comfortable. But the ways all these wonderful people employ may not be what you want. Eventually, of course, a conservator (or guardian) could be appointed by a court. A public agency can request designation of a conservator and, if your family cannot be located, the conservator may be a public agency.

What If I Can't Sign a Directive: What to Do When Someone Is Already Incapacitated

What if you don't have a chance to plan for your own or a loved one's death? What if you are responsible for a person who has suffered a severe stroke, is already in late-stage dementia, or becomes severely disabled from a traumatic brain injury? Laws and programs exist for these situations, too.

If the impairment is gradual, it may be possible to employ many planning measures already discussed. This depends on the degree of impairment the person has experienced and their legal ability to sign documents. If the impairment or incapacity is sudden and permanent, it is imperative that the responsible person—spouse, child, grandchild, a favorite niece or nephew, long-time friend or companion, or other individual—seek guidance quickly from an attorney, hospital social work staff, and accountant or financial planner. The person's own physician as well as the hospital medical personnel should also be consulted. Several legal mechanisms are available, the most common being the conservatorship.

Questions to ask if you are responsible for an incapacitated person include:

- What is the prognosis?
- Has the person prepared and signed advance directives?
- Who would the person most want to take responsibility?
- Would he or she want that responsibility shared, perhaps among more than one adult child?
- Does the hospital provide an ethics committee or other staff that can help you sort through options for care decisions?
- What are the person's financial assets?
- Do they have Medicare, medical or long-term care insurance, or other specialized insurance plans for hospital or illness coverage?

- Are they eligible for Medicaid?

Some aspects of an incapacitated person's financial affairs could be handled through joint tenancy of property, community property (husband and wife) provisions, and representative payees. Joint tenancy is the registration of various assets, such as real estate or bank accounts, in the names of two or more joint tenants. Potential problems include the ability of one joint tenant to withdraw money from a jointly held account without the other's knowledge and possible adverse tax and estate planning consequences. While a spouse can manage the community property owned with an incapacitated spouse, court approval may be required for transactions including sales of real property, borrowing money, signing leases, or giving gifts of property. Also, many states do not have community property laws. A representative payee can be named for a person who receives only governmental benefits, such as Social Security or SSI. The payee, who can be a trustworthy relative, friend, or professional, manages the person's funds. The most effective means of handling an incapacitated person's affairs is the conservatorship or guardianship.

Conservatorships or Guardianships

A judicial procedure that appoints someone to take charge of an incapacitated person's legal, financial, and personal affairs may be called a "conservatorship," "guardianship," or some other term in your state. The term "conservatorship" is used in this text.

A conservatorship may be established after a relative, friend, or public official petitions the court for appointment of a "conservator." The petition must contain information on why the individual (the "conservatee") cannot manage his or her financial affairs or make decisions concerning his or her personal care. An investigation is conducted under the court's direction to determine if the individual is truly incapacitated and whether appointment of a conservator is justified. The court holds hearings and determines whether or not the conservatorship is required. The types of special powers to be granted to the conservator are decided.

Advantages of a conservatorship include a higher degree of protection for the conservatee than with other mechanisms. The conservator must file reports and inventories and accountings with the court. A court investigator also visits the conservatee regularly to determine if a conservatorship continues to be necessary. Disadvantages include the costs of the legal proceedings and the cumbersome requirements to return to court for approval of various transactions. Also, the details of a conservatorship become part of a public record, a loss of privacy that many find intolerable.

The two types of conservatorship are "of the estate" and "of the person."

- Conservator of the Estate: In this type of conservatorship, the conservator handles the financial and legal affairs of the con- servatee. The conservator collects the person's assets, pays bills, makes investments, etc. However, court supervision must be sought for some transactions, such as the purchase or sale of real property, borrowing money, or "gifting" of assets.

- Conservator of the Person: Decisions about medical care, food, clothing, and residence are made by this type of conservator. In the case of mental health facility placement, however, special requirements must be followed.

Mental Illness or Developmental Disability

If the person for whom decisions must be made has a mental illness or developmental disability, various federal and state laws apply. No one can be committed to a mental institution, for example, without specific legal proceedings.

A Special Model for Dementia

A study published in the *Journal of the American Medical Association* (July, 2000) reported that doctors often fail to acknowledge the final stages of Alzheimer's disease and other forms of dementia as a terminal illness. This can mean that patients are subjected to invasive procedures rather than comfort care. One problem area discussed in the study is the administration of pain medication to dementia patients. The study found that less pain relief is often prescribed for dementia patients than may be needed because the patient is unable to communicate the presence of pain. Treatment models developed for dementia patients suggest hospice and comfort care, rather than life-prolonging treatments, might be more appropriate in the end-stages of the disease. This would mean that in the event of a hip fracture, pneumonia, localized infection, or other treatable condition, treatments might be withheld in favor of medications and methods that bring comfort and ease.

There is much that we can plan and attend to in advance of our own death. We can make our wishes known about where we want to be, who we want to be with, and what we want to happen to us and around us.

We can set up ways to pay the costs of care and even pay for our own funeral. But financial and legal planning and medical advance directives must be made with the knowledge that someday other people will have to implement our wishes and live with the results. For that reason our plans should, when possible, allow for flexibility and trust in the discretion of our surrogates.

Part Six

Caregiver Concerns

Chapter 45

Caring for a Person with AD or Dementia

Caring for a person with Alzheimer disease at home is a difficult task and can become overwhelming at times. Each day brings new challenges as the caregiver copes with changing levels of ability and new patterns of behavior. Research has shown that caregivers themselves often are at increased risk for depression and illness, especially if they do not receive adequate support from family, friends, and the community.

One of the biggest struggles caregivers face is dealing with the difficult behaviors of the person they are caring for. Dressing, bathing, eating—basic activities of daily living—often become difficult to manage for both the person with Alzheimer disease and the caregiver. Having a plan for getting through the day can help caregivers cope. Many caregivers have found it helpful to use strategies for dealing with difficult behaviors and stressful situations. Through trial and error you will find that some of the following tips work, while others do not. Each person with Alzheimer disease is unique and will respond differently, and each person changes over the course of the disease. Do the best you can, and remind yourself to take breaks.

Dealing with the Diagnosis

Finding out that a loved one has Alzheimer disease can be stressful, frightening, and overwhelming. As you begin to take stock of the situation, here are some tips that may help:

From "Caregiver Guide," by the National Institute on Aging (NIA, www.nia .nih.gov), part of the National Institutes of Health, March 2010.

- Ask the doctor any questions you have about Alzheimer disease. Find out what treatments might work best to alleviate symptoms or address behavior problems.

- Contact organizations such as the Alzheimer's Association and the Alzheimer's Disease Education and Referral (ADEAR) Center for more information about the disease, treatment options, and caregiving resources. Some community groups may offer classes to teach caregiving, problem-solving, and management skills.

- Find a support group where you can share your feelings and concerns. Members of support groups often have helpful ideas or know of useful resources based on their own experiences. Online support groups make it possible for caregivers to receive support without having to leave home. The Alzheimer's Association and other organizations sponsor support groups.

- Study your day to see if you can develop a routine that makes things go more smoothly. If there are times of day when the person with Alzheimer disease is less confused or more cooperative, plan your routine to make the most of those moments. Keep in mind that the way the person functions may change from day to day, so try to be flexible and adapt your routine as needed.

- Consider using adult day care or respite services to ease the day-to-day demands of caregiving. These services allow you to have a break while knowing that the person with Alzheimer disease is being well cared for.

- Begin to plan for the future. This may include getting financial and legal documents in order, investigating long-term care options, and determining what services are covered by health insurance and Medicare.

Communication

Trying to communicate with a person who has Alzheimer disease can be a challenge. Both understanding and being understood may be difficult.

- Choose simple words and short sentences and use a gentle, calm tone of voice.

- Avoid talking to the person with Alzheimer disease like a baby or talking about the person as if he or she weren't there.

- Minimize distractions and noise—such as the television or radio—to help the person focus on what you are saying.

- Make eye contact and call the person by name, making sure you have his or her attention before speaking.

- Allow enough time for a response. Be careful not to interrupt.

- If the person with Alzheimer disease is struggling to find a word or communicate a thought, gently try to provide the word he or she is looking for.

- Try to frame questions and instructions in a positive way.

- Be open to the person's concerns, even if he or she is hard to understand.

Bathing

While some people with Alzheimer disease don't mind bathing, for others it is a frightening, confusing experience. Advance planning can help make bath time better for both of you.

- Plan the bath or shower for the time of day when the person is most calm and agreeable. Be consistent. Try to develop a routine.

- Respect the fact that bathing is scary and uncomfortable for some people with Alzheimer disease. Be gentle and respectful. Be patient and calm.

- Tell the person what you are going to do, step by step, and allow him or her to do as much as possible.

- Prepare in advance. Make sure you have everything you need ready and in the bathroom before beginning. Draw the bath ahead of time.

- Be sensitive to the temperature. Warm up the room beforehand if necessary and keep extra towels and a robe nearby. Test the water temperature before beginning the bath or shower.

- Minimize safety risks by using a handheld showerhead, shower bench, grab bars, and nonskid bath mats. Never leave the person alone in the bath or shower.

- Try a sponge bath. Bathing may not be necessary every day. A sponge bath can be effective between showers or baths.

Dressing

For someone who has Alzheimer disease, getting dressed presents a series of challenges—choosing what to wear, getting some clothes off and other clothes on, and struggling with buttons and zippers. Minimizing the challenges may make a difference.

- Try to have the person get dressed at the same time each day so he or she will come to expect it as part of the daily routine.

- Encourage the person to dress himself or herself to whatever degree possible. Plan to allow extra time so there is no pressure or rush.

- Allow the person to choose from a limited selection of outfits. If he or she has a favorite outfit, consider buying several identical sets.

- Store some clothes in another room to reduce the number of choices. Keep only one or two outfits in the closet or dresser.

- Arrange the clothes in the order they are to be put on to help the person move through the process.

- Hand the person one item at a time or give clear, step-by-step instructions if the person needs prompting.

- Choose clothing that is comfortable, easy to get on and off, and easy to care for. Elastic waists and Velcro® enclosures minimize struggles with buttons and zippers.

Eating

Eating can be a challenge. Some people with Alzheimer disease want to eat all the time, whereas others have to be encouraged to maintain a good diet.

- View mealtimes as opportunities for social interaction and success for the person with Alzheimer disease. Try to be patient and avoid rushing, and be sensitive to confusion and anxiety.

- Aim for a quiet, calm, reassuring mealtime atmosphere by limiting noise and other distractions.

- Maintain familiar mealtime routines, but adapt to the person's changing needs.

- Give the person food choices, but limit the number of choices. Try to offer appealing foods that have familiar flavors, varied textures, and different colors.

- Serve small portions or several small meals throughout the day. Make healthy snacks, finger foods, and shakes available. In the earlier stages of dementia, be aware of the possibility of overeating.

- Choose dishes and eating tools that promote independence. If the person has trouble using utensils, use a bowl instead of a plate, or offer utensils with large or built-up handles. Use straws or cups with lids to make drinking easier.

- Encourage the person to drink plenty of fluids throughout the day to avoid dehydration.

- As the disease progresses, be aware of the increased risk of choking because of chewing and swallowing problems.

- Maintain routine dental checkups and daily oral health care to keep the mouth and teeth healthy.

Activities

What to do all day? Finding activities that the person with Alzheimer disease can do and is interested in can be a challenge. Building on current skills generally works better than trying to teach something new.

- Don't expect too much. Simple activities often are best, especially when they use current abilities.

- Help the person get started on an activity. Break the activity down into small steps and praise the person for each step he or she completes.

- Watch for signs of agitation or frustration with an activity. Gently help or distract the person to something else.

- Incorporate activities the person seems to enjoy into your daily routine and try to do them at a similar time each day.

- Try to include the person with Alzheimer disease in the entire activity process. For instance, at mealtimes, encourage the person to help prepare the food, set the table, pull out the chairs, or put away the dishes. This can help maintain functional skills, enhance feelings of personal control, and make good use of time.

- Take advantage of adult day services, which provide various activities for the person with Alzheimer disease, as well as an opportunity for caregivers to gain temporary relief from tasks associated with caregiving. Transportation and meals often are provided.

Exercise

Incorporating exercise into the daily routine has benefits for both the person with Alzheimer disease and the caregiver. Not only can it improve health, but it also can provide a meaningful activity for both of you to share.

• Think about what kind of physical activities you both enjoy, perhaps walking, swimming, tennis, dancing, or gardening. Determine the time of day and place where this type of activity would work best.

• Be realistic in your expectations. Build slowly, perhaps just starting with a short walk around the yard, for example, before progressing to a walk around the block.

• Be aware of any discomfort or signs of overexertion. Talk to the person's doctor if this happens.

• Allow as much independence as possible, even if it means a less-than-perfect garden or a scoreless tennis match.

• See what kinds of exercise programs are available in your area. Senior centers may have group programs for people who enjoy exercising with others. Local malls often have walking clubs and provide a place to exercise when the weather is bad.

• Encourage physical activities. Spend time outside when the weather permits. Exercise often helps everyone sleep better.

Incontinence

As the disease progresses, many people with Alzheimer disease begin to experience incontinence, or the inability to control their bladder and/or bowels. Incontinence can be upsetting to the person and difficult for the caregiver. Sometimes incontinence is due to physical illness, so be sure to discuss it with the person's doctor.

• Have a routine for taking the person to the bathroom and stick to it as closely as possible. For example, take the person to the bathroom every 3 hours or so during the day. Don't wait for the person to ask.

• Watch for signs that the person may have to go to the bathroom, such as restlessness or pulling at clothes. Respond quickly.

- Be understanding when accidents occur. Stay calm and reassure the person if he or she is upset. Try to keep track of when accidents happen to help plan ways to avoid them.

- To help prevent nighttime accidents, limit certain types of fluids—such as those with caffeine—in the evening.

- If you are going to be out with the person, plan ahead. Know where restrooms are located, and have the person wear simple, easy-to-remove clothing. Take an extra set of clothing along in case of an accident.

Sleep Problems

For the exhausted caregiver, sleep can't come too soon. For many people with Alzheimer disease, however, the approach of nighttime may be a difficult time. Many people with Alzheimer disease become restless, agitated, and irritable around dinnertime, often referred to as "sundowning" syndrome. Getting the person to go to bed and stay there may require some advance planning.

- Encourage exercise during the day and limit daytime napping, but make sure that the person gets adequate rest during the day because fatigue can increase the likelihood of late afternoon restlessness.

- Try to schedule physically demanding activities earlier in the day. For example, bathing could be done in the morning, or the largest family meal could be served at midday.

- Set a quiet, peaceful tone in the evening to encourage sleep. Keep the lights dim, eliminate loud noises, even play soothing music if the person seems to enjoy it.

- Try to keep bedtime at a similar time each evening. Developing a bedtime routine may help.

- Limit caffeine.

- Use night-lights in the bedroom, hall, and bathroom if the darkness is frightening or disorienting.

Hallucinations and Delusions

As the disease progresses, a person with Alzheimer disease may experience hallucinations and/or delusions. Hallucinations are when the person sees, hears, smells, tastes, or feels something that is not there.

- Delusions are false beliefs that the person thinks are real. Sometimes hallucinations and delusions are signs of physical illness. Keep track of what the person is experiencing and discuss it with the doctor.

- Avoid arguing with the person about what he or she sees or hears. Try to respond to the feelings he or she is expressing. Comfort the person if he or she is afraid.

- Try to distract the person to another topic or activity. Sometimes moving to another room or going outside for a walk may help.

- Turn off the television set when violent or disturbing programs are on. The person with Alzheimer disease may not be able to distinguish television programming from reality.

- Make sure the person is safe and does not have access to anything he or she could use to harm anyone.

- Discuss with the doctor any illness the person has had or medicines he or she is taking. Sometimes an illness or medicine may cause hallucinations or delusions.

Wandering

Keeping the person safe is one of the most important aspects of caregiving. Some people with Alzheimer disease have a tendency to wander away from their home or their caregiver. Knowing how to limit wandering can protect a person from getting lost.

- Make sure that the person carries some kind of identification or wears a medical bracelet.

- Consider enrolling the person in the Alzheimer's Association Safe Return program if the program is available in your area. If the person gets lost and is unable to communicate adequately, identification will alert others to the person's medical condition.

- Notify neighbors and local authorities in advance that the person has a tendency to wander.

- Keep a recent photograph or videotape of the person with Alzheimer disease to assist police if the person becomes lost.

- Keep doors locked. Consider a keyed deadbolt or an additional lock up high or down low on the door. If the person can open a lock because it is familiar, a new latch or lock may help.

• Install an "announcing system" that chimes when the door opens.

Home Safety

Caregivers of people with Alzheimer disease often have to look at their homes through new eyes to identify and correct safety risks. Creating a safe environment can prevent many stressful and dangerous situations.

• Install secure locks on all outside windows and doors, especially if the person is prone to wandering. Remove the locks on bathroom doors to prevent the person from accidentally locking himself or herself in.

• Use childproof latches on kitchen cabinets and anyplace where cleaning supplies or other chemicals are kept.

• Label medications and keep them locked up. Also make sure knives, lighters and matches, and guns are secured and out of reach.

• Keep the house free from clutter. Remove scatter rugs and anything else that might contribute to a fall.

• Make sure lighting is good both inside and outside the home.

• Be alert to and address kitchen-safety issues, such as the person forgetting to turn off the stove after cooking. Consider installing an automatic shut-off switch on the stove to prevent burns or fire.

• Be sure to secure or put away anything that could cause danger, both inside and outside the home.

Driving

Making the decision that a person with Alzheimer disease is no longer safe to drive is difficult, and it needs to be communicated carefully and sensitively. Even though the person may be upset by the loss of independence, safety must be the priority.

• Look for clues that safe driving is no longer possible, including getting lost in familiar places, driving too fast or too slow, disregarding traffic signs, or getting angry or confused.

• Be sensitive to the person's feelings about losing the ability to drive, but be firm in your request that he or she no longer do so. Be consistent—don't allow the person to drive on "good days" but forbid it on "bad days."

- Ask the doctor to help. The person may view the doctor as an authority and be willing to stop driving. The doctor also can contact the Department of Motor Vehicles and request that the person be reevaluated.

- If necessary, take the car keys. If just having keys is important to the person, substitute a different set of keys.

- If all else fails, disable the car or move it to a location where the person cannot see it or gain access to it.

- Ask family or friends to drive the person or find out about services that help people with disabilities get around their community.

Visiting the Doctor

It is important that the person with Alzheimer disease receive regular medical care. Advance planning can help the trip to the doctor's office go more smoothly.

- Try to schedule the appointment for the person's best time of day. Also, ask the office staff what time of day the office is least crowded.

- Let the office staff know in advance that this person may be confused because of Alzheimer disease. Ask them for help to make the visit go smoothly.

- Don't tell the person about the appointment until the day of the visit or even shortly before it is time to go. Be positive and matter of fact.

- Bring along something for the person to eat and drink and any materials or activities that he or she enjoys.

- Have a friend or another family member go with you on the trip, so that one of you can be with the person while the other speaks with the doctor.

- Take a brief summary listing the person's medical history, primary care doctor, and current medications.

Coping with Holidays

Holidays are bittersweet for many Alzheimer disease caregivers. The happy memories of the past contrast with the difficulties of the present, and extra demands on time and energy can seem overwhelming. Finding a balance between rest and activity can help.

- Keep or adapt family traditions that are important to you. Include the person with Alzheimer disease as much as possible.

- Recognize that things will be different, and be realistic about what you can do.

- Encourage friends and family to visit. Limit the number of visitors at one time, and try to schedule visits during the time of day when the person is at his or her best.

- Avoid crowds, changes in routine, and strange places that may cause confusion or agitation.

- Do your best to enjoy yourself. Try to find time for the holiday things you like to do.

- Ask a friend or family member to spend time with the person while you are out.

- At larger gatherings such as weddings or family reunions, try to have a space available where the person can rest, be alone, or spend some time with a smaller number of people, if needed.

Visiting a Person with Alzheimer Disease

Visitors are important to people with Alzheimer disease. They may not always remember who the visitors are, but the human connection has value. Here are some ideas to share with someone who is planning to visit a person with the disease.

- Plan the visit for the time of day when the person with Alzheimer disease is at his or her best.

- Consider bringing along an activity, such as something familiar to read or photo albums to look at, but be prepared to skip it if necessary.

- Be calm and quiet. Avoid using a loud tone of voice or talking to the person as if he or she were a child.

- Respect the person's personal space and don't get too close.

- Try to establish eye contact and call the person by name to get his or her attention.

- Remind the person who you are if he or she doesn't seem to recognize you.

- Don't argue if the person is confused. Respond to the feelings you hear being communicated, and distract the person to a different topic if necessary.

455

- Remember not to take it personally if the person doesn't recognize you, is unkind, or responds angrily. He or she is reacting out of confusion.

Choosing a Nursing Home

For many caregivers, there comes a point when they are no longer able to take care of their loved one at home. Choosing a residential care facility—a group home, assisted living facility, or nursing home—is a big decision, and it can be hard to know where to start.

- It's helpful to gather information about services and options before the need actually arises. This gives you time to explore fully all the possibilities before making a decision.

- Determine what facilities are in your area. Doctors, friends and relatives, hospital social workers, and religious organizations may be able to help you identify specific facilities.

- Make a list of questions you would like to ask the staff. Think about what is important to you, such as activity programs, transportation, or special units for people with Alzheimer disease.

- Contact the places that interest you and make an appointment to visit. Talk to the administration, nursing staff, and residents.

- Observe the way the facility runs and how residents are treated. You may want to drop by again unannounced to see if your impressions are the same.

- Find out what kinds of programs and services are offered for people with Alzheimer disease and their families. Ask about staff training in dementia care, and check to see what the policy is about family participation in planning patient care.

- Check on room availability, cost and method of payment, and participation in Medicare or Medicaid. You may want to place your name on a waiting list even if you are not ready to make an immediate decision about long-term care.

- Once you have made a decision, be sure you understand the terms of the contract and financial agreement. You may want to have a lawyer review the documents with you before signing.

- Moving is a big change for both the person with Alzheimer disease and the caregiver. A social worker may be able to help you plan for and adjust to the move. It is important to have support during this difficult transition.

Chapter 46

Long-Distance Caregiving

Five years ago, Dave's mother moved from their old house in Philadelphia to an apartment that was closer to his sister in Baltimore. Before the move, the 30-minute drive to visit his mom wasn't a big deal, and Dave had lunch with her weekly. Sometimes they'd go to a ballgame together. After the move, neither Dave nor his mom expected much to change—what was another hour or so of drive time? But as time passed, the trip seemed to get longer, time together was harder to arrange, and as a result, they saw less of each other. Then his mom's health began to slide. When Dave's sister called to say their mom had fallen and broken her hip, Dave needed and wanted to help. Should he offer to hire a nurse? Should he take a week off work and help out himself? After all the years his mom had devoted to caring for the family, what could Dave do from far away to help her—and his sister?

The answer for Dave, and for so many families faced with similar situations, is encouraging. Long-distance caregivers can be helpful no matter how far away they live. This text focuses on some issues that are unique to long-distance caregiving. You will also find other information that is important to know whether you live next door or across the country.

But what is long-distance caregiving? It can be helping Aunt Lilly sort through her medical bills or thinking about how to make the most of a weekend visit with Mom. It can include checking the references of

---

Excerpted from "So Far Away: Twenty Questions for Long-Distance Caregivers," by the National Institute on Aging (NIA, www.nia.nih.gov), part of the National Institutes of Health, August 2010.

an aide who's been hired to help your grandfather or trying to take the pressure off your sister who lives in the same town as both your aging parents and her aging in-laws. This text often refers to caregiving for aging parents, but in fact, it offers tips you can use no matter who you are caring for—an older relative, family friend, or neighbor.

What does a long-distance caregiver do? How many other people are trying to help out from a distance, like me?

If you live an hour or more away from a person who needs care, you can think of yourself as a long-distance caregiver. This kind of care can take many forms—from helping with finances or money management to arranging for in-home care; from providing respite care for a primary caregiver to creating a plan in case of emergencies.

Many long-distance caregivers act as information coordinators, helping aging parents understand the confusing maze of new needs, including home health aides, insurance benefits and claims, and durable medical equipment.

Caregiving, no matter where the caregiver lives, is often long-lasting and ever-expanding. For the long-distance caregiver, what may start out as an occasional social phone call to share family news can eventually turn into regular phone calls about managing household bills, getting medical information, and arranging for grocery deliveries. What begins as a monthly trip to check on Mom may become a larger project to move her to a new home or nursing facility closer to where you live.

If you are a long-distance caregiver, you are definitely not alone. There may be as many as 7 million people in your same situation in the United States. In the past, caregivers have been primarily working women in mid-life with other family responsibilities. That's changing. More and more men are getting involved; in fact, surveys show that men now represent almost 40 percent of caregivers. Anyone, anywhere can be a long-distance caregiver. Gender, income, age, social status, employment—none of these prevent you from taking on at least some caregiving responsibilities and possibly feeling some of the satisfaction.

How will I know if help is needed? Uncle Simon sounds fine on the phone. How can I know that he really is?

Sometimes, your relative will ask for help. Or, the sudden start of a severe illness will make it clear that assistance is needed. But, when you live far away, some detective work might be in order to uncover possible signs that support or help is needed.

A phone call is not always the best way to tell whether or not an older person needs help handling daily activities. Uncle Simon might not want to worry his nephew, Brad, who lives a few hours away, or he might not want to admit that he's often too tired to cook an entire meal. But how can Brad know this? If he calls at dinner and asks "what's cooking," Brad might get a sense that dinner is a bowl of cereal. If so, he might want to talk with his uncle and offer some help. With Simon's okay, Brad might contact people who see his uncle regularly—neighbors, friends, doctors, or local relatives, for example—and ask them to call Brad if they have concerns about Simon. Brad might also ask if he could check in with them periodically. When Brad spends a weekend with his uncle, he should look around for possible trouble areas—it's easier to disguise problems during a short phone call than during a longer visit.

Brad can make the most of his visit if he takes some time in advance to develop a list of possible problem areas he wants to check out while visiting his uncle. That's a good idea for anyone in this type of situation. Of course, it may not be possible to do everything in one trip—but make sure that any potentially dangerous situations are taken care of as soon as possible. If you can't correct everything on your list, see if you can arrange for someone else to finish up.

In addition to safety issues and the overall condition of the house, try to determine the older person's mood and general health status. Sometimes people confuse depression in older people with normal aging. A depressed older person might brighten up for a phone call or short visit, but it's harder to hide serious mood problems during an extended visit.

What can I really do from far away? My sister lives pretty close to our parents and has gradually been doing more and more for them. I'm halfway across the country. I'd like to help them and my sister, but I don't feel comfortable just jumping in.

Many long-distance caregivers provide emotional support and occasional respite to a primary caregiver. Staying in contact with your parents by phone or e-mail might also take some pressure off your sister. Long-distance caregivers can play a part in arranging for professional caregivers, hiring home health and nursing aides, or locating care in an assisted living facility or nursing home (also known as a skilled nursing facility). Some long-distance caregivers find they can be helpful by handling things online—for example, researching health problems or medicines, paying bills, or keeping family and friends updated. Some long-distance caregivers help a parent pay for care, while others step in to manage finances.

Caregiving is not easy for anyone, not for the caregiver and not for the care recipient. There are sacrifices and adjustments for everyone. When you don't live where the care is needed, it may be especially hard to feel that what you are doing is enough and that what you are doing is important. It often is.

How can my family decide who does what? My brother lives closest to our grandmother, but he's uncomfortable coordinating her medical care.

This is a question that many families have to work out. You could start by setting up a family meeting and, if your grandmother is capable, include her in the discussion. This is best done when there is not an emergency. A calm conversation about what kind of care is needed in the present and might be called for in the future can avoid a lot of confusion. Ask your grandmother what she wants. Use her wishes as the basis for a plan. Decide who will be responsible for which tasks. Many families find the best first step is to name a primary caregiver, even if one is not needed immediately. That way the primary caregiver can step in if there is a crisis.

Think about your schedules and how to adapt them to give respite to a primary caregiver or to coordinate holiday and vacation times. One family found that it worked to have the long-distance caregiver come to town while the primary caregiver was on a family vacation. Many families report that offering appreciation, reassurance, and positive feedback to the primary caregiver is an important, but sometimes forgotten contribution.

How can I know my strengths and set limits?

If you decide to work as a family team, it makes sense to agree in advance how your efforts can complement one another. Ideally, each of you will be able to take on tasks best suited to your skills or interests. For example, who is available to help Mom get to the grocery store each week? Who can help Dad organize his move to an assisted living facility? After making these kinds of decisions, remember that over time responsibilities may need to be revised to reflect changes in the situation, your parent's needs, and each family member's abilities and limitations. Be realistic about how much you can do and what you are willing to do.

When thinking about your strengths, consider what you are particularly good at and how those skills might help in the current situation:

- Are you good at finding information, keeping people up-to-date on changing conditions, and offering cheer, whether on the phone or with a computer?

- Are you good at supervising and leading others?

- Are you comfortable speaking with medical staff and interpreting what they say to others?

- Is your strongest suit doing the numbers—paying bills, keeping track of bank statements, and reviewing insurance policies and reimbursement reports?

- Are you the one in the family who can fix anything, while no one else knows the difference between pliers and a wrench?
  When reflecting on your limits, consider:

- How often, both mentally and financially, can you afford to travel?

- Are you emotionally prepared to take on what may feel like a reversal of roles between you and your parent—taking care of your parent instead of your parent taking care of you? Can you continue to respect your parent's independence?

- Can you be both calm and assertive when communicating from a distance?

- How will your decision to take on caregiving responsibilities affect your work and home life?

What is a geriatric care manager, and how can I find one? A friend of mine thought that having a professional "on the scene" to help my dad would take some of the pressure off me.

Professional care managers are usually licensed nurses or social workers who specialize in geriatrics. Some families hire a geriatric care manager to evaluate and assess a parent's needs and to coordinate care through community resources. The cost of an initial evaluation varies and may be expensive, but depending on your family circumstances, geriatric care managers might offer a useful service. They are a sort of "professional relative" to help you and your family to identify needs and how to meet them. These professionals can also help by leading family discussions about sensitive subjects.

When interviewing a geriatric care manager, you might want to ask:

- Are you a licensed geriatric care manager?

- Are you a member of the National Association of Professional Geriatric Care Managers?

- How long have you been providing care management services?

- Are you available for emergencies around the clock?

- Does your company also provide home care services?

- How will you communicate information to me?

- What are your fees? Will you provide information on fees in writing prior to starting services?

- Can you provide references?

The National Association of Professional Geriatric Care Managers, www.caremanager.org, can help you find a care manager near your family member's community. You can also call or write the Eldercare Locator for recommendations. In some cases, support groups for diseases related to aging may be able to recommend geriatric care managers who have assisted other families.

My friends who have been caregivers say that a lot of what they did was organizing paperwork. Is that a good way to be helpful?

Yes. That's one way that a long-distance caregiver can be a big help. An important part of effective caregiving depends on keeping a great deal of information in order and up-to-date. Often, long-distance caregivers will need access to a parent's personal, health, financial, and legal records. If you have ever tried to gather and organize your own personal information, you know what a chore it can be. Getting all this material together is a lot of work at first, and from far away it can seem even more challenging. But once you have gathered everything together, many other caregiving tasks will be easier. Maintaining current information about your parent's health and medical care, as well as finances, home ownership, and other legal issues, lets you get a handle on what is going on and allows you to respond more quickly if there is a crisis.

If you do not see your parent often, one visit may not be enough time for you to get all the paperwork organized. Instead, try to focus on gathering the essentials first; you can fill in the blanks as you go along. You might begin by talking to your parent and his or her primary caregiver about the kinds of records that need to be pulled together. If a primary caregiver is already on the scene, chances are that some of the information has already been assembled. Talk about any missing information or documentation and how you might help to organize the records. It is also a good idea to check at the same time to make sure that all financial matters, including wills and life insurance policies, are in order. It will also help if someone also has a durable power of attorney (the legal document naming one person to handle financial and property issues for another).

Your parents may be reluctant to share personal information with you. Explain that you are not trying to invade their privacy or take over their personal lives—you are only trying to assemble what will be needed in the event of an emergency. Assure them that you will respect their privacy, and then keep your promise. If your parents are still uncomfortable, ask if they would be willing to work with an attorney (some lawyers specialize in elder affairs) or perhaps with another trusted family member or friend.

What information should a caregiver keep track of?

The answer to this question is different for every family. You might want to help organize the following information and update it as needed. This list is just a starting point.

- Full legal name and residence
- Birth date and place, birth certificate
- Social Security and Medicare numbers
- Employer(s) and dates of employment
- Education and military records
- Sources of income and assets; investment income (stocks, bonds, property)
- Insurance policies, bank accounts, deeds, investments, and other valuables
- Most recent income tax return

- Money owed, to whom, and when payments are due
- Credit card account names and numbers
- Safe deposit box key and information
- Will, beneficiary information
- Durable power of attorney
- Living will and/or durable power of attorney for health care
- Where cash or other valuables might be kept in the home

My parents are in their 70s and have not said anything about their future healthcare preferences. Since they are still relatively healthy, do we need to talk about that now?

For most of us, talking with people about the kind of medical care they would want if they are seriously ill and unable to make decisions can be difficult. But, when the conversation is with someone close to you, it can be many times harder for everyone. Yet, it's important to be prepared, especially in case of unexpected illness.

As a long-distance caregiver, you might want to wait until you are face to face with your parents, rather than try to handle this sensitive subject on the phone. During a visit, you could try saying that you have just made your living will, or you could tell them you've chosen someone to make your healthcare decisions. A friend or neighbor's illness might also jumpstart a conversation about healthcare preferences. For some families, a conversation about, for example, who would like Grandma's china could be a gentle way to start the discussion. Would you rather begin on a less personal note? Discussing a TV show, newspaper article, or movie might be the way to start.

When talking about medical care, assure your parents that as long as they are alert, they will be the ones to make decisions. But documenting their healthcare wishes is important. Healthcare providers can't know your parents' preferences unless they are included in their medical records. Having these wishes on the record allows your parents to receive the care they want. It may also help avoid some of the conflicts that can occur when family members disagree over treatment decisions.

Advance care planning is often done through an advance directive, which includes verbal and written instructions about future medical care. There are two types of advance directives—a living will and a durable power of attorney for health care. A living will states in writing what kinds of life-sustaining medical treatments, if any, a person wants if he or she is unable to speak or respond and at risk of dying.

A durable power of attorney for health care names someone to make medical decisions in that same type of situation. This person, called a healthcare proxy, can decide on care based on what he or she knows the patient would want. It is vital for your parents to discuss their wishes with the healthcare proxy.

Naming a healthcare proxy is an extremely important decision. Living nearby is not a requirement to be a healthcare proxy, also called "healthcare agent" or "surrogate." Even a long-distance caregiver can be one. Most people ask a close friend or family member to be their healthcare proxy. Some people turn to a trusted member of the clergy or a lawyer. Whoever is chosen should be able to understand the treatment choices, know your parents' values, and support their decisions.

Advance directives are not set in stone. You might want to let your parents know that they can revise and update their instructions as often as they wish. Patients and caregivers should discuss these decisions—and any changes in them—and keep the healthcare team informed. Consider giving copies of advance directives to all caregivers and to your brothers and sisters. Keep a copy at home as well. Because state laws vary, check with your Area Agency on Aging, your state department of aging, or a lawyer for more information.

How can I find information about financial assistance for my parents who live across the country from me? They saved money for retirement, but the cost of their medical care is really high, and they are worried.

You and your parents are not alone in worrying about how much medical care costs. These expenses can use up a significant part of monthly income, even for families who thought they had saved enough. Your parents may be eligible for some healthcare benefits. As a long-distance caregiver, one way you can be helpful is by learning more about possible sources of financial help and then assisting your parents in applying for aid as appropriate. The internet can be a helpful tool in this search.

There are several federal and state programs that provide help with healthcare-related costs. Here is an overview to help you get started. The Centers for Medicare & Medicaid Services (CMS), the federal agency responsible for Medicare, offers several programs. Over time, the benefits and eligibility requirements of these programs can change and differ from state to state, so it is best to check with CMS, www.cms.gov, or the individual programs directly for the most recent information. People on fixed incomes who have limited resources may qualify for Medicaid, www.cms.gov/home/medicaid.asp. This program covers the costs of medical care for people of all ages who have limited income and meet other eligibility requirements.

Under Medicare, some states have PACE, Program of All-Inclusive Care for the Elderly, www.pace4you.org. This is a program providing care and services to people who otherwise would need care in a nursing home. SHIP, the State Health Insurance Counseling and Assistance Program, www.medicare.gov/Contacts/staticpages/ships.aspx, offers counseling and assistance to people and their families on Medicare, Medicaid, and Medigap matters.

If your parent is eligible for veterans benefits, don't forget to check with the Department of Veterans Affairs (VA), www.va.gov. Or, get in touch with the VA medical center nearest you.

For information about other federal, state, and local government benefits, go to www.govbenefits.gov. If you don't have a computer, call 800-FED-INFO (800-333-4636).

The National Council on Aging website, www.benefitscheckup.org, is another good place to start. By providing some general information about your parent, you can see a list of possible benefits you might want to explore. You don't have to give the name, address, or Social Security number in order to use this service.

If prescription medicines cost too much, ask the doctor if there is a less expensive medication or a generic choice. Learn more about Medicare insurance for prescription drugs at www.medicare.gov/find-a-plan/questions/home.aspx or call Medicare or SHIP. Also, the Partnership for Prescription Assistance, www.pparx.org, can provide a list of patient assistance programs supported by pharmaceutical companies.

Chapter 47

Coping with Challenging Behaviors

Section 47.1

Understanding Challenging Behaviors

"Caregiver's Guide to Understanding Dementia Behaviors," © 2008 Family
Caregiver Alliance. Reprinted with permission. To view the complete text
of this article including recommendations for further reading and related
organizations and websites, visit www.caregiver.org.

Caring for a loved one with dementia poses many challenges for
families and caregivers. People with dementia from conditions such as
Alzheimer's and related diseases have a progressive brain disorder that
makes it more and more difficult for them to remember things, think
clearly, communicate with others, or take care of themselves. In addition,
dementia can cause mood swings and even change a person's personality
and behavior. This text provides some practical strategies for dealing
with the troubling behavior problems and communication difficulties
often encountered when caring for a person with dementia.

Ten Tips for Communicating with a Person with Dementia

We aren't born knowing how to communicate with a person with
dementia—but we can learn. Improving your communication skills will
help make caregiving less stressful and will likely improve the quality
of your relationship with your loved one. Good communication skills
will also enhance your ability to handle the difficult behavior you may
encounter as you care for a person with a dementing illness.

1. Set a positive mood for interaction. Your attitude and body lan-
    guage communicate your feelings and thoughts stronger than
    your words. Set a positive mood by speaking to your loved one
    in a pleasant and respectful manner. Use facial expressions,
    tone of voice, and physical touch to help convey your message
    and show your feelings of affection.

2. Get the person's attention. Limit distractions and noise—turn
    off the radio or TV, close the curtains or shut the door, or move
    to quieter surroundings. Before speaking, make sure you have

her attention; address her by name, identify yourself by name and relation, and use nonverbal cues and touch to help keep her focused. If she is seated, get down to her level and maintain eye contact.

3. State your message clearly. Use simple words and sentences. Speak slowly, distinctly, and in a reassuring tone. Refrain from raising your voice higher or louder; instead, pitch your voice lower. If she doesn't understand the first time, use the same wording to repeat your message or question. If she still doesn't understand, wait a few minutes and rephrase the question. Use the names of people and places instead of pronouns or abbreviations.

4. Ask simple, answerable questions. Ask one question at a time; those with yes or no answers work best. Refrain from asking open-ended questions or giving too many choices. For example, ask, "Would you like to wear your white shirt or your blue shirt?" Better still, show her the choices—visual prompts and cues also help clarify your question and can guide her response.

5. Listen with your ears, eyes, and heart. Be patient in waiting for your loved one's reply. If she is struggling for an answer, it's okay to suggest words. Watch for nonverbal cues and body language, and respond appropriately. Always strive to listen for the meaning and feelings that underlie the words.

6. Break down activities into a series of steps. This makes many tasks much more manageable. You can encourage your loved one to do what he can, gently remind him of steps he tends to forget, and assist with steps he's no longer able to accomplish on his own. Using visual cues, such as showing him with your hand where to place the dinner plate, can be very helpful.

7. When the going gets tough, distract and redirect. When your loved one becomes upset, try changing the subject or the environment. For example, ask him for help or suggest going for a walk. It is important to connect with the person on a feeling level, before you redirect. You might say, "I see you're feeling sad—I'm sorry you're upset. Let's go get something to eat."

8. Respond with affection and reassurance. People with dementia often feel confused, anxious, and unsure of themselves. Further, they often get reality confused and may recall

things that never really occurred. Avoid trying to convince them they are wrong. Stay focused on the feelings they are demonstrating (which are real) and respond with verbal and physical expressions of comfort, support, and reassurance. Sometimes holding hands, touching, hugging, and praise will get the person to respond when all else fails.

9. Remember the good old days. Remembering the past is often a soothing and affirming activity. Many people with dementia may not remember what happened 45 minutes ago, but they can clearly recall their lives 45 years earlier. Therefore, avoid asking questions that rely on short-term memory, such as asking the person what they had for lunch. Instead, try asking general questions about the person's distant past—this information is more likely to be retained.

10. Maintain your sense of humor. Use humor whenever possible, though not at the person's expense. People with dementia tend to retain their social skills and are usually delighted to laugh along with you.

Handling Troubling Behavior

Some of the greatest challenges of caring for a loved one with dementia are the personality and behavior changes that often occur. You can best meet these challenges by using creativity, flexibility, patience, and compassion. It also helps to not take things personally and maintain your sense of humor.

To start, consider these ground rules:

We cannot change the person. The person you are caring for has a brain disorder that shapes who he has become. When you try to control or change his behavior, you'll most likely be unsuccessful or be met with resistance. It's important to:

• Try to accommodate the behavior, not control the behavior. For example, if the person insists on sleeping on the floor, place a mattress on the floor to make him more comfortable.

• Remember that we can change our behavior or the physical environment. Changing our own behavior will often result in a change in our loved one's behavior.

Check with the doctor first. Behavioral problems may have an underlying medical reason: Perhaps the person is in pain or experiencing

470

an adverse side effect from medications. In some cases, like incontinence or hallucinations, there may be some medication or treatment that can assist in managing the problem.

Behavior has a purpose. People with dementia typically cannot tell us what they want or need. They might do something, like take all the clothes out of the closet on a daily basis, and we wonder why. It is very likely that the person is fulfilling a need to be busy and productive. Always consider what need the person might be trying to meet with their behavior—and, when possible, try to accommodate them.

Behavior is triggered. It is important to understand that all behavior is triggered—it doesn't occur out of the blue. It might be something a person did or said that triggered a behavior or it could be a change in the physical environment. The root to changing behavior is disrupting the patterns that we create. Try a different approach, or try a different consequence.

What works today, may not tomorrow. The multiple factors that influence troubling behaviors and the natural progression of the disease process means that solutions that are effective today may need to be modified tomorrow—or may no longer work at all. The key to managing difficult behaviors is being creative and flexible in your strategies to address a given issue.

Get support from others. You are not alone—there are many others caring for someone with dementia. Call your local Area Agency on Aging, the local chapter of the Alzheimer's Association, or a Caregiver Resource Center to find support groups, organizations, and services that can help you. Expect that, like the loved one you are caring for, you will have good days and bad days. Develop strategies for coping with the bad days.

The following is an overview of the most common dementia-associated behaviors with suggestions that may be useful in handling them.

Wandering

People with dementia walk, seemingly aimlessly, for a variety of reasons, such as boredom, medication side effects, or to look for "something" or someone. They also may be trying to fulfill a physical need—thirst, hunger, a need to use the toilet, or exercise. Discovering the triggers for wandering are not always easy, but they can provide insights to dealing with the behavior.

- Make time for regular exercise to minimize restlessness.

- Consider installing new locks that require a key. Position locks high or low on the door; many people with dementia will not think to look beyond eye level. Keep in mind fire and safety concerns for all family members; the lock(s) must be accessible to others and not take more than a few seconds to open.

- Try a barrier like a curtain or colored streamer to mask the door. A "stop" sign or "do not enter" sign also may help.

- Place a black mat or paint a black space on your front porch; this may appear to be an impassable hole to the person with dementia.

- Add "child-safe" plastic covers to doorknobs.

- Consider installing a home security system or monitoring system designed to keep watch over someone with dementia. Also available are new digital devices that can be worn like a watch or clipped on a belt that use global positioning systems (GPS) or other technology to track a person's whereabouts or locate him if he wanders off.

- Put away essential items such as the confused person's coat, purse, or glasses. Some individuals will not go out without certain articles.

- Have your relative wear an ID bracelet and sew ID labels in their clothes. Always have a current photo available should you need to report your loved one missing. Consider leaving a copy on file at the police department or registering the person with the Alzheimer's Association Safe Return program.

- Tell neighbors about your relative's wandering behavior and make sure they have your phone number.

Incontinence

The loss of bladder or bowel control often occurs as dementia progresses. Sometimes accidents result from environmental factors; for example, someone can't remember where the bathroom is located or can't get to it in time. If an accident occurs, your understanding and reassurance will help the person maintain dignity and minimize embarrassment.

- Establish a routine for using the toilet. Try reminding the person or assisting her to the bathroom every 2 hours.

472

- Schedule fluid intake to ensure the confused person does not become dehydrated. However, avoid drinks with a diuretic effect like coffee, tea, cola, or beer. Limit fluid intake in the evening before bedtime.

- Use signs (with illustrations) to indicate which door leads to the bathroom.

- A commode, obtained at any medical supply store, can be left in the bedroom at night for easy access.

- Incontinence pads and products can be purchased at the pharmacy or supermarket. A urologist may be able to prescribe a special product or treatment.

- Use easy-to-remove clothing with elastic waistbands or Velcro closures, and provide clothes that are easily washable.

Agitation

Agitation refers to a range of behaviors associated with dementia, including irritability, sleeplessness, and verbal or physical aggression. Often these types of behavior problems progress with the stages of dementia, from mild to more severe. Agitation may be triggered by a variety of things, including environmental factors, fear, and fatigue. Most often, agitation is triggered when the person experiences "control" being taken from him.

- Reduce caffeine intake, sugar, and junk food.

- Reduce noise, clutter, or the number of persons in the room.

- Maintain structure by keeping the same routines. Keep household objects and furniture in the same places. Familiar objects and photographs offer a sense of security and can suggest pleasant memories.

- Try gentle touch, soothing music, reading, or walks to quell agitation. Speak in a reassuring voice. Do not try to restrain the person during a period of agitation.

- Keep dangerous objects out of reach.

- Allow the person to do as much for himself as possible—support his independence and ability to care for himself.

- Acknowledge the confused person's anger over the loss of control in his life. Tell him you understand his frustration.

- Distract the person with a snack or an activity. Allow him to forget the troubling incident. Confronting a confused person may increase anxiety.

Repetitive Speech or Actions (Perseveration)

People with dementia will often repeat a word, statement, question, or activity over and over. While this type of behavior is usually harmless for the person with dementia, it can be annoying and stressful to caregivers. Sometimes the behavior is triggered by anxiety, boredom, fear, or environmental factors.

- Provide plenty of reassurance and comfort, both in words and in touch.

- Try distracting with a snack or activity.

- Avoid reminding them that they just asked the same question. Try ignoring the behavior or question and distract the person into an activity.

- Don't discuss plans with a confused person until immediately prior to an event.

- You may want to try placing a sign on the kitchen table, such as, "Dinner is at 6:30" or "Lois comes home at 5:00" to remove anxiety and uncertainty about anticipated events.

- Learn to recognize certain behaviors. An agitated state or pulling at clothing, for example, could indicate a need to use the bathroom.

Paranoia

Seeing a loved one suddenly become suspicious, jealous, or accusatory is unsettling. Remember, what the person is experiencing is very real to them. It is best not to argue or disagree. This, too, is part of the dementia—try not to take it personally.

- If the confused person suspects money is "missing," allow her to keep small amounts of money in a pocket or handbag for easy inspection.

- Help them look for the object and then distract them into another activity. Try to learn where the confused person's favorite hiding places are for storing objects, which are frequently assumed to be "lost." Avoid arguing.

- Take time to explain to other family members and home-helpers that suspicious accusations are a part of the dementing illness.

- Try nonverbal reassurances like a gentle touch or hug. Respond to the feeling behind the accusation and then reassure the person. You might try saying, "I see this frightens you; stay with me, I won't let anything happen to you."

Sleeplessness/Sundowning

Restlessness, agitation, disorientation, and other troubling behavior in people with dementia often get worse at the end of the day and sometimes continue throughout the night. Experts believe this behavior, commonly called sundowning, is caused by a combination of factors, such as exhaustion from the day's events and changes in the person's biological clock that confuse day and night.

- Increase daytime activities, particularly physical exercise. Discourage inactivity and napping during the day.

- Watch out for dietary culprits, such as sugar, caffeine, and some types of junk food. Eliminate or restrict these types of foods and beverages to early in the day. Plan smaller meals throughout the day, including a light meal, such as half a sandwich, before bedtime.

- Plan for the afternoon and evening hours to be quiet and calm; however, structured, quiet activity is important. Perhaps take a stroll outdoors, play a simple card game, or listen to soothing music together.

- Turning on lights well before sunset and closing the curtains at dusk will minimize shadows and may help diminish confusion. At minimum, keep a nightlight in the person's room, hallway, and bathroom.

- Make sure the house is safe: Block off stairs with gates, lock the kitchen door, and/or put away dangerous items.

- As a last resort, consider talking to the doctor about medication to help the agitated person relax and sleep. Be aware that sleeping pills and tranquilizers may solve one problem and create another, such as sleeping at night but being more confused the next day.

- It's essential that you, the caregiver, get enough sleep. If your loved one's nighttime activity keeps you awake, consider asking a friend or relative, or hiring someone, to take a turn so that you can get a good night's sleep. Catnaps during the day also might help.

Eating/Nutrition

Ensuring that your loved one is eating enough nutritious foods and drinking enough fluids is a challenge. People with dementia literally begin to forget that they need to eat and drink. Complicating the issue may be dental problems or medications that decrease appetite or make food taste "funny." The consequences of poor nutrition are many, including weight loss, irritability, sleeplessness, bladder or bowel problems, and disorientation.

- Make meal and snack times part of the daily routine and schedule them around the same time every day. Instead of three big meals, try five or six smaller ones.

- Make mealtimes a special time. Try flowers or soft music. Turn off loud radio programs and the TV.

- Eating independently should take precedence over eating neatly or with "proper" table manners. Finger foods support independence. Pre-cut and season the food. Try using a straw or a child's "sippy cup" if holding a glass has become difficult. Provide assistance only when necessary and allow plenty of time for meals.

- Sit down and eat with your loved one. Often they will mimic your actions and it makes the meal more pleasant to share it with someone.

- Prepare foods with your loved one in mind. If they have dentures or trouble chewing or swallowing, use soft foods or cut food into bite-size pieces.

- If chewing and swallowing are an issue, try gently moving the person's chin in a chewing motion or lightly stroking their throat to encourage them to swallow.

- If loss of weight is a problem, offer nutritious high-calorie snacks between meals. Breakfast foods high in carbohydrates are often preferred. On the other hand, if the problem is weight gain, keep high-calorie foods out of sight. Instead, keep handy fresh fruits, veggie trays, and other healthy low-calorie snacks.

Bathing

People with dementia often have difficulty remembering "good" hygiene, such as brushing teeth, toileting, bathing, and regularly changing their clothes. From childhood we are taught these are highly private and personal activities; to be undressed and cleaned by another can feel frightening, humiliating, and embarrassing. As a result, bathing often causes distress for both caregivers and their loved ones.

- Think historically of your loved one's hygiene routine—did she prefer baths or showers? Mornings or nights? Did she have her hair washed at the salon or do it herself? Was there a favorite scent, lotion, or talcum powder she always used? Adopting—as much as possible—her past bathing routine may provide some comfort. Remember that it may not be necessary to bathe every day—sometimes twice a week is sufficient.

- If your loved one has always been modest, enhance that feeling by making sure doors and curtains are closed. Whether in the shower or the bath, keep a towel over her front, lifting to wash as needed. Have towels and a robe or her clothes ready when she gets out.

- Be mindful of the environment, such as the temperature of the room and water (older adults are more sensitive to heat and cold) and the adequacy of lighting. It's a good idea to use safety features such as non-slip floor bath mats, grab-bars, and bath or shower seats. A hand-held shower might also be a good feature to install. Remember—people are often afraid of falling. Help them feel secure in the shower or tub.

- Never leave a person with dementia unattended in the bath or shower. Have all the bath things you need laid out beforehand. If giving a bath, draw the bath water first. Reassure the person that the water is warm—perhaps pour a cup of water over her hands before she steps in.

- If hair washing is a struggle, make it a separate activity. Or, use a dry shampoo.

- If bathing in the tub or shower is consistently traumatic, a towel bath provides a soothing alternative. A bed bath has traditionally been done with only the most frail and bed-ridden patients, soaping up a bit at a time in their beds, rinsing off with a basin of water, and drying with towels. A growing number of nurses in and out of facilities, however, are beginning to recognize its value and a variation—the "towel bath"—for others as well, including people with dementia who find bathing in the tub or shower uncomfortable or unpleasant. The towel bath uses a large bath towel and washcloths dampened in a plastic bag of warm water and no-rinse soap. Large bath-blankets are used to keep the patient covered, dry, and warm while the dampened towel and washcloths are massaged over the body. For more information, see the book *Bathing Without a Battle,* or visit www .bathingwithoutabattle.unc.edu.

Additional Problem Areas

- Dressing is difficult for most dementia patients. Choose loose-fitting, comfortable clothes with easy zippers or snaps and minimal buttons. Reduce the person's choices by removing seldom-worn clothes from the closet. To facilitate dressing and support independence, lay out one article of clothing at a time, in the order it is to be worn. Remove soiled clothes from the room. Don't argue if the person insists on wearing the same thing again.

- Hallucinations (seeing or hearing things that others don't) and delusions (false beliefs, such as someone is trying to hurt or kill another) may occur as the dementia progresses. State simply and calmly your perception of the situation, but avoid arguing or trying to convince the person their perceptions are wrong. Keep rooms well-lit to decrease shadows, and offer reassurance and a simple explanation if the curtains move from circulating air or a loud noise such as a plane or siren is heard. Distractions may help. Depending on the severity of symptoms, you might consider medication.

- Sexually inappropriate behavior, such as masturbating or undressing in public, lewd remarks, unreasonable sexual demands, even sexually aggressive or violent behavior, may occur during the course of the illness. Remember, this behavior is caused by the disease. Talk to the doctor about possible treatment plans. Develop an action plan to follow before the behavior occurs, i.e., what you will say and do if the behavior happens at home, around other adults or children. If you can, identify what triggers the behavior.

- Verbal outbursts such as cursing, arguing, and threatening often are expressions of anger or stress. React by staying calm and reassuring. Validate your loved one's feelings and then try to distract or redirect his attention to something else.

- "Shadowing" is when a person with dementia imitates and follows the caregiver, or constantly talks, asks questions, and interrupts. Like sundowning, this behavior often occurs late in the day and can be irritating for caregivers. Comfort the person with verbal and physical reassurance. Distraction or redirection might also help. Giving your loved one a job such as folding laundry might help to make her feel needed and useful.

• People with dementia may become uncooperative and resistant to daily activities such as bathing, dressing, and eating. Often this is a response to feeling out of control, rushed, afraid, or confused by what you are asking of them. Break each task into steps and, in a reassuring voice, explain each step before you do it. Allow plenty of time. Find ways to have them assist to their ability in the process, or follow with an activity that they can perform.

Section 47.2

Depression and Anxiety Often Present in People with Dementia

It's well known that people with dementia often suffer from anxiety and depression, but now researchers are realizing that symptoms of depression and anxiety actually wax and wane as cognitive dysfunction increases.

The cognitive changes of dementia—impairment of memory, learning, attention, and concentration—can also occur in people who are depressed, making the diagnosis of dementia more difficult. In fact, depression and cognitive decline often occur together.

Now a study in the journal *Dementia and Geriatric Cognitive Disorders* (Volume 24, page 213) shows that symptoms of depression and anxiety actually wax and wane as cognitive dysfunction increases.

The researchers compared four groups in various stages of cognitive decline from a community-based sample and a clinical sample of older people diagnosed with Alzheimer's. The prevalence of anxiety and depression symptoms among people in various stages of cognitive decline was established, then analyses were conducted to determine differences between the levels of cognitive functioning.

Anxiety symptoms were noted in 8.6% of people with good cognitive functioning, rising to 11.8% in those with moderate functioning and dropping to 10.7% in those with poor functioning. Similarly, depressive symptoms were found in 8.9% of those with good functioning, 22.1% of those with moderate functioning, and 21.1% of those with poor functioning. Of those diagnosed with Alzheimer's disease, only 6% had anxiety and 16.7% suffered from depression.

The increase in depression and anxiety symptoms earlier in the course of cognitive decline may be attributed to individuals noticing the decrease in functioning, while in later cognitive decline (and Alzheimer's) anxiety and depression may appear to decrease due to lack of awareness.

Chapter 48

Techniques for Communicating with Someone with Dementia

"It's not what you say, but how you say it." This expression holds doubly true when communicating with individuals with dementia.

Alzheimer's disease or related illnesses impair a person's ability to understand words and to speak. However, they can still benefit from non-verbal communication—body language, voice tone, and facial expressions. As the individual's ability to process verbal information declines, the importance of how caregivers communicate with them, verbally and non-verbally, increases.

Here are some tips to enhance interactions:

- Remember that the individual with dementia might be feeling confused, anxious, irritable and depressed, and suffering from low self-esteem.

- Speak clearly, slowly, and in a calm and friendly tone.

- Be aware of body language. Individuals with dementia are very receptive to body language. They are often able to detect if a person's body language depicts happiness, anger, or other emotions, and then mimic the cues they see. If a frustrated caregiver, for example, gives off a certain negative energy, the individual with the disease might mirror back the emotion and respond with an equal amount of anger or impatience.

"Communication: Techniques," © 2010 Alzheimer's Foundation of America (www.alzfdn.org). Reprinted with permission.

- Use visual cues, pointing to things to show what you mean. Instead of saying, "Please brush your teeth," pick up the toothbrush and demonstrate, for instance.

- Make certain that the person with dementia has the best chance of seeing and hearing you. This involves checking that the person is wearing glasses and hearing aids, if necessary, and that talking occurs in a quiet environment.

- Approach the individual from the front. An unexpected touch or drawing near from behind may startle and upset the person.

- Before asking the individual to do something, address the person by name to get his attention. While you are speaking, maintain eye contact to help him focus.

- Ask only one question at a time and allow time for an answer. If he does not seem to understand, repeat the question using the same wording. If this does not work, after a few minutes, rephrase it.

- Allow the individual adequate time to respond in conversation or when performing an activity. Rushing will increase confusion.

- If the individual repeatedly asks a question, keep in mind that he cannot remember the response you have just given him. Instead of answering the question after a second or third repetition, reassure the individual in some way—everything is fine, you will be with him, you will help him.

- Eliminate distractions, such as the TV or radio, when talking to the person with dementia.

- Avoid statements that sound negative. For example, instead of "Don't go outside," say, "Stay inside."

- Use humor whenever possible, though not at the individual's expense.

- Break down all tasks into simple steps. Tell the individual one step at a time what to do. Giving too many directions at once or too quickly will increase confusion. If the individual gets upset and becomes uncooperative, stop and try again later.

- Keep on talking, even when a person may no longer be verbal. Chat about things that mattered to the person and mention names of family and friends. Even if communication is one-sided, it can loudly show that you care.

Communication also plays a big role in behavior management.

Assess the situation. Once you have observed the person's behavior, try to find out what might have caused it. Ask yourself questions such as "Why is my loved one upset?" or "What happened in the last few minutes that could have prompted this behavior?" Also, do a basic evaluation to cover all your bases: Consider that the person could be cold, hungry, in pain, bored, threatened, sleepy, frightened, etc. Once you assess the root cause of this behavior, you can communicate accordingly.

Offer comfort. Caregivers can provide comfort or reassurance through validation—a technique that allows the person to stay in the moment without being proven wrong or brought back to reality. For instance, if an older man becomes upset because he cannot find his mother, an effective response might be: "I know you miss your mother very much, and she loves you, too. You were always your mother's pride and joy." This will help the individual feel understood and safe.

Distraction is a powerful tool that diverts a person's attention and can help minimize disruptive behaviors. Since individuals with dementia have a very small window of short-term memory, changing the subject will help the individual focus on something positive while leaving sadness or anger behind. Any distraction topic could work, as long as it is pleasant for the individual with the illness. This could range from the weather outside, to the painting on the wall, to the wedding story that the individual loves to tell over and over again. During a state of agitation, a caregiver might say "I can tell you are upset, but always know that your family loves you dearly. In fact, we really miss those family dinners we had every Sunday. Why don't you tell me all about that time you surprised us with a pot roast?"

Chapter 49

Planning the Day for Someone with Dementia

Activities and the Person with Dementia

Activities are the "things that we do," like getting dressed, doing chores, playing cards—even paying bills. They can be active or passive, done alone or with others. Activities represent who we are and what we're about.

A person with dementia will eventually need assistance from a caregiver to organize the day. Planned activities can enhance the person's sense of dignity and self-esteem by giving more purpose and meaning to his or her life.

Activities structure time. They can make the best of a person's abilities, enhance quality of life, and facilitate relaxation. Activities can also reduce behavior like wandering or agitation.

Both the person with dementia and the caregiver can enjoy the sense of security and togetherness that activities can provide.

Types of Activities

Daily Routines

- Chores: Dusting, sweeping, doing laundry

"Activities at Home," is reprinted with permission of the Alzheimer's Association. For additional information, call the Alzheimer's Association toll-free helpline, 800-272-3900, or visit their website at www.alz.org. © 2010 Alzheimer's Association. All rights reserved.

- Mealtime: Preparing food, cooking, eating
- Personal care: Bathing, shaving, getting dressed

Other Activities

- Creative: Painting, playing the piano
- Intellectual: Reading a book, doing crossword puzzles
- Physical: Taking a walk, playing catch
- Social: Having coffee, talking, playing cards
- Spiritual: Praying, singing a hymn
- Spontaneous: Going out to dinner, visiting friends
- Work-related: Making notes, typing, fixing something

Planning Activities

The strategies for planning activities focus on the:

- person;
- activity;
- approach;
- place.

Person

Planning activities for the person with dementia is best when you continually explore, experiment, and adjust. Consider the person's likes and dislikes; strengths and abilities; and interests. As the disease progresses, keep activities flexible, and be ready to make adjustments.

Keep the person's skills and abilities in mind: He or she may be able to play simple songs learned on the piano years ago. Bring these types of skills into daily activities.

Pay special attention to what the person enjoys: Take note when the person seems happy, anxious, distracted, or irritable. Some people enjoy watching sports, while others may be frightened by the fast pace or noise.

Consider if the person begins activities without direction: Does he or she set the table before dinner or begin sweeping the kitchen floor mid-morning? If so, you may wish to plan these activities as part of the daily routine.

Be aware of physical problems: Does he or she get tired quickly or have difficulty seeing, hearing, or performing simple movements? If so, you may want to avoid certain activities.

Activity

Focus on enjoyment, not achievement: Find activities that build on remaining skills and talents. A professional artist might become frustrated over the declining quality of work, but an amateur might enjoy a new opportunity for self-expression.

Encourage involvement in daily life: Activities that help the individual feel like a valued part of the household—like setting the table, wiping counter tops, or emptying wastebaskets—provide a sense of success and accomplishment.

Relate activity to work life: A former office worker might enjoy activities that involve organizing, like putting coins in a holder, helping to assemble a mailing, or making a "to do" list. A farmer or gardener will probably take pleasure in working in the yard.

Look for favorites: The person who always enjoyed drinking coffee and reading the newspaper may still find these activities enjoyable, even if he or she is no longer able to completely understand what the newspaper says.

Change activities as needed: Try to be flexible and acknowledge the person's changing interests and abilities.

Consider time of day: Caregivers may find they have more success with certain activities at specific times of day, such as bathing and dressing in the morning. Keep in mind that your typical daily routine may need to change somewhat.

Adjust activities to stages of the disease: As the disease progresses, you may want to introduce more repetitive tasks. Be prepared for the person to eventually take a less active role in activities.

Approach

Offer support and supervision: You may need to show the person how to perform the activity and provide simple, step-by-step directions.

Concentrate on the process, not the result: Does it really matter if the towels are folded properly? Not really. What matters is that you were able to spend time together, and the person feels as if he or she has helped do something useful.

Be flexible: When the person insists that he or she doesn't want to do something, it may be because he or she can't do it or fears doing it. Don't force it. If the person insists on doing it a different way, let it happen, and fix it later.

Be realistic and relaxed: Don't be concerned about filling every minute of the day with an activity. The person with Alzheimer's needs a balance of activity and rest, and may need more frequent breaks and varied tasks.

Help get the activity started: Most people with dementia still have the energy and desire to do things but may lack the ability to organize, plan, initiate, and successfully complete the task.

Break activities into simple, easy-to-follow steps: Too many directions at once often overwhelm a person with dementia. Focus on one task at a time.

Assist with difficult parts of the task: If you're cooking, and the person can't measure the ingredients, finish the measuring and say, "Would you please stir this for me?"

Let the individual know he or she is needed: Ask, "Could you please help me?" Be careful, however, not to place too many demands upon the person.

Stress a sense of purpose: If you ask the person to make a card, he or she may not respond. But, if you say that you're sending a special get-well card to a friend, the person may enjoy working on this task with you.

Don't criticize or correct the person: If the person enjoys a harmless activity, even if it may seem insignificant or meaningless to you, you should encourage the person to continue.

Encourage self-expression: Include activities that allow the person a chance for expression. These types of activities could include painting, drawing, music, or conversation.

Involve the person through the use of conversation: While you're polishing shoes, washing the car, or cooking dinner, talk to the person about what you're doing. Even if the person cannot respond, he or she is likely to benefit from your communication.

Substitute an activity for a behavior: If a person with dementia rubs his or her hand on a table, put a cloth in his or her hand, and encourage the person to wipe the table. Or, if the person is moving his or her feet on the floor, play some music so the person can tap them to the beat.

Try again later: If something isn't working, it may just be the wrong time of day or the activity may be too complicated. Try again later, or adapt the activity.

Place

Make activities safe: Modify a workshop by removing toxic materials and dangerous tools so an activity such as sanding a piece of wood can be safe and pleasurable.

Change your surroundings to encourage activities: Place in key locations scrapbooks, photo albums, or old magazines that help the person reminisce.

Minimize distractions that can frighten or confuse: A person with dementia may not be able to recall familiar sounds and places or may feel uncomfortable in certain settings.

Creating a Daily Plan

Consider how you organize your own day when planning the day for the person with dementia. There are times when you want variety and other times when you welcome routine. The challenge for caregivers is to find activities that provide meaning and purpose, as well as pleasure.

Begin by thinking about the past week. Try keeping a daily journal, and make notes about:

- Which activities worked best and which didn't? Why?

- Were there times when there was too much going on or too little to do?

- Were spontaneous activities enjoyable, or did they create anxiety and confusion?

Use what you've learned to set up a written daily plan. A planned day allows you to spend less time and energy trying to figure out what to do from moment to moment. Allow yourself and the person with dementia some flexibility for spontaneous activities, as well as time to rest.

Effective activities:

- bring meaning, purpose, joy, and hope to the person's life;
- use the person's skills and abilities;
- give the person a sense of normalcy;
- involve family and friends;
- are dignified and appropriate for adults;
- are enjoyable.

Example of a Daily Plan

Morning

- Wash, brush teeth, get dressed
- Prepare and eat breakfast
- Have coffee and make conversation
- Discuss the newspaper, try a craft project, reminisce about old photos
- Take a break, have some quiet time
- Do some chores together
- Take a walk, play an active game

Afternoon

- Prepare and eat lunch, read mail, wash dishes
- Listen to music, do crossword puzzles, watch TV
- Do some gardening, take a walk, visit a friend
- Take a short break or nap

Evening

- Prepare and eat dinner, clean up the kitchen
- Reminisce over coffee and dessert
- Play cards, watch a movie, give a massage
- Take a bath, get ready for bed, read a book

Measuring the Plan's Success

To decide how the daily plan is working, think about how the person responds to each activity and how well it meets your needs.

The success of an activity can vary from day to day. In general, if the person seems bored, distracted, or irritable, it may be time to introduce another activity or to take time out for rest.

Oftentimes, structured and pleasant activities reduce agitation and improve mood. The type of activity and how well it's completed are not as important as the joy and sense of accomplishment the person gets from doing it.

Ten Quick Tips: Activities at Home

1. Be flexible and patient.

2. Encourage involvement in daily life.

3. Avoid correcting the person.

4. Help the person remain as independent as possible.

5. Offer opportunities for choice.

6. Simplify instructions.

7. Establish a familiar routine.

8. Respond to the person's feelings.

9. Simplify, structure, and supervise.

10. Provide encouragement and praise.

Chapter 50

Safety Issues for People with AD

Chapter Contents

Section 50.1

Safety at Home

Excerpted from "Home Safety for People with Alzheimer's Disease,"
by the National Institute on Aging (NIA, www.nia.nih.gov), part of
the National Institutes of Health, March 2010.

People with Alzheimer disease become increasingly unable to take
care of themselves. However, the disease progresses differently in each
person. As a caregiver, you face the ongoing challenge of adapting to
each change in the person's behavior and functioning. The following
general principles may be helpful.

1. **Think prevention.** It is very difficult to predict what a person with Alzheimer disease might do. Just because something
    has not yet occurred does not mean it should not be cause for
    concern. Even with the best-laid plans, accidents can happen.
    Therefore, checking the safety of your home will help you take
    control of some of the potential problems that may create hazardous situations.

2. **Adapt the environment.** It is more effective to change
    the environment than to change most behaviors. While some
    Alzheimer disease behaviors can be managed with special
    medications prescribed by a doctor, many cannot. You can
    make changes in an environment to decrease the hazards
    and stressors that accompany these behavioral and
    functional changes.

3. **Minimize danger.** By minimizing danger, you can maximize
    independence. A safe environment can be a less restrictive environment where the person with Alzheimer disease can experience increased security and more mobility.

Is It Safe to Leave the Person with Alzheimer Disease Alone?

This issue needs careful evaluation and is certainly a safety concern.
The following points may help you decide.

Does the person with Alzheimer disease:

- become confused or unpredictable under stress?

- recognize a dangerous situation, for example, fire?

- know how to use the telephone in an emergency?

- know how to get help?

- stay content within the home?

- wander and become disoriented?

- show signs of agitation, depression, or withdrawal when left alone for any period of time?

- attempt to pursue former interests or hobbies that might now warrant supervision, such as cooking, appliance repair, or woodworking?

You may want to seek input and advice from a health care professional to assist you in these considerations. As Alzheimer disease progresses, these questions will need ongoing evaluation.

Home Safety Room by Room

Prevention begins with a safety check of every room in your home. Use the following room-by-room checklist to alert you to potential hazards and to record any changes you need to make. You can buy products or gadgets necessary for home safety at stores carrying hardware, electronics, medical supplies, and children's items.

Keep in mind that it may not be necessary to make all of the suggested changes. This text covers a wide range of safety concerns that may arise, and some modifications may never be needed. It is important, however, to re-evaluate home safety periodically as behavior and abilities change.

Your home is a personal and precious environment. As you go through this checklist, some of the changes you make may impact your surroundings positively, and some may affect you in ways that may be inconvenient or undesirable. It is possible, however, to strike a balance. Caregivers can make adaptations that modify and simplify without severely disrupting the home. You may want to consider setting aside a special area for yourself, a space off-limits to anyone else and arranged exactly as you like. Everyone needs private, quiet time, and as a caregiver, this becomes especially crucial.

A safe home can be a less stressful home for the person with Alzheimer disease, the caregiver, and family members. You don't have to make these changes alone. You may want to enlist the help of a friend, professional, or community service such as the Alzheimer's Association.

Throughout the Home

- Display emergency numbers and your home address near all telephones.

- Use an answering machine when you cannot answer phone calls, and set it to turn on after the fewest number of rings possible. A person with Alzheimer disease often may be unable to take messages or could become a victim of telephone exploitation. Turn ringers on low to avoid distraction and confusion. Put all portable and cell phones and equipment in a safe place so they will not be easily lost.

- Install smoke alarms and carbon monoxide detectors in or near the kitchen and all sleeping areas. Check their functioning and batteries frequently.

- Avoid the use of flammable and volatile compounds near gas appliances. Do not store these materials in an area where a gas pilot light is used.

- Install secure locks on all outside doors and windows.

- Hide a spare house key outside in case the person with Alzheimer disease locks you out of the house.

- Avoid the use of extension cords if possible by placing lamps and appliances close to electrical outlets. Tack extension cords to the baseboards of a room to avoid tripping.

- Cover unused electrical outlets with childproof plugs.

- Place red tape around floor vents, radiators, and other heating devices to deter the person with Alzheimer disease from standing on or touching them when hot.

- Check all rooms for adequate lighting.

- Place light switches at the top and the bottom of stairs.

- Stairways should have at least one handrail that extends beyond the first and last steps. If possible, stairways should be carpeted or have safety grip strips. Put a gate across the stairs if the person has balance problems.

- Keep all medications (prescription and over-the-counter) locked. Each bottle of prescription medicine should be clearly labeled with the person's name, name of the drug, drug strength, dosage frequency, and expiration date. Child-resistant caps are available if needed.

- Keep all alcohol in a locked cabinet or out of reach of the person with Alzheimer disease. Drinking alcohol can increase confusion.

- If smoking is permitted, monitor the person with Alzheimer disease while he or she is smoking. Remove matches, lighters, ashtrays, cigarettes, and other means of smoking from view. This reduces fire hazards, and with these reminders out of sight, the person may forget the desire to smoke.

- Avoid clutter, which can create confusion and danger. Throw out or recycle newspapers and magazines regularly. Keep all areas where people walk free of furniture.

- Keep plastic bags out of reach. A person with Alzheimer disease may choke or suffocate.

- Remove all guns and other weapons from the home or lock them up. Installing safety locks on guns or remove ammunition and firing pins.

- Lock all power tools and machinery in the garage, workroom, or basement.

- Remove all poisonous plants from the home. Check with local nurseries or contact the poison control center (800-222-1222) for a list of poisonous plants.

- Make sure all computer equipment and accessories, including electrical cords, are kept out of the way. If valuable documents or materials are stored on a home computer, protect the files with passwords and back up the files. Password protect access to the internet, and restrict the amount of online time without supervision. Consider monitoring computer use by the person with Alzheimer disease, and install software that screens for objectionable or offensive material on the internet.

- Keep fish tanks out of reach. The combination of glass, water, electrical pumps, and potentially poisonous aquatic life could be harmful to a curious person with Alzheimer disease.

Outside Approaches to the House

- Keep steps sturdy and textured to prevent falls in wet or icy weather.

- Mark the edges of steps with bright or reflective tape.

- Consider installing a ramp with handrails as an alternative to the steps.

- Eliminate uneven surfaces or walkways, hoses, and other objects that may cause a person to trip.

- Restrict access to a swimming pool by fencing it with a locked gate, covering it, and closely supervising it when in use.

- In the patio area, remove the fuel source and fire starters from any grills when not in use, and supervise use when the person with Alzheimer disease is present.

- Place a small bench or table by the entry door to hold parcels while unlocking the door.

- Make sure outside lighting is adequate. Light sensors that turn on lights automatically as you approach the house may be useful. They also may be used in other parts of the home.

- Prune bushes and foliage well away from walkways and doorways.

- Consider a No Soliciting sign for the front gate or door.

Entryway

- Remove scatter rugs and throw rugs.

- Use textured strips or nonskid wax on hardwood and tile floors to prevent slipping.

Kitchen

- Install childproof door latches on storage cabinets and drawers designated for breakable or dangerous items. Lock away all household cleaning products, matches, knives, scissors, blades, small appliances, and anything valuable.

- If prescription or nonprescription drugs are kept in the kitchen, store them in a locked cabinet.

- Remove scatter rugs and foam pads from the floor.

- Install safety knobs and an automatic shut-off switch on the stove.

- Do not use or store flammable liquids in the kitchen. Lock them in the garage or in an outside storage unit.

- Keep a night-light in the kitchen.

- Remove or secure the family junk drawer. A person with Alzheimer disease may eat small items such as matches, hardware, erasers, plastics, etc.

- Remove artificial fruits and vegetables or food-shaped kitchen magnets, which might appear to be edible.

- Insert a drain trap in the kitchen sink to catch anything that may otherwise become lost or clog the plumbing.

- Consider disconnecting the garbage disposal. People with Alzheimer disease may place objects or their own hands in the disposal.

Bedroom

- Anticipate the reasons a person with Alzheimer disease might get out of bed, such as hunger, thirst, going to the bathroom, restlessness, and pain. Try to meet these needs by offering food and fluids and scheduling ample toileting.

- Use a night-light.

- Use a monitoring device (like those used for infants) to alert you to any sounds indicating a fall or other need for help. This also is an effective device for bathrooms.

- Remove scatter rugs and throw rugs.

- Remove portable space heaters. If you use portable fans, be sure that objects cannot be placed in the blades.

- Be cautious when using electric mattress pads, electric blankets, electric sheets, and heating pads, all of which can cause burns and fires. Keep controls out of reach.

- If the person with Alzheimer disease is at risk of falling out of bed, place mats next to the bed, as long as they do not create a greater risk of accident.

- Use transfer or mobility aids.

- If you are considering using a hospital-type bed with rails and/or wheels, read the Food and Drug Administration's up-to-date safety information at http://www.fda.gov/MedicalDevices/Products andMedicalProcedures/GeneralHospitalDevicesandSupplies/HospitalBeds/default.htm.

Bathroom

- Do not leave a severely impaired person with Alzheimer disease alone in the bathroom.

- Remove the lock from the bathroom door to prevent the person with Alzheimer disease from getting locked inside.

- Place nonskid adhesive strips, decals, or mats in the tub and shower. If the bathroom is uncarpeted, consider placing these strips next to the tub, toilet, and sink.

- Use washable wall-to-wall bathroom carpeting to prevent slipping on wet tile floors.

- Use a raised toilet seat with handrails, or install grab bars beside the toilet.

- Install grab bars in the tub/shower. A grab bar in contrasting color to the wall is easier to see.

- Use a foam rubber faucet cover (often used for small children) in the tub to prevent serious injury should the person with Alzheimer disease fall.

- Use a plastic shower stool and a hand-held shower head to make bathing easier.

- In the shower, tub, and sink, use a single faucet that mixes hot and cold water to avoid burns.

- Set the water heater at 120 degrees Fahrenheit to avoid scalding tap water.

- Insert drain traps in sinks to catch small items that may be lost or flushed down the drain.

- Store medications (prescription and nonprescription) in a locked cabinet. Check medication dates and throw away outdated medications.

- Remove cleaning products from under the sink, or lock them away.

- Use a night-light.

- Remove small electrical appliances from the bathroom. Cover electrical outlets.

- If a man with Alzheimer disease uses an electric razor, have him use a mirror outside the bathroom to avoid water contact.

Living Room

- Clear electrical cords from all areas where people walk.

- Remove scatter rugs or throw rugs. Repair or replace torn carpet.

- Place decals at eye level on sliding glass doors, picture windows, or furniture with large glass panels to identify the glass pane.

- Do not leave the person with Alzheimer disease alone with an open fire in the fireplace. Consider alternative heating sources.

- Keep matches and cigarette lighters out of reach. Keep the remote controls for the television, DVD player, and stereo system out of sight.

Laundry Room

- Keep the door to the laundry room locked if possible.

- Lock all laundry products in a cabinet.

- Remove large knobs from the washer and dryer if the person with Alzheimer disease tampers with machinery.

- Close and latch the doors and lids to the washer and dryer to prevent objects from being placed in the machines.

Garage/Shed/Basement

- Lock access to all garages, sheds, and basements if possible.

- Inside a garage or shed, keep all potentially dangerous items, such as tools, tackle, machines, and sporting equipment either locked away in cabinets or in appropriate boxes/cases.

- Secure and lock all motor vehicles and keep them out of sight if possible. Consider covering vehicles, including bicycles, that

501

are not frequently used. This may reduce the possibility that the person with Alzheimer disease will think about leaving.

- Keep all toxic materials, such as paint, fertilizers, gasoline, or cleaning supplies, out of view. Either put them in a high, dry place, or lock them in a cabinet.

- If the person with Alzheimer disease is permitted in a garage, shed, or basement, preferably with supervision, make sure the area is well lit and that stairs have a handrail and are safe to walk up and down. Keep walkways clear of debris and clutter, and place overhanging items out of reach.

Home Safety Behavior by Behavior

Although a number of behavior and sensory problems may accompany Alzheimer disease, not every person will experience the disease in exactly the same way. As the disease progresses, particular behavioral changes can create safety problems. The person with Alzheimer disease may or may not have these symptoms. However, should these behaviors occur, the following safety recommendations may help reduce risks.

Wandering

- Remove clutter and clear the pathways from room to room to prevent falls and allow the person with Alzheimer disease to move about more freely.

- Make sure floors provide good traction for walking or pacing. Use nonskid floor wax or leave floors unpolished. Secure all rug edges, eliminate throw rugs, or install nonskid strips. The person with Alzheimer disease should wear nonskid shoes or sneakers.

- Place locks high or low on exit doors so they are out of direct sight.

- Consider installing double locks that require a key. Keep a key for yourself, and hide one near the door for emergency exit purposes.

- Use loosely fitting doorknob covers so that the cover turns instead of the actual knob. Due to the potential hazard they could cause if an emergency exit is needed, locked doors and doorknob covers should be used only when a caregiver is present.

- Install safety devices found in hardware stores to limit how much windows can be opened.

- If possible, secure the yard with fencing and a locked gate. Use door alarms such as loose bells above the door or devices that ring when the doorknob is touched or the door is opened.

- Divert the attention of the person with Alzheimer disease away from using the door by placing small scenic posters on the door; placing removable gates, curtains, or brightly colored streamers across the door; or wallpapering the door to match any adjoining walls.

- Place STOP, DO NOT ENTER, or CLOSED signs on doors in strategic areas.

- Keep shoes, keys, suitcases, coats, hats, and other signs of departure out of sight.

- Obtain a medical identification bracelet for the person with Alzheimer disease with the words "memory loss" inscribed along with an emergency telephone number. Place the bracelet on the person's dominant hand to limit the possibility of removal, or solder the bracelet closed. Check with the local Alzheimer's Association about the Safe Return program.

- Place labels in garments to aid in identification.

- Keep an article of the person's worn, unwashed clothing in a plastic bag to aid in finding someone with the use of dogs.

- Notify neighbors of the person's potential to wander or become lost.

- Alert them to contact you or the police immediately if the individual is seen alone and on the move.

- Give local police, neighbors, and relatives a recent photo of the person with Alzheimer disease, along with the person's name and pertinent information, as a precaution should he or she become lost. Keep extra photos on hand.

- Consider making an up-to-date home video of the person with Alzheimer disease.

- Do not leave a person with Alzheimer disease who has a history of wandering unattended.

Rummaging/Hiding Things

- Lock up all dangerous or toxic products or place them out of the person's reach.

- Remove all old or spoiled food from the refrigerator and cupboards. A person with Alzheimer disease may rummage for snacks but may lack the judgment or taste to rule out spoiled foods.

- Simplify the environment by removing clutter or valuable items that could be misplaced, lost, or hidden by the person with Alzheimer disease. These include important papers, checkbooks, charge cards, and jewelry.

- If your yard has a fence with a locked gate, place the mailbox outside the gate. People with Alzheimer disease often hide, lose, or throw away mail. If this is a serious problem, consider obtaining a post office box.

- Create a special place for the person with Alzheimer disease to rummage freely or sort (for example, a chest of drawers, a bag of selected objects, or a basket of clothing to fold or unfold). Often, safety problems occur when the person with Alzheimer disease becomes bored or does not know what to do.

- Provide the person with Alzheimer disease a safe box, treasure chest, or cupboard to store special objects.

- Close access to unused rooms, thereby limiting the opportunity for rummaging and hiding things.

- Search the house periodically to discover hiding places. Once found, these hiding places can be discreetly and frequently checked.

- Keep all trash cans covered or out of sight. The person with Alzheimer disease may not remember the purpose of the container or may rummage through it.

- Check trash containers before emptying them in case something has been hidden there or accidentally thrown away.

Hallucinations, Illusions, and Delusions

Due to complex changes occurring in the brain, people with Alzheimer disease may see or hear things that have no basis in reality. Hallucinations involve hearing, seeing, smelling, or feeling things that are not really there. For example, a person with Alzheimer disease may see children playing in the living room when no children exist. Illusions differ from hallucinations because the person with Alzheimer disease is misinterpreting something that actually does exist. Shadows on the

504

wall may look like people, for example. Delusions are false beliefs that the person thinks are real. For example, stealing may be suspected but cannot be verified.

It is important to seek medical evaluation if a person with Alzheimer disease has ongoing disturbing hallucinations, illusions, or delusions. Discuss with the doctor any illnesses the person has and medicines he or she is taking. An illness or medicine may cause hallucinations or delusions. Often, these symptoms can be treated with medication or behavior management techniques. With all of these symptoms, the following environmental adaptations also may be helpful.

- Paint walls a light color to reflect more light. Use solid colors, which are less confusing to an impaired person than a patterned wall. Large, bold prints (for example, florals in wallpaper or drapes) may cause confusing illusions.

- Make sure there is adequate lighting, and keep extra bulbs handy in a secured place. Dimly lit areas may produce confusing shadows or difficulty with interpreting everyday objects.

- Reduce glare by using soft light or frosted bulbs, partially closing blinds or curtains, and maintaining adequate globes or shades on light fixtures.

- Remove or cover mirrors if they cause the person with Alzheimer disease to become confused or frightened.

- Ask if the person can point to a specific area that is producing confusion. Perhaps one particular aspect of the environment is being misinterpreted.

- Vary the home environment as little as possible to minimize the potential for visual confusion. Keep furniture in the same place.

- Avoid violent or disturbing television programs. The person with Alzheimer disease may believe a story is real.

- Do not confront the person with Alzheimer disease who becomes aggressive. Withdraw and make sure you have access to an exit as needed.

Special Occasions/Gatherings/Holidays

When celebrations, special events, or holidays include large numbers of people, remember that large groups may cause a person with Alzheimer disease some confusion and anxiety. The person with

Alzheimer disease may find some situations easier and more pleasurable than others.

- Large gatherings, weddings, family reunions, or picnics may cause anxiety. Consider having a more intimate gathering with only a few people in your home. Think about having friends and family visit in small groups rather than all at once. If you are hosting a large group, remember to prepare the person with Alzheimer disease ahead of time. Try to have a space available where he or she can rest, be alone, or spend some time with a smaller number of people, if needed.

- Consider simplifying your holidays around the home and remember that you already may have more responsibilities than in previous years. For example, rather than cooking an elaborate dinner at Thanksgiving or Christmas, invite family and friends for a potluck dinner. Instead of elaborate decorations, consider choosing a few select items to celebrate holidays. Make sure holiday decorations do not significantly alter the environment, which might confuse the person with Alzheimer disease.

- Holiday decorations, such as Christmas trees, lights, or menorahs, should be secured so that they do not fall or catch on fire. Anything flammable should be monitored at all times, and extra precautions should be taken so that lights or anything breakable are fixed firmly, correctly, and out of the way of those with Alzheimer disease.

- As suggested by most manufacturers, candles of any size should never be lit without supervision. When not in use, they should be put away. Try to avoid clutter in general, especially in walkways, during the holidays.

Impairment of the Senses

Alzheimer disease can cause changes in a person's ability to interpret what he or she can see, hear, taste, feel, or smell. The person with Alzheimer disease should be evaluated periodically by a physician for any such changes that may be correctable with glasses, dentures, hearing aids, or other devices.

Vision

People with Alzheimer disease may experience a number of changes in visual abilities. For example, they may lose their ability to comprehend visual images. Although there is nothing physically wrong with their eyes, people with Alzheimer disease may no longer be able to interpret accurately what they see because of brain changes. Also, their sense of perception and depth may be altered. These changes can cause safety concerns.

- Create color contrast between floors and walls to help the person see depth. Floor coverings are less visually confusing if they are a solid color.

- Use dishes and placemats in contrasting colors for easier identification.

- Mark the edges of steps with brightly colored strips of tape to outline changes in height.

- Place brightly colored signs or simple pictures on important rooms (the bathroom, for example) for easier identification.

- Be aware that a small pet that blends in with the floor or lies in walkways may be a hazard. The person with Alzheimer disease may trip over the pet.

Smell

A loss of or decrease in smell often accompanies Alzheimer disease.

- Install smoke detectors and check them frequently. The person with Alzheimer disease may not smell smoke or may not associate it with danger.

- Keep refrigerators clear of spoiled foods.

Touch

People with Alzheimer disease may experience loss of sensation or may no longer be able to interpret feelings of heat, cold, or discomfort.

- Adjust water heaters to 120 degrees Fahrenheit to avoid scalding tap water. Most hot water heaters are set at 150 degrees, which can cause burns.

- Color code separate water faucet handles, with red for hot and blue for cold.

- Place a sign on the oven, coffee maker, toaster, crock-pot, iron, and other potentially hot appliances that says DO NOT TOUCH or STOP! VERY HOT. The person with Alzheimer disease should not use appliances without supervision. Unplug appliances when not in use.

- Use a thermometer to tell you if bath water is too hot or too cold.

- Remove furniture or other objects with sharp corners or pad the corners to reduce potential for injury.

Taste

People with Alzheimer disease may lose taste sensitivity. As their judgment declines, they also may place dangerous or inappropriate things in their mouths.

- Keep all condiments such as salt, sugar, or spices hidden if you see the person with Alzheimer disease using excess amounts. Too much salt, sugar, or spice can be irritating to the stomach or cause other health problems.

- Remove or lock up medicine cabinet items such as toothpaste, perfume, lotions, shampoos, rubbing alcohol, and soap, which may look and smell like food to the person with Alzheimer disease.

- Consider a childproof latch on the refrigerator, if necessary.

- Keep the toll-free poison control number (800-222-1222) by the telephone. Keep a bottle of ipecac (vomit-inducing agent) available, but use only with instructions from poison control or 911.

- Keep pet litter boxes inaccessible to the person with Alzheimer disease. Do not store pet food in the refrigerator.

- Learn the Heimlich maneuver or other techniques to use in case of choking. Check with your local Red Cross chapter for more information and instruction.

- If possible, keep a spare set of dentures. If the person keeps removing dentures, check for correct fit.

Hearing

People with Alzheimer disease may have normal hearing, but they may lose their ability to interpret what they hear accurately. This loss may result in confusion or overstimulation.

- Avoid excessive noise in the home such as having the stereo and the TV on at the same time.

- Be sensitive to the amount of noise outside the home, and close windows or doors, if necessary.

- Avoid large gatherings of people in the home if the person with Alzheimer disease shows signs of agitation or distress in crowds. If the person wears a hearing aid, check the batteries and functioning frequently.

Driving

Driving is a complex activity that demands quick reactions, alert senses, and split-second decision making. For a person with Alzheimer disease, driving becomes increasingly difficult. Memory loss, impaired judgment, disorientation, impaired visual and spatial perception, slow reaction time, certain medications, diminished attention span, and inability to recognize cues such as stop signs and traffic lights can make driving particularly hazardous.

People with Alzheimer disease who continue to drive can be a danger to themselves, their passengers, and the community at large. As the disease progresses, they lose driving skills and must stop driving. Unfortunately, people with Alzheimer disease often cannot recognize when they should no longer drive. This is a tremendous safety concern. It is extremely important to have the impaired person's driving abilities carefully evaluated.

Often, the caregiver or a family member, neighbor, or friend is the first to become aware of the safety hazards of someone with Alzheimer disease behind the wheel. If a person with Alzheimer disease experiences one of more of the following problems, it may be time to limit or stop driving.

Does the person with Alzheimer disease:

- get lost while driving in a familiar location?

- fail to observe traffic signals?

- drive at an inappropriate speed?

- become angry, frustrated, or confused while driving?

- make slow or poor decisions?

Please do not wait for an accident to happen. Take action immediately.

Explaining to the person with Alzheimer disease that he or she can no longer drive can be extremely difficult. Loss of driving privileges may represent a tremendous loss of independence, freedom, and identity. It is a significant concern for the person with Alzheimer disease and the caregiver. The issue of not driving may produce anger, denial, and grief in the person with Alzheimer disease, as well as guilt and anxiety in the caregiver. Family and concerned professionals need to be both sensitive and firm. Above all, they should be persistent and consistent. The doctor of a person with Alzheimer disease can assist the family with the task of restricting driving. Talk with the doctor about your concerns.

Most people will listen to their doctor. Ask the doctor to advise the person with Alzheimer disease to reduce his or her driving, go for a driving evaluation or test, or stop driving altogether. An increasing number of states have laws requiring physicians to report Alzheimer disease and related disorders to the Department of Motor Vehicles. The Department of Motor Vehicles then is responsible for retesting the at-risk driver. Testing should occur regularly, at least yearly.

When dementia impairs driving and the person with Alzheimer disease continues to insist on driving, a number of different approaches may be necessary.

- Work as a team with family, friends, and professionals, and use a single, simple explanation for the loss of driving ability such as: "You have a memory problem, and it is no longer safe to drive," "You cannot drive because you are on medication," or "The doctor has prescribed that you no longer drive."

- Ask the doctor to write on a prescription pad DO NOT DRIVE. Ask the doctor to write to the Department of Motor Vehicles or Department of Public Safety saying this person should no longer drive. Show the letter to the person with Alzheimer disease as evidence.

- Offer to drive or ask a friend or family member to drive.

- Walk when possible, and make these outings special events.

- Use public transportation or any special transportation provided by community organizations. Ask about senior discounts or transportation coupons. The person with Alzheimer disease should not take public transportation unsupervised.

- Park the car at a friend's home.

- Hide the car keys.

- Exchange car keys with a set of unusable keys. Some people with Alzheimer disease are in the habit of carrying keys.

510

- Place a large note under the car hood requesting that any mechanic call you before doing work requested by the person with Alzheimer disease.

- Have a mechanic install a "kill switch" or alarm system that disengages the fuel line to prevent the car from starting.

- Consider selling the car and putting aside for taxi fares the money saved from insurance, repairs, and gasoline.

- Do not leave a person with Alzheimer disease alone in a parked car.

Natural Disaster Safety

Natural disasters come in many forms and degrees of severity. They seldom give warning, and they call upon good judgment and the ability to follow through with crisis plans. People with Alzheimer disease are at a serious disadvantage. Their impairments in memory and reasoning severely limit their ability to act appropriately in crises.

It is always important to have a plan of action in case of fire, earthquake, flood, tornado, or other disasters. Specific home safety precautions may apply and environmental changes may be needed. The American Red Cross is an excellent resource for general safety information and preparedness guides for comprehensive planning. If there is a person with Alzheimer disease in the home, the following precautions apply:

- Get to know your neighbors, and identify specific individuals who would be willing to help in a crisis. Formulate a plan of action with them should the person with Alzheimer disease be unattended during a crisis.

- Give neighbors a list of emergency phone numbers of caregivers, family members, and primary medical resources.

- Educate neighbors beforehand about the person's specific disabilities, including inability to follow complex instructions, memory loss, impaired judgment, and probable disorientation and confusion. Give examples of some of the simple one-step instructions that the person may be able to follow.

- Have regular emergency drills so that each member of the household has a specific task. Realize that the person with Alzheimer disease cannot be expected to hold any responsibility in the crisis plan and that someone will need to take primary responsibility for supervising the individual.

- Always have at least an extra week's supply of any medical or personal hygiene items critical to the person's welfare, such as the following:

  - Food and water

  - Medications

  - Incontinence undergarments

  - Hearing aid batteries

- Keep an extra pair of the person's eyeglasses on hand.

- Be sure that the person with Alzheimer disease wears an identification bracelet stating "memory loss" should he or she become lost or disoriented during the crisis. Contact your local Alzheimer's Association chapter and enroll the person in the Safe Return program.

- Under no circumstances should a person with Alzheimer disease be left alone following a natural disaster. Do not count on the individual to stay in one place while you go to get help. Provide plenty of reassurance.

Who Would Take Care of the Person with Alzheimer Disease If Something Happened to You?

It is important to have a plan in case of your own illness, disability, or death.

- Consult a lawyer about setting up a living trust, durable power of attorney for health care and finances, and other estate planning tools.

- Consult with family and close friends to decide who will take responsibility for the person with Alzheimer disease. You also may want to seek information about your local public guardian's office, mental health conservator's office, adult protective services, or other case management services. These organizations may have programs to assist the person with Alzheimer disease in your absence.

- Maintain a notebook for the responsible person who will assume caregiving. Such a notebook should contain the following information:

  - Emergency phone numbers

- Current problem behaviors and possible solutions

- Ways to calm the person with Alzheimer disease

- Assistance needed with toileting, feeding, or grooming

- Favorite activities or food

- Preview board and care or long-term care facilities in your community and select a few as possibilities. Share this information with the responsible person. If the person with Alzheimer disease is no longer able to live at home, the responsible person will be better able to carry out your wishes for long-term care.

Conclusion

Home safety takes many forms. This text focuses on the physical environment and specific safety concerns. But the home environment also involves the needs, feelings, and lifestyles of you the caregiver, your family, and the person with Alzheimer disease. Disability affects all family members, and it is crucial to maintain your emotional and physical welfare in addition to ensuring a safe environment.

We encourage you to make sure you have quiet time, time out, and time to take part in something you enjoy. Protect your own emotional and physical health. Your local Alzheimer's Association chapter can help you with the support and information you may need as you address this very significant checkpoint in your home safety list. You are extremely valuable. As you take on a commitment to care for a person with Alzheimer disease, please take on the equally important commitment to care for yourself.

Section 50.2

MedicAlert® and the Safe Return® Program

"MedicAlert + Safe Return," is reprinted with permission of the Alzheimer's Association. For additional information, call the Alzheimer's Association toll-free helpline, 800-272-3900, or visit their website at www.alz.org. © 2007 Alzheimer's Association. All rights reserved.

The Alzheimer's Association and MedicAlert have formed an alliance to improve the safety of individuals with Alzheimer's or related dementia. MedicAlert® + Alzheimer's Association Safe Return® is a 24-hour nationwide emergency response service for individuals with Alzheimer's or a related dementia that wander or who have a medical emergency.

How MedicAlert + Safe Return Works

If an individual with Alzheimer's or related dementia wanders and becomes lost, caregivers can call the 24-hour emergency response line (800-625-3780) to report it. A community support network will be activated, including local Alzheimer's Association chapters and law enforcement agencies, to help reunite the family member or caregiver with the person who wandered. With this enhanced service, critical medical information will be provided to emergency responders when needed.

MedicAlert + Safe Return Features

- One identification product (bracelet or necklace) that serves two purposes. It provides emergency medical information and assists in the event of a wandering incident.

- The member's personal health record lists medical conditions, medications, and allergies and can be updated 24 hours a day through a private online account or by calling the toll-free number during business hours.

- A national database that includes a member's photo and emergency contact information to help reunite the lost person with his or her caregivers.

- The MedicAlert + Safe Return hotline activates the resources of law enforcement, medical professionals, and the local chapter staff to assist the member when an incident—either wandering or medical emergency—occurs.

Cost for MedicAlert + Safe Return products

The enrollment fee is $49.95 with an annual renewal fee of $25. The enrollment kit includes 24-hour emergency response system, ID jewelry (bracelet or necklace), personalized emergency wallet card, personal health record, and "6 steps to a Safe Return refrigerator magnet," which provides useful tips when someone is missing.

Companion caregiver jewelry can be purchased for $25 with an annual renewal fee of $25, which includes everything listed above.

For safety and peace of mind, enroll in MedicAlert + Safe Return today: Call 888-572-8566 (6 a.m.–7 p.m. [PST] Monday–Friday and 8 a.m.–5 p.m. [PST] Saturday) or online at www.alz.org.

Section 50.3

Caring for Someone with Dementia in a Disaster

From "Caring for Someone with Dementia in a Disaster," by the Federal Emergency Management Agency (FEMA, www.fema.gov), August 11, 2010.

If You Know a Disaster Is about to Occur

- Get yourself and the person with Alzheimer disease to a safe place.

- Alert others (friends, family, and medical personnel) to the fact that you are changing locations, and give them your contact information. Contact them as regularly as you can as you move.

- Be sure there are people other than the primary caregiver who have copies of the person with dementia's medical history, medications, and physician information.

- Purchase extra medications.

Advance Preparations

Safe Return

As a precaution, register your loved one in the Alzheimer's Association Safe Return program.

- Safe Return is an identification and support program that provides assistance for a person with Alzheimer disease who wanders off and becomes lost, either locally or far from home.

- If you are already registered in Safe Return, make sure personal contact information, medicines needed, and doctor information are updated with the program.

Emergency Kit

Consider preparing an emergency kit in advance. Keep it in a watertight container and store it in an easily accessible location. Your emergency kit might include the following:

516

- Flotation devices, such as Floaties armbands
- Easy on/off clothes (a couple of sets)
- Velcro shoes/sneakers
- Back-up eyeglasses
- Incontinence products
- Wipes
- Lotion (good for soothing the person)
- Pillow, toy, or something else to hug
- Favorite items or foods and liquid meals
- Supplies of medication
- Extra identification items for the person, such as an ID bracelet or clothing tags
- Copies of legal documents, such as power of attorney
- Copies of medical documents that indicate the person's condition and current medications
- Copies of insurance and Social Security cards
- Zippered bags to hold medications and documents
- Physician's name, address, and phone numbers
- Alzheimer's Association phone number and address and Safe Return phone number
- Recent picture of the person with dementia

Tips for If You Are Relocated

In an emergency, people with dementia and their caregivers may find themselves uprooted or displaced to alternative living arrangements. Extra care and attention must be made to ensure the health and safety of the people with dementia. The change of location, plus unfamiliar noises and activities, may cause them increased stress and confusion. And certain behaviors of persons with Alzheimer disease may puzzle or alarm others.

Be Calm and Supportive

- Remain flexible, patient, and calm—a person with dementia will respond to the tone you set.

- Respond to an emotion being expressed by the person. Ask "Are you feeling frightened?" Offer your hand or a hug.

- Don't leave the person with Alzheimer disease alone. Don't ask a stranger to watch the person. A person who doesn't understand Alzheimer disease and its effects, and who doesn't know you or the person, won't understand how to react in a difficult situation.

Create a Safe Environment

- Try to spend extra time with the person to help him or her adjust to the new environment.

- As much as possible, try to maintain daily routines.

- Use simple sentences to indicate the need to stay where you are. Divert attention to a new topic. For example, "I know you want to go home. For now, we need to stay here. Let's see if we can get some lunch."

- As appropriate, inform people around you that the person has memory loss.

- Limit news media exposure to the disaster.

Take Care of Your Loved One and Yourself

- Ensure proper nutrition and hydration.

- Make it a priority to find a doctor and pharmacy.

- Find a good listener—seek spiritual support.

Section 50.4

Understanding Elder Abuse

From "Why Should I Care about Elder Abuse?" by the
National Center on Elder Abuse (NCEA, www.ncea.aoa.gov),
part of the Administration on Aging, March 3, 2010.

Elder abuse is an under recognized problem with devastating and even life-threatening consequences.

Every day, headlines throughout the United States paint a grim picture of seniors who have been abused, neglected, and exploited, often by people they trust the most. Abusers may be spouses, family members, personal acquaintances, professionals in positions of trust or opportunistic strangers who prey on the vulnerable.

How big is the problem? No one really knows. Relatively few cases are identified, as elders often are reluctant to report the mistreatment. Experts estimate that only one in six cases or fewer are reported, which means that very few seniors who have been abused get the help they need.

One thing is for certain: Elder abuse can happen to any older individual—your neighbor, your loved one—it can even happen to you.

What Is Elder Abuse?

In general, elder abuse refers to intentional or neglectful acts by a caregiver or trusted individual that lead to, or may lead to, harm of a vulnerable elder. Physical abuse, neglect, emotional or psychological abuse, verbal abuse and threats, financial abuse and exploitation, sexual abuse, and abandonment are considered forms of elder abuse. In many states, self-neglect is also considered mistreatment.

Who Is at Risk?

Elder abuse can occur anywhere—in the home, in nursing homes, or other institutions. It affects seniors across all socioeconomic groups, cultures, and races. Based on available information, women and "older" elders are more likely to be victimized. Dementia is a significant risk factor. Mental health and substance abuse issues—of both abusers and victims—are risk factors. Isolation can also contribute to risk.

Types of Elder Abuse

- **Physical abuse:** Use of force to threaten or physically injure a vulnerable elder

- **Emotional abuse:** Verbal attacks, threats, rejection, isolation, or belittling acts that cause or could cause mental anguish, pain, or distress to a senior

- **Sexual abuse:** Sexual contact that is forced, tricked, threatened, or otherwise coerced upon a vulnerable elder, including anyone who is unable to grant consent

- **Exploitation:** Theft, fraud, misuse or neglect of authority, and use of undue influence as a lever to gain control over an older person's money or property

- **Neglect:** A caregiver's failure or refusal to provide for a vulnerable elder's safety and physical or emotional needs

- **Abandonment:** Desertion of a frail or vulnerable elder by anyone with a duty of care

- **Self-neglect:** An inability to understand the consequences of one's own actions or inaction, which leads to, or may lead to, harm or endangerment

Warning Signs

- **Physical abuse:** Slap marks, unexplained bruises, most pressure marks, and certain types of burns or blisters, such as cigarette burns

- **Neglect:** Pressure ulcers, filth, lack of medical care, malnutrition, or dehydration

- **Emotional abuse:** Withdrawal from normal activities, unexplained changes in alertness, or other unusual behavioral changes

- **Sexual abuse:** Bruises around the breasts or genital area and unexplained sexually transmitted diseases

- **Financial abuse/exploitation:** Sudden change in finances and accounts, altered wills and trusts, unusual bank withdrawals, checks written as loans or gifts, and loss of property

What Can I Do to Prevent Elder Abuse?

- **Report suspected mistreatment to your local adult protective services agency or law enforcement:** Although a situation may have already been investigated, if you believe circumstances are getting worse, continue to speak out.

- **Keep in contact:** Talk with your older friends, neighbors, and relatives. Maintaining communication will help decrease isolation, a risk factor for mistreatment. It will also give them a chance to talk about any problems they may be experiencing.

- **Be aware of the possibility of abuse:** Look around and take note of what may be happening with your older neighbors and acquaintances. Do they seem lately to be withdrawn, nervous, fearful, sad, or anxious, especially around certain people, when they have not seemed so in the past?

- **Contact your local Area Agency on Aging office to identify local programs and sources of support**, such as Meals on Wheels. These programs help elders to maintain health, well-being, and independence—a good defense against abuse.

- **Volunteer:** There are many local opportunities to become involved in programs that provide assistance and support for seniors.

- Observe **World Elder Abuse Awareness Day:** Elder abuse is a global issue. Contact your local aging services organizations to find out how your community will observe World Day. Help to raise awareness by talking about the issue.

- **Learn more about the issue:** Visit the National Center on Elder Abuse website at www.ncea.aoa.gov.

What Should I Do If I Suspect Elder Abuse?

Report your concerns. Remember: Most cases of elder abuse go undetected. Don't assume that someone has already reported a suspicious situation.

To report suspected abuse in the community, contact your local adult protective services agency. For state reporting numbers, visit the NCEA website at www.ncea.aoa.gov or call the Eldercare Locator at 800-677-1116.

If you or someone you know is in a life-threatening situation or immediate danger, contact 911 or the local police or sheriff.

To report suspected abuse in a nursing home or long-term care facility, contact your state specific agency. To find the listing, visit the Long-Term Care Ombudsman website: www.ltcombudsman.org.

Remember: You do not need to prove that abuse is occurring; it is up to the professionals to investigate the suspicions.

Chapter 51

Dementia, Caregiving, and Controlling Frustration

The Stresses of Caregiving

Caring for an individual with Alzheimer's disease or a related dementia can be challenging and, at times, overwhelming. Frustration is a normal and valid emotional response to many of the difficulties of being a caregiver. While some irritation may be part of everyday life as a caregiver, feeling extreme frustration can have serious consequences for you or the person you care for. Frustration and stress may negatively impact your physical health or cause you to be physically or verbally aggressive towards your loved one. If your caregiving situation is causing you extreme frustration or anger, you may want to explore some new techniques for coping.

When you are frustrated, it is important to distinguish between what is and what is not within your power to change. Frustration often arises out of trying to change an uncontrollable circumstance. As a caregiver of someone with dementia, you face many uncontrollable situations. Normal daily activities—dressing, bathing, and eating—may become sources of deep frustration for you. Behaviors often associated with dementia, like wandering or asking questions repeatedly, can be frustrating for caregivers but are uncontrollable behaviors for people with dementia. Unfortunately, you cannot simply change the behavior of a person suffering from dementia.

When dealing with an uncontrollable circumstance, you do control one thing: How you respond to that circumstance.

In order to respond without extreme frustration, you will need to:

- learn to recognize the warning signs of frustration;
- intervene to calm yourself down physically;
- modify your thoughts in a way that reduces your stress;
- learn to communicate assertively;
- learn to ask for help.

Warning Signs of Frustration

If you can recognize the warning signs of frustration, you can intervene and adjust your mood before you lose control. Some of the common warning signs of frustration include:

- shortness of breath;
- knot in the throat;
- stomach cramps;
- chest pains;
- headache;
- compulsive eating;
- excessive alcohol consumption;
- increased smoking;
- lack of patience;
- desire to strike out.

Calming Down Physically

When you become aware of the warning signs of frustration, you can intervene with an immediate activity to help you calm down. This gives you time to look at the situation more objectively and to choose how to respond in a more controlled way.

When you feel yourself becoming frustrated, try counting from one to ten slowly and taking a few deep breaths. If you are able, take a brief walk or go to another room and collect your thoughts. It is better to leave the situation, even for a moment, than to lose control or react in a way you will regret. If you think someone may be offended when you leave the room, you can tell that person you need to go to the restroom. You can also try calling a friend, praying, meditating, singing, listening to music, or taking a bath. Try experimenting with different responses to find out what works best for you and the person you care for.

The regular practice of relaxation techniques can also help prepare you for frustrating circumstances. If possible, try the following relaxation exercise for at least 10 minutes each day: Sit in a comfortable position in a quiet place. Take slow, deep breaths and relax the tension in your body. While you continue to take slow, deep breaths, you may want to imagine a safe and restful place and repeat a calming word or phrase.

Modifying Your Thoughts

As you take time out to collect your thoughts, try rethinking your situation in ways that reduce frustration. How you think often affects how you feel. Of course, feelings of frustration arise from difficult circumstances. If, however, you analyze your response to a frustrating situation, you will usually find some form of maladaptive—or negative—thinking that has the effect of increasing your frustration, preventing you from looking at your situation objectively, or finding a better way to deal with it.

Below are six major types of unhelpful thought patterns common among caregivers. Following each unhelpful thought pattern is an example of an adaptive—or more helpful—thought that can be used as self-defense against frustration. Familiarizing yourself with the unhelpful thought patterns and the adaptive responses can help you control your frustration.

Over-generalization: You take one negative situation or characteristic and multiply it. For example, you're getting ready to take the person in your care to a doctor's appointment when you discover the car battery has died. You then conclude, "This always happens; something always goes wrong."

Adaptive response: "This does not happen all the time. Usually my car is working just fine. At times things don't happen the way I would like, but sometimes they do."

Discounting the positive: You overlook the good things about your circumstances and yourself. For example, you might not allow yourself to feel good about caregiving by thinking, "I could do more" or "anyone could do what I do."

Adaptive response: "Caregiving is not easy. It takes courage, strength, and compassion to do what I do. I am not always perfect, but I do a lot and I am trying to be helpful."

Jumping to conclusions: You reach a conclusion without having all the facts. You might do this in two ways:

- Mind-reading: We assume that others are thinking negative thoughts about us. For example, a friend doesn't return a phone call, and we assume that he or she is ignoring us or doesn't want to talk to us. Adaptive response: "I don't know what my friend is thinking. For all I know, she didn't get the message. Maybe she is busy or just forgot. If I want to know what she is thinking, I will have to ask her."

- Fortune-telling: You predict a negative outcome in the future. For example, you will not try adult day care because you assume the person in your care will not enjoy it. You think, "He will never do that. Not a chance!" Adaptive response: "I cannot predict the future. I don't think he is going to like it, but I won't know for sure unless I try."

"Should" statements: You try to motivate yourself using statements such as "I should call mother more often" or "I shouldn't go to a movie because Mom might need me." What you think you "should" do is in conflict with what you want to do. You end up feeling guilty, depressed, or frustrated.

Adaptive response: "I would like to go to a movie. It's okay for me to take a break from caregiving and enjoy myself. I will ask a friend or neighbor to check in on Mom."

Labeling: You identify yourself or other people with one characteristic or action. For example, you put off doing the laundry and think, "I am lazy."

Adaptive response: "I am not lazy. Sometimes I don't do as much as I could, but that doesn't mean I am lazy. I often work hard and do the best that I can. Even I need a break sometimes."

Personalizing: You take responsibility for a negative occurrence that is beyond your control. For example, you might blame yourself when the person in your care requires hospitalization or placement in a facility.

Adaptive response: "Mom's condition has gotten to the point where I can no longer take care of her myself. It is her condition and not my shortcomings that require her to be in a nursing home."

Using the "Triple-Column Technique": Unhelpful thought patterns are usually ingrained reactions or habits. To modify your negative thoughts, you will have to learn to recognize them, know why they are false, and talk back to them.

One helpful way to practice using more adaptive thinking processes is to use the "triple-column technique." Draw two lines down the center of a piece of paper to divide the paper into thirds. When you are feeling frustrated, take a personal "time out" and write your negative thoughts in the first column. In the second column, try to identify the type of unhelpful pattern from the six examples above. In the third column, talk back to your negative thoughts with a more positive point of view.

Communicating Assertively

Good communication can reduce frustration by allowing you to express yourself while helping others to understand your limits and needs. Assertive communication is different from passive or aggressive communication. When you communicate passively, you may be keeping your own needs and desires inside to avoid conflict with others. While this may seem easier on the surface, the long-term result may be that others feel they can push you around to get their way.

When you communicate aggressively, you may be forcing your needs and desires onto others. While this allows you to express your feelings, aggressive communication generally makes others more defensive and less cooperative.

When you communicate assertively, you express your own needs and desires while respecting the needs and desires of others. Assertive communication allows both parties to engage in a dignified discussion about the issue at hand.

Keys to assertive communication are:

- respecting your own feelings, needs and desires;

- standing up for your feelings without shaming, degrading, or humiliating the other person;

- using "I" statements rather than "you" statements. For example, say, "I need a break" or "I would like to talk to you and work this out" instead of "You are irresponsible" or "You never help out!"

- not using "should" statements. For example, say, "It's important to me that promises be kept," instead of "You should keep your promise."

The Critical Step: Asking for Help

You cannot take on all the responsibilities of caregiving by yourself. It is essential that you ask for and accept help. Discuss your needs with family members and friends who might be willing to share caregiving responsibilities. People will not realize you need help if you do not explain your situation and ask for assistance. Remember, you have the right to ask for help and express your needs.

When to Say "Yes"

Don't be afraid to say "Yes" if someone offers to help. Say "Yes" at the moment a person offers to help rather than saying "maybe" and waiting until you are in a fix. Have a list handy of errands or tasks you need help with. Keep in mind that people feel useful and gratified when they are able to help others.

When to Say "No"

Often, caregivers are pulled in multiple directions. In addition to the demands of caregiving, you may feel compelled to meet the demands of your immediate and extended family, your friends, and your employer. Learn how to say "No" to the demands of others when you are overwhelmed or need a break. It is your right to say "No" to extra demands on your time without feeling guilty.

Learning Effective Communication Techniques for Dementia Caregiving

Many families find it frustrating to communicate with a loved one who has dementia. The person with dementia may repeat questions over and over or mistake you for someone else. It is important to remember that the person with dementia cannot control behavior caused by their disease. They do not need to be corrected or grounded in "reality." You can distract them or just agree with them as a way to reduce your frustration.

It can be helpful, however, to learn more about dementia and effective communication techniques which will ease your frustration. For example, use simple, direct statements, and place yourself close when speaking to a person with a cognitive disorder. Try not to argue about unimportant things such as what the date is. Allow extra time to accomplish tasks such as dressing. Remember, people with dementia often react more to our feelings than our words. Finding ways to be calm can help you to gain cooperation. See FCA's Fact Sheet: Behavior Management Strategies (Dementia) [http://www.caregiver.org/caregiver/jsp/content_node.jsp?nodeid=391] for more helpful strategies.

Self-Care to Prevent Frustration

Caregiving can be tiring and stressful. When you're caring for others, it's easy to forget to care for yourself. While it may be difficult to find time to focus on yourself and your needs, it is very important that you do so to prevent frustration and burnout. FCA's Fact Sheet: Taking Care of YOU: Self-Care for Caregivers [http://www.caregiver.org/caregiver/jsp/content_node.jsp?nodeid=847] offers additional information.

Here are three steps to taking better care of you:

Make Time for Yourself

You may feel guilty about needing or wanting time out for rest, socialization, and fun. However, everyone deserves regular and ongoing breaks from work, including caregivers. "Respite" providers can give you the opportunity to take the breaks you need. Respite breaks may be provided by in-home help, adult day care, "friendly visitor" programs, friends and neighbors, or other means. The important point is to allow yourself to take a break from caregiving.

Take Care of Yourself

Although caregiving may make it difficult to find time for yourself, it is important to eat well, exercise, get a good night's sleep, and attend to your own medical needs. When you do not take care of yourself, you are prone to increased anxiety, depression, frustration, and physical distress that will make it more difficult to continue providing care.

Seek Outside Support

Sharing your feelings with a counselor, pastor, a support group, or with another caregiver in a similar situation can be a great way to release stress and get helpful advice. You may want to contact the organizations under "Resources" at http://www.caregiver.org/caregiver/jsp/content_node.jsp?nodeid=891 or look in the community services section at the front of the Yellow Pages, under "Counseling" or "Senior Services" to find services to help you get some caregiver support. The FCA Fact Sheet on Community Care Options [http://www.caregiver.org/caregiver/jsp/content_node.jsp?nodeid=1992] also offers information.

Chapter 52

Respite Care: Giving Caregivers a Break

What is respite care?

Millions of Americans provide unpaid assistance each year to elderly family, friends, and neighbors to help them remain in their own homes and communities for as long as possible. Sometimes these caregivers need time off to relax or take care of other responsibilities. This is where respite care can be helpful. It provides the family caregivers with the break they need, and also ensures that their elderly loved one is still receiving the attention that he or she needs.

Respite care is not all the same. Respite can vary in time from part of a day to several weeks. Respite encompasses a wide variety of services including traditional home-based care, as well as adult day care, skilled nursing, home health, and short-term institutional care. More specifically respite care may take any one of the following forms:

- **Adult day care:** These programs are designed to provide care and companionship for frail and disabled persons who need assistance or supervision during the day. The program offers relief to family members or caregivers and allows them the freedom to go to work, handle personal business, or just relax while knowing their relative is well cared for and safe.

Excerpted from "Respite Care," by the Administration on Aging (www.elder care.gov), part of the U.S. Department of Health and Human Services, September 21, 2010.

- **Informal and volunteer respite care:** This is as simple as it sounds. It is accepting help from other family members, friends, neighbors, or church volunteers who offer to stay with the elderly individual while you go to the store or run other errands. Sometimes your local church group or area agency on aging (AAA) will even run a formal "Friendly Visitor Program" in which volunteers may be able to provide basic respite care, as well. Many communities have formed either Interfaith Caregiver or Faith in Action Programs where volunteers from faith-based communities are matched with caregivers to provide them with some relief.

- **In-home respite care:** Generally speaking, in-home respite care involves the following four types of services for the more impaired older person:

  - Companion services to help the family caregiver supervise, entertain, or just visit with the senior when he or she is lonely and wants company

  - Homemaker services to assist with housekeeping chores, preparing meals, or shopping

  - Personal care services to help the aged individual bathe, get dressed, go to the bathroom, and/or exercise

  - Skilled care services to assist the family caregiver in tending to the senior's medical needs, such as when administering medications

How do you pay for respite?

The cost of respite care varies with the type of agency and the services needed, but federal and/or state programs may help to pay for it. Long term care insurance policies may cover some of the cost of respite care. Your local AAA will have more information on whether financial assistance is available, depending on your situation and where you live.

Can the National Family Caregiver Support Program offer respite?

The enactment of the Older Americans Act Amendments of 2000 (Public Law 106-501) established an important program, the National Family Caregiver Support Program (NFCSP). Funds have been allocated to states to work in partnership with area agencies on aging and local and community service providers to put into place multi-faceted systems of support for family caregivers. A specific component of these systems is respite. That could include, for example, respite care provided in a home, an adult day-care program, or over a weekend in a nursing home or an assisted living facility. For more information on the NFCSP visit the Administration on Aging website at http://aoa .gov/AoARoot/AoA_Programs/HCLTC/Caregiver/index.aspx.

How can I ensure that respite care is quality care?

When evaluating a respite care program, family members should check to see if it is licensed by the state where they live (where required) and if the caregivers have the qualifications necessary for the job. They can ask respite care program managers the following questions to assess their credentials:

- Are families limited to a certain number of hours for services needed?

- Can the provider take care of more than one person at a time?

- Can family members meet and interview the people who will be providing the respite care?

- Does the program provide transportation for the caregiver/ senior?

- Does the program keep an active file on the senior's medical condition and other needs? Is there a written care plan?

- How are the caregivers screened for their jobs?

- How are the caregivers trained? Do they receive extra training, where appropriate, to meet specific family needs?

- How are the caregivers supervised and evaluated?

- How much does the respite care cost? What is included in the fee?

- How far ahead of time do family members have to call to arrange services?

- How do the caregivers handle emergencies? What instructions do they receive to prepare them for unexpected situations (being snowed in or losing power during a thunderstorm, for example)?

- How is the program evaluated? Are family members contacted for their feedback? If so, review their comments.

Second, when interviewing an in-home respite care aide, you may want to ask these questions:

- Are you insured?

- Do you have any references? What are they?

- Do you have any special skills that might help you with this job?

- Have you ever worked with someone in the same medical condition as my loved one?

- How would you handle the following situation? (Cite examples of challenges you have encountered as a family caregiver.)

- What is your background and training?

- What are your past experiences in providing respite care?

- When are you available? Do you have a back-up/assistant if you are unable to come when expected?

- Who can I talk to at your agency if I am concerned about something?

- Why are you interested in this job?

- Why did you leave your last job?

Chapter 53

Hiring In-Home Care Providers

What is home health care?

Home health care helps seniors live independently for as long as possible, given the limits of their medical condition. It covers a wide range of services and can often delay the need for long-term nursing home care.

More specifically, home health care may include occupational and physical therapy, speech therapy, and even skilled nursing. It may involve helping the elderly with activities of daily living such as bathing, dressing, and eating. Or it may include assistance with cooking, cleaning, other housekeeping jobs, and monitoring one's daily regimen of prescription and over-the-counter medications.

At this point, it is important to understand the difference between home health care and home care services. Although they sound the same (and home health care may include some home care services), home health care is more medically oriented. While home care typically includes chore and housecleaning services, home health care usually involves helping seniors recover from an illness or injury. That is why the people who provide home health care are often licensed practical nurses, therapists, or home health aides. Most work for home health agencies, hospitals, or public health departments that are licensed by the state.

Excerpted from "Home Health Care," by the Administration on Aging (www.eldercare.gov), part of the U.S. Department of Health and Human Services, September 21, 2010.

How do I make sure that home health care is quality care?

As with any important purchase, it is always a good idea to talk with friends, neighbors, and your local area agency on aging to learn more about the home health care agencies in your community. In looking for a home health care agency, the following 20 questions can be used to help guide your search:

- How long has the agency been serving this community?

- Does the agency have any printed brochures describing the services it offers and how much they cost? If so, get one.

- Is the agency an approved Medicare provider?

- Is the quality of care certified by a national accrediting body such as the Joint Commission for the Accreditation of Healthcare Organizations?

- Does the agency have a current license to practice (if required in the state where you live)?

- Does the agency offer seniors a Patients' Bill of Rights that describes the rights and responsibilities of both the agency and the senior being cared for?

- Does the agency write a plan of care for the patient (with input from the patient, his or her doctor, and family), and update the plan as necessary?

- Does the care plan outline the patient's course of treatment, describing the specific tasks to be performed by each caregiver?

- How closely do supervisors oversee care to ensure quality?

- Will agency caregivers keep family members informed about the kind of care their loved one is getting?

- Are agency staff members available around the clock, 7 days a week, if necessary?

- Does the agency have a nursing supervisor available to provide on-call assistance 24 hours a day?

- How does the agency ensure patient confidentiality?

- How are agency caregivers hired and trained?

- What is the procedure for resolving problems when they occur, and who can I call with questions or complaints?

- How does the agency handle billing?

- Is there a sliding fee schedule based on ability to pay, and is financial assistance available to pay for services?

- Will the agency provide a list of references for its caregivers?

- Who does the agency call if the home health care worker cannot come when scheduled?

- What type of employee screening is done?

When purchasing home health care directly from an individual provider (instead of through an agency), it is even more important to screen the person thoroughly. This should include an interview with the home health caregiver to make sure that he or she is qualified for the job. You should request references. Also, prepare for the interview by making a list of any special needs the senior might have. For example, you would want to note whether the elderly patient needs help getting into or out of a wheelchair. Clearly, if this is the case, the home health caregiver must be able to provide that assistance. The screening process will go easier if you have a better idea of what you are looking for first.

Another thing to remember is that it always helps to look ahead, anticipate changing needs, and have a backup plan for special situations. Since every employee occasionally needs time off (or a vacation), it is unrealistic to assume that one home health care worker will always be around to provide care. Seniors or family members who hire home health workers directly may want to consider interviewing a second part-time or on-call person who can be available when the primary caregiver cannot be. Calling an agency for temporary respite care also may help to solve this problem.

In any event, whether you arrange for home health care through an agency or hire an independent home health care aide on an individual basis, it helps to spend some time preparing for the person who will be doing the work. Ideally, you could spend a day with him or her, before the job formally begins, to discuss what will be involved in the daily routine. If nothing else, tell the home health care provider (both verbally and in writing) the following things that he or she should know about the senior:

- Illnesses/injuries and signs of an emergency medical situation

- Likes and dislikes

- Medications and how and when they should be taken

537

- Need for dentures, eyeglasses, canes, walkers, etc.
- Possible behavior problems and how best to deal with them
- Problems getting around (in or out of a wheelchair, for example, or trouble walking)
- Special diets or nutritional needs
- Therapeutic exercises

In addition, you should give the home health care provider more information about the following:

- Clothing the senior may need (if/when it gets too hot or too cold)
- How you can be contacted (and who else should be contacted in an emergency)
- How to find and use medical supplies and medications
- When to lock up the apartment/house and where to find the keys
- Where to find food, cooking utensils, and serving items
- Where to find cleaning supplies
- Where to find light bulbs and flash lights, and where the fuse box is located (in case of a power failure)
- Where to find the washer, dryer, and other household appliances (as well as instructions for how to use them)

Although most states require that home health care agencies perform criminal background checks on their workers and carefully screen job applicants for these positions, the actual regulations will vary depending on where you live.

Therefore, before contacting a home health care agency, you may want to call your local area agency on aging or department of public health to learn what laws apply in your state.

How can I pay for home health care?

The cost of home health care varies across states and within states. In addition, costs will fluctuate depending on the type of health care professional required. Home care services can be paid for directly by the patient and his or her family members, or through a variety of public and private sources. Sources for home health care funding include Medicare, Medicaid, the Older Americans Act, the Veterans' Administration, and private insurance.

Medicare is the largest single payer of home care services. The Medicare program will pay for home health care if all of the following conditions are met:

• The patient must be homebound and under a doctor's care.

• The patient must need skilled nursing care, or occupational, physical, or speech therapy, on at least an intermittent basis (that is, regularly but not continuously).

• The services provided must be under a doctor's supervision and performed as part of a home health care plan written specifically for that patient.

• The patient must be eligible for the Medicare program and the services ordered must be medically reasonable and necessary.

• The home health care agency providing the services must be certified by the Medicare program.

To get help with your Medicare questions, call 800-MEDICARE (800-633-4227, TTY/TDD: 877-486-2048 for the speech and hearing impaired) or look on the internet at www.medicare.gov.

Chapter 54

Choosing a Nursing Home

Follow these steps to find the nursing home that is best for you:

- Step 1: Find nursing homes in your area.

- Step 2: Compare the quality of nursing homes you are considering. Look at health inspection and fire safety inspection reports, nursing home staffing rates, quality measures and other important information such as how many stars they received on their quality rating.

- Step 3: Visit the nursing homes you are interested in, or have someone visit for you.

- Step 4: Choose the nursing home that meets your needs.

Step 1: Find Nursing Homes in Your Area

- Medicare's Nursing Home Compare web tool has information to help you find and compare nursing homes. Visit www.medicare .gov/NHCompare. You can search by nursing home name, city, county, state, or ZIP code.

- Ask people you trust, like your doctor, family, friends, neighbors, or clergy if they have had personal experience with nursing homes. They may be able to recommend a nursing home for you.

Excerpted from "Guide to Choosing a Nursing Home," by the Centers for Medicare and Medicaid Services (www. medicare.gov), September 20, 2010.

- If you are in the hospital, ask the hospital's discharge planner or social worker for a list of local nursing homes. They should be able to help you find an available bed. Some nursing homes work together with hospitals, and some are independent.

- Visit or call your local social service agency or hospital. Ask to speak to a social worker or case manager who can help you find a nursing home in your area.

- Contact your local Agency on Aging to ask for a list of long-term care choices in your area.

Step 2: Compare the Quality of the Nursing Homes You Are Considering

It is important to compare the care that nursing homes give in order to make your best nursing home decision. One way to compare nursing homes is to look at the information about nursing home quality on the Nursing Home Compare website. Visit www.medicare.gov and select "Compare Nursing Homes in Your Area," or visit www.medicare.gov/NHCompare.

The Nursing Home Compare website has information about the nursing homes in the country that are certified to participate in Medicare and/or Medicaid. You can compare the nursing homes you are considering using the Five Star Quality Rating, detailed information on health inspections, nursing home staffing, quality measures, and fire safety inspections. Maps and directions are also available.

NOTE: Information on Nursing Home Compare isn't an endorsement or advertisement for any nursing home. You should use a variety of resources when choosing a nursing home. Don't rely only on the nursing home's star rating to make a final decision. Visit the nursing homes you're considering if at all possible, or have someone visit for you.

Nursing Home Compare's Five Star Quality Rating System

The Five Star Quality Rating System on Nursing Home Compare is designed to do the following:

1. Give you easy-to-use information to help you choose a nursing home for yourself or others

2. Give you information about the care in nursing homes where you or family members already live

3. Help you talk to nursing home staff about the quality of care

4. Help nursing homes with their quality improvement efforts

Nursing homes are rated on these three areas—health inspections, nursing home staffing information, and quality measures. These ratings are combined for an overall quality rating. Information about fire safety inspections is included on Nursing Home Compare to give consumers more information about a nursing home's overall quality.

Health Inspections

To be part of the Medicare and Medicaid programs (that is, be a certified provider), nursing homes have to meet over 150 requirements (regulatory standards) Congress set to protect nursing home residents. These requirements cover a wide range of topics, from protecting residents from physical or mental abuse and inadequate care, to the safe storage and preparation of food.

The Centers for Medicare & Medicaid Services (CMS) has contracts with state governments to do health inspections and fire safety inspections of these certified nursing homes and investigate complaints about nursing home care. The health inspection team consists of trained inspectors, including at least one registered nurse. These inspections take place, on average, about once a year, but may be done more often if the nursing home is performing poorly.

Using the requirements, the state inspection team looks at many aspects of life in the nursing home including the following:

*   The care of residents and the processes used to give that care

*   How the staff and residents interact

*   The nursing home environment

In addition, inspectors review the residents' clinical records, interview some residents and family members about their life in the nursing home, and interview caregivers and administrative staff.

Using the information about health inspections on Nursing Home Compare, you can see what health and safety standards a nursing home failed to meet during recent health inspections.

Nursing Home Staffing

Federal law requires all certified nursing homes to provide enough staff to adequately care for residents; however, there is no current federal standard for the best staffing levels.

The nursing home must have at least one licensed Registered Nurse (RN) for at least 8 straight hours a day, 7 days a week, and other nursing staff such as an RN or Licensed Practical Nurse/Licensed Vocational Nurse (LPN/LVN) on duty 24 hours per day. Certain states may have additional staffing requirements.

Certified Nursing Assistants (CNAs) are generally on staff 24 hours per day. They work under a licensed nurse to help residents with daily activities like eating and bathing. All full-time CNAs must have completed a competency evaluation program or a nurse assistant training within 4 months of their permanent employment. They must also take continuing education training each year.

Some nursing homes might require more staff due to the conditions of their residents, along with other factors such as whether the nursing home has special care units.

The staffing numbers on Nursing Home Compare are based on information reported by the nursing home. They represent staffing levels for a 2-week period prior to the time of the state inspection. You should be cautious when interpreting staffing data. Although the data is checked for unusual reporting issues, there is no system to fully verify the accuracy of the staffing data that nursing homes report.

Quality Measures

Nursing homes regularly collect certain assessment information about their residents' health, physical functioning, mental status, and general well-being, using a form called the Minimum Data Set. Nursing homes report this information to Medicare. Medicare uses some of the assessment information to measure the quality of certain aspects of nursing home care, like whether residents have gotten their flu shots, are in pain, or are losing weight. These measures of care are called "quality measures."

Medicare posts each nursing home's ratings for these quality measures on Nursing Home Compare. The quality measures were selected because they show important ways nursing homes differ from one another.

The quality measures on Nursing Home Compare were chosen because they can be measured, and are valid and reliable. However, they aren't benchmarks, thresholds, guidelines, or standards of care. They are based on care provided to the population of residents in a facility, not to any individual resident, and aren't appropriate for use in a lawsuit.

The quality measures are based on the best research currently available. As this research continues, scientists will keep improving the quality measures on Nursing Home Compare.

Fire Safety Inspections

Fire safety specialists inspect nursing homes to see if they meet Life Safety Code (LSC) standards. The LSC is a set of fire protection requirements designed to provide a reasonable degree of safety from fire.

The Fire Safety inspection covers a wide range of aspects of fire protection, including construction, protection, and operational features designed to provide safety from fire, smoke, and panic. When an inspection team finds that a home doesn't meet a specific LSC regulation, it issues a deficiency citation. Using the information about fire safety inspections on Nursing Home Compare, you can see what fire safety standards a nursing home failed to meet, the level of potential harm, the number of residents this affected, and the date of correction.

Important: While comparing nursing homes, it may be important for you to contact the nursing home to find out about their sprinkler system. Federal Rules indicate that by 2013, all older nursing homes must be fully equipped with sprinklers.

Other ways to find out about nursing home quality:

- Ask friends and other people you know for nursing home recommendations.

- Call your Long-Term Care Ombudsman. The Ombudsman program helps nursing home residents solve problems by acting on their behalf. Ombudsmen do the following:

  - Visit nursing homes and speak with residents throughout the year to make sure residents' rights are protected.

  - Discuss general information about nursing homes and nursing home care.

  - Work to solve problems with your nursing home care, including financial issues.

  - May help you compare the nursing home's strengths and weaknesses. Ask them questions like how many complaints they have gotten about a nursing home, what kind of complaints they were, and if the problems were resolved.

- Call the local office of consumer affairs for your state. Ask if they have information on the quality of nursing homes. Look in the blue pages of your telephone book for their phone number.

- Call your state health department or state licensing agency. Ask if they have information on the quality of nursing homes. Look in the blue pages of your telephone book for their phone number.

A friend, family member, or your local library or senior center may be able to help you find the information on Nursing Home Compare if you don't have a computer. You can also call 800-MEDICARE (800-633-4227) and a customer service representative will read this information to you. TTY users should call 877-486-2048. You can get a printed copy in the mail. It takes about 3 weeks.

Resident-Directed Care and the Culture Change Movement

There is a growing, nationwide movement among many nursing homes to change the nursing home culture from rigid institutional living to living in a setting more like a home. Nursing homes involved in this "culture change" practice resident-directed or resident-centered care, which promotes much greater resident choice over their schedules (getting up, going to sleep, method and timing of bathing), and their activities. It also involves changes to the building environment to enhance the residents' quality of life.

Many homes involved in this culture change have "households" within their former living units, which include small groups of residents—usually less than 20. This group of residents has the same staff assigned to them, and has activities and meals together. Each household has a kitchen, dining room, and living room space.

A small number of homes have sets of free-standing houses on-campus that contain approximately 10–12 residents each, with private rooms and settings much more like that of a large, private home. Other homes have remodeled their buildings to include more private rooms and a new style of "privacy-enhanced, shared rooms" which have a partial wall separating each resident's half of a room.

Whether in small houses or households in larger buildings, the consistent assignment of staff permits the nursing home staff to develop close relationships with each resident to more fully meet their needs and preferences, and help them to attain their highest level of well-being and functioning. Some homes have been unable to remodel into households but have embraced the principles of culture change with consistent staffing and much greater resident choice over daily life.

Often culture changing homes have resident dogs and cats, and some permit a resident to bring in his or her own pet, with staff or volunteers assisting the resident with pet care. Other homes have connections to a day care setting in which elders and the children interact regularly. For more information on resident-directed care and the culture change movement, contact the Pioneer Network, a non-profit organization that serves as the focal point of the movement. Visit www.pioneernetwork.net for more information.

Step 3: Visit the Nursing Homes You Are Interested In

Before you make a decision about a nursing home, visit the nursing homes that interest you whenever possible. A visit gives you the chance to see the residents, staff, and the nursing home setting. It also allows you to ask questions of the nursing home staff, and talk with the residents and their family members.

If you can't visit the nursing home yourself, you may want to get a family member or friend to visit for you. If a family member or friend can't visit for you, you can call for information. However, a visit gives you a better way to see the quality of care and life of the residents.

Before you visit, consider what is important to you:

Quality of Life

- Will you be treated in a respectful way?

- Can you participate in social, recreational, religious, or cultural activities that are important to you? Can you decide when you want to participate?

- Do you get to choose what time to get up, go to sleep, and bathe?

- Can you get food and drinks that you like at any time? What if you don't like the food that is served?

- Can you have visitors anytime?

- Is transportation provided to community activities?

- Can you bring your pet?

- Can you decorate your living space any way you want?

- Will you have privacy for visits or personal care?

Quality of Care

- Will you be included in planning your care? Will your interests and preferences be included in the care plan? Will you be able to change the plan if you feel there is a need? Will you be able to choose which of your family member or friends will be involved in the planning process? Will you get a copy of your care plan?

- Are there enough staff so you get the care you need?

- Who are the doctors that will care for you? Can you still see your personal doctors?

- Does the nursing home's inspection report show quality of care problems (deficiencies)?

- What did the quality information on "Nursing Home Compare" show about how well this nursing home cares for its residents? Visit www.medicare.gov/NHCompare.

- Does the nursing home participate in quality improvement initiatives such as the Advancing Excellence for America's Nursing Homes?

- What care improvement goals is the nursing home working on?

- What kind of progress is the nursing home making on those goals?

Location

- Is the nursing home close to your family and friends so they can visit often?

Availability

- Is a bed available now, or can you add your name to a waiting list? Remember, nursing homes don't have to accept all applicants, but they must comply with Civil Rights laws that prohibit discrimination based on race, color, national origin, disability, age, or religion under certain conditions.

Staffing

- Will you have the same staff people take care of you most of the time or do they change from day to day?

- Ask the staff to show you the information they are required to post about the number of licensed and unlicensed nursing staff.

- Do the Certified Nursing Assistants (CNAs) work with a reasonable number of residents on each shift (day and night) and during meals?

- Is there a doctor available?

- Are therapy staff available?

- Is there a social worker available? Can you meet him or her?

Religious and Cultural Preferences

- Does the nursing home offer the religious or cultural support you need?

- Do they provide any special diet your faith practice requires?

Language

- Is your primary language spoken at the nursing home by staff or residents?

- If not, is an interpreter available?

Policies

- What are the resident policies you must follow? (Policies are rules that all residents must follow.) For example, smoking may not be allowed in the nursing home.

Security

- Does the nursing home provide a safe environment?

- Is there a guard at the door? Does this make you feel better or worse about a nursing home?

- Is the nursing home locked at night?

- Are there special personal monitoring devices to alert staff if a resident becomes confused and wanders in the facility?

Preventive Care

- Does the nursing home make sure that residents get preventive care to help keep them healthy?

- Does the nursing home have a screening program for immunizations such as flu (influenza) and pneumonia?

Hospitals

- Does the nursing home have an arrangement with a nearby hospital for emergencies?

- Can your doctor care for you at that hospital?

Accredited (Accreditation)

- Is the nursing home accredited by a state-approved accreditation organization? Being accredited means the nursing home meets certain additional standards for care that the state-approved accreditation organization sets.

Licensing

- Are the nursing home and current administrator licensed in your state? This means that they have met certain standards set by a state or local government agency.

Certified (Certification)

If you are getting skilled care, and Medicare or Medicaid is paying for your care, make sure the nursing home is Medicare and Medicaid certified. This means the nursing home has passed an inspection survey done by the state survey agency. If they are certified, make sure they have not recently lost their certification or are about to lose their certification. Medicare and Medicaid will only pay for care in a certified nursing home. Being certified isn't the same as being accredited. Also, some nursing homes set aside only a few beds for Medicare or Medicaid residents.

Services

- What services does the nursing home provide? Does the nursing home have the services you need (like skilled or custodial care)?

Charges and Fees

Nursing homes must tell you in writing about their services, charges, and fees before you move into the home. Get a copy of the fee schedule to find out which services are available, which are included in your monthly fee, and which services cost extra. Then, compare nursing home costs.

- Is there a basic fee for room, meals, and personal care?
- Are there extra charges for other services or care for special medical needs?

The Health Inspection and Fire Safety Inspection Reports

Ask the staff for the health inspection and fire safety inspection reports. The inspection report tells you how well the nursing home meets federal health and safety requirements. The nursing home must have the report of the most recent federal or state survey of the facility available for you to look at.

Resident, Family, and Staff Satisfaction

Talk to staff, residents, and family members if you can. Ask them if they are satisfied with the nursing home and its services.

Important Things to Know When Visiting a Nursing Home

- Before you go, call and make an appointment.

- Don't be afraid to ask questions.

- Ask the staff to explain anything you see and hear that you don't understand. For example, if you hear a person calling out, it may be because they are confused, and not because they are being hurt or neglected.

- Ask who to call if you have further questions, and write down the name and phone number.

- Talk to residents and family members about the care and their experience.

- Don't go into resident rooms or care areas without asking the resident and nursing home staff first. Residents have a right to privacy.

- After your visit, write down any questions you still have about the nursing home or how the nursing home will meet your needs.

Visit Again

Visit the nursing home a second time, on a different day and at a different time than when you first visited. Staffing can be different at different times of the day and on weekends.

Try to visit during the late morning or midday. This allows you to see the residents when they are out of bed, eating, and going to activities.

Go to Resident/Family Council Meetings

Ask a nursing home staff member if you can get permission to attend a resident council and/or family council meeting. These councils are usually organized and managed by the residents' families to address concerns and improve the quality of care and life for the residents.

Here are some questions you can ask a council member:

- What improvements were made in the quality of life for residents in the last year?

- What are the plans for future improvements?

- How has the nursing home responded to recommendations for improvement?

- Who does the council report to?

- How does membership on the council work?

- Who sets the agendas for meetings?

- How are decisions made (for example, by voting, consensus, or does one person make them)?

Step 4: Choose the Nursing Home That Meets Your Needs

When you have all the information about the nursing homes you are interested in, talk with people who understand your personal and health care needs. This might include your family, friends, doctor, clergy, spiritual advisor, hospital discharge planner, or social worker.

If you find more than one nursing home you like with a bed available, use all the information you get to compare them. Trust your senses. If you didn't like what you saw on a visit, like if the facility wasn't clean or if you weren't comfortable talking to the nursing home staff, you may want to choose another nursing home. If you felt that the residents were treated well, the facility was clean, and the staff was helpful, you might feel better about choosing that nursing home.

If you are helping someone, keep the person you are helping involved in making the decision as much as possible. People who are involved from the beginning are better prepared when they move into a nursing home. If the person you are helping isn't alert or able to communicate well, keep his or her values and preferences in mind.

Important: If you visit a nursing home that you don't like, look at other options if available. Quality care is important. If you are in a hospital, talk to the hospital discharge planner or your doctor before you decide not to go to a nursing home that has an available bed. They may be able to help you find a more suitable nursing home, or arrange for other care, like short-term homecare, until a bed is available at another nursing home you choose. However, you may be responsible for paying the bill for any additional days you stay in the hospital.

Moving is difficult. However, an extra move may be better for you than choosing to stay at a facility that isn't right for you. Be sure to explain to your doctor or discharge planner why you aren't happy with a facility they may be recommending.

Once in the nursing home, if you find that you don't like the nursing home you chose, you can move to another facility with an available bed. The nursing home you leave may require that you let them know ahead of time that you are planning to leave. Talk to the nursing home staff about their rules for leaving. If you don't follow the rules for leaving, you may have to pay extra fees.

Chapter 55

Hospitalization and AD

A new environment filled with strange sights, odors and sounds, a change in the daily routine, medications and tests, and the disease process itself can all be factors that increase confusion, anxiety, and agitation in a hospitalized individual with Alzheimer disease. This text will help you to meet the needs of these patients. In it you will find facts about Alzheimer disease, communication tips, personal care techniques, suggestions for working with behaviors, and environmental factors to consider in the emergency room (ER) and in the hospital room.

When hospitalization occurs, the best option for the individual with Alzheimer disease is the constant presence of a family member or a trusted friend. Because this may not always be possible, this text hopes to serve as a guide in helping you understand and practice the many facets of care for your patient with memory disorder.

Remember, family members are your most valuable resource for information about the individual and the caregiving techniques that work best.

Alzheimer Disease: Just the Facts

- Alzheimer disease attacks the brain and causes problems with memory, thinking, and behavior.

From "Acute Hospitalization and Alzheimer's Disease: A Special Kind of Care," by the National Institute on Aging (NIA, www.nia.nih.gov), part of the National Institutes of Health, February 5, 2009.

- Most people diagnosed with Alzheimer disease are over age 65, but it can occur in people in their 40s and 50s.

- Symptoms include gradual memory loss, decreased ability to perform routine tasks, disorientation, problems with language skills, poor judgment, and personality changes.

- The time from the beginning of symptoms until death ranges from 3 to 20 years; the average is 8 years.

- There is no single test to identify Alzheimer disease. A complete medical evaluation for diagnosis is essential.

- A thorough evaluation will provide a correct diagnosis of possible or probable Alzheimer disease 90 percent of the time.

- There is no cure for Alzheimer disease at present. There are FDA (U.S. Food and Drug Administration)-approved drug treatments, designed specifically for memory symptoms occurring in mild to moderate stages of Alzheimer disease.

- The causes of Alzheimer disease are not known. Suspected causes include genes and environmental exposure.

Communicating with an Alzheimer disease patient can be challenging, but remember, decreased verbal communication does not mean decreased awareness. Most patients are very aware and feel a great deal of distress about their increased loss of ability.

General Rules of Thumb

Reality orientation does not work. Instead, use memory aids such as labeling objects (i.e., closet, bathroom). Be aware that as Alzheimer disease progresses, an individual's ability to name objects and use words decreases.

Simplify the environment for Alzheimer disease patients. Eliminate distracting noises such as the radio, TV, or loud conversation.

Do not use the in-room intercom to communicate. The patient may be frightened or confused by hearing a voice only.

Communication Tips

- Always begin by identifying yourself and calling the patient's name.

- Always approach from the front.

- Maintain good eye contact.

- Use short, simple sentences.

- Speak slowly.

- Be specific. Use the name of the person or object instead of "this" or "they."

- Keep tone of voice low and pleasant.

- Keep facial expression warm and friendly.

- Use non-verbal cues—a reassuring touch, a smile, a demonstration stating the emotion.

- Give the person plenty of time to respond to your question (20 seconds).

- Always repeat your question exactly the same way.

- Use concrete language.

- State in positive terms. Constant use of "no" or commands increases resistance.

- Don't test the patient's memory. Erase the words, "Don't you remember?" from your vocabulary.

- Give directions simply and one at a time.

- When helping with personal care, tell the patient what you are doing each step of the way. Add occasional social or reassuring comments to avoid "task-focused talk" only.

- Do not appear rushed or tense. The patient will become tense and agitated.

- Listen to the patient. Try to find the key thought and take note of the feeling or emotion being expressed along with the spoken word.

- Reassure through words. Remind the patient who you are and that you will take care of him.

- Sometimes asking a "Why" question can get to the reason behind a repetitive question and decrease its occurrence. (i.e., "Why are you concerned about what time it is?")

In the Emergency Room: Assessment Tips

- Do not leave the patient alone. A family member, trusted caregiver, or friend should be present at all times.

- Continuous cueing to the environment (place) and activity may be necessary. A family member can assist with this and offer reassurance as well.

- Obtain patient's history from a close relative or caregiver.

- Pay close attention to the caregiver's description of the patient's usual level of consciousness. Increased dementia or the onset of delirium can be a sign of acute physical illness or metabolic distress.

- Perform a complete head-to-toe assessment. The patient may not be able to automatically identify painful or affected areas to you.

- Before every communication with the patient, make sure you have his attention by calling his name and making direct eye contact with him.

- Your eyes should be level with the patient's eyes.

- Ask simple "yes" and "no" questions. Allow ample response time (at least 20 seconds).

- Watch for non-verbal communication of pain or discomfort such as grimacing, guarding, or anger.

- Apologize each time you cause pain and avoid repeating painful exams.

- In short, simple statements, tell the patient what you are doing, why, and that you will be finished soon. Repeat this throughout the examination.

- Never talk about the patient to others as if he is not in the room.

My Patient Has Alzheimer Disease: General Guidelines

For an Alzheimer disease patient, the trauma or ailment that preceded hospitalization, the strange new environment, the disrupted daily routine, and the influence of medications can all be factors for increased confusion and decreased ability.

There are a number of things you can do to reassure your patient. You should do the following:

- Provide a consistent, predictable routine. Ask the primary caregiver for the patient's usual routine and follow it as closely as possible.

- Encourage the use of security objects from home (i.e., favorite pillow or quilt).

- Provide care by the same nurses and nursing assistants as much as possible.

- Avoid surrounding the patient with several doctors and medical students at one time.

- Evaluate the patient for sources of potential pain and discomfort. Even though he may be experiencing pain, the patient will probably not verbally complain.

- When possible, schedule tests at a time of day when the patient is at his best and not fatigued.

- Discontinue asking orientation questions once the patient's level of comprehension is established.

- Use good communication techniques.

- Schedule at least two rest periods—a half hour after morning care and an hour in early afternoon. Rest is important.

- Post rest period times on the patient's door. Use a big "Resting" or "Do Not Disturb" sign during the actual rest period.

- Limit visitors to one or two at a time.

- Cue the patient for sleep by darkening and quieting the room.

- Avoid using physical restraints. They do not prevent falls. Injuries from falls while the patient is restrained are often more serious.

Room Service: Assessing the Environment

- Avoid numerous room changes. Change increases confusion and anxiety.

- Avoid placing the patient in a room located in a high noise, high traffic area.

- Keep the television off until the patient turns it on or requests it.

- Remove artwork containing people or animals if the patient interprets them as real-life intruders.

- Keep lighting as free of shadows and glare as possible.

- Avoid clutter. It can increase confusion, agitation, and the risk of falls.

- If the patient can understand written words, then large, bold lettered signs can serve as cues to the bathroom, closet, and personal items.

Providing the Essentials: Comfort and Safety

Comfort

- Always communicate a sense of security, caring, and respect.

- Each staff/patient interaction should include touch, eye contact, orienting information, and an activity the patient can successfully perform.

- Eyeglasses, dentures, and hearing aids can enhance the patient's communication. Offer to assist the patient with placement of these devices. Be aware in some instances the patient is more comfortable without them.

- If the patient has a comfort item, something that makes him feel secure, make sure it is within reach.

Safety

- Provide a safe, structured environment.

- Provide consistent staff to attend the patient.

- Place the patient in a room that allows easy and careful observation.

- Place bed in low position.

- Don't leave anything at the bedside that might harm the patient.

- Elopement precautions: Place the patient in a room where he has to pass the nursing station in order to reach an exit. Have a photo of the patient on file.

Positive Approaches to Personal Care: Activities of Daily Living

Eating

- Do not ask the patient to fill out a menu. Ask the family about food preferences.

- Simplify the food tray. Keep small, colored dishes on the unit to allow for smaller portions and the ability to offer one or two food items at a time.

- Smaller, more frequent meals may work better for the patient than the standard three large meals.

- Cueing the patient to eat by using verbal reminders along with a light touch to the forearm increases food intake.
- Finger foods, cups with lids, and broad-handled utensils may make mealtime easier for the patient.
- Late-stage patients may chew, but need frequent reminders to swallow.
- Plate guards and bibs with pockets catch spills and protect the patient's clothing.
- Offer the patient fluids frequently throughout the day. Ask the caregiver what the patient prefers to drink and the type of drinking container used at home.

Oral Hygiene

- Brush the patient's teeth at least twice a day.
- For less impaired patients, apples and other fresh fruits aid with oral hygiene.

Bathing

- Bathe the patient at his "best" time of day.
- If possible, bathe the patient at the time he normally bathes at home.
- Avoid using the shower. A hand-held showerhead provides better control of the water.
- Allow the patient to do as much as possible. Break down the task into simple steps using verbal and visual cues.
- When assisting the patient, give the bath slowly. To avoid agitation, tell the patient what you are going to do one step at a time.
- Use soft music, talking, or snacks as pleasant distractions.
- Keep the patient warm. During a bed bath, cover body parts except the parts that are being washed.
- Sounds amplify off tile walls. Running water can sound frightening.
- Be flexible. A "bird bath" may be more acceptable to the patient.

Toileting

- Clear a path to the toilet or commode.

- Place bed in view of toilet.

- To help cue the patient, place a picture of a toilet or a written sign on bathroom door.

- Place your patient on a 2-hour toileting schedule.

- Use a nightlight to make it easier for the patient to find the toilet in the middle of the night.

- Observe your patient for constipation. Ask questions about abdominal discomfort. Watch for non-verbal signs of discomfort such as grimacing or clutching. Do not ask the patient if he has had a bowel movement.

The Art of Camouflage: Protecting Tubes and Dressings

Reduce the number of tubes as quickly as possible while considering patient safety. Make remaining tubes as unobtrusive as possible.

- Nasogastric tubes (of small diameter): Tape to the side of the face, place tube behind patient's ear, and fasten to shoulder area of the gown with a safety pin.

- Central venous pressure lines: Can remain under the gown with a point of departure through the sleeve.

- Peripheral intravenous line: Can be wrapped in bandage gauze to prevent access or can be placed high on dominant arm. Dress patient in long-sleeved gown with cuff (like an operating room gown) and run tubing up the arm and out the neck of the gown.

- Foley catheters: Should be run directly from the area of insertion to the end of the bed to prevent accidental pulling by the patient. Patient should wear undergarments to minimize access to the catheter.

- Foley catheter in men: Should be taped to the abdomen.

- Picks at dressing: Consult with your occupational therapist to develop hand splints (like those used for patients with burns or rheumatoid arthritis) that maintain alignment and mobility but eliminate the pincer grasp, thus eliminating the ability to pick at the dressing.

Tips for Working with Behaviors

General Guidelines

- Think of behaviors (no matter how unusual) as communication signals from the patient that there is a problem or unmet need. Try to figure out that signal.

- Remain calm.

- Protect the patient both physically and from embarrassment.

- Offer reassurance and appropriate assistance.

Changes in Sleep Patterns

Possible Causes

- Medications

- Pain

- Not enough activity during the day

- Can't find the bathroom

- Too hot or too cold

- May be hungry

Possible Strategies

- Review medications for possible side effect of restlessness.

- Evaluate your patient for pain and treat if needed.

- Provide nightlights to aid the patient in finding the bathroom. Make sure the pathway is clear and well lit.

- Attend to toilet needs right before bedtime.

- Continue the patient's at-home bedtime routine as much as possible.

- Limit beverages containing caffeine in the afternoon and evening.

- If the patient wakes up at night, let him walk around (in sight) or sit at the nursing station until he is tired.

Confusion

Possible Causes

- Unfamiliar environment
- Medications
- Environment too noisy
- Unfamiliar or difficult task
- Unable to understand directions

Possible Strategies

- Identify any potential dangers in the environment.
- Use pictures (symbols) instead of written signs to assist the patient with locating his room and bathroom.
- Decrease noise level if possible by avoiding paging systems and buzzing call lights.
- Place the patient's name in large block letters on the door to his room.
- Review medications for side effect of confusion.
- Simplify tasks. Break them down into smaller steps.
- Simplify communication. Use short sentences and avoid lengthy explanations.
- Ask the family member/caregiver about the comfort strategies used at home.

Wandering

Possible Causes

- Patient is stressed and anxious
- Lifestyle related—previous work role or habits
- Looking for security
- Pain
- Searching for something familiar

Possible Strategies

- Ask the caregiver where and when the patient usually wanders. Find out what strategies have worked at home.
- Place the patient in a room that is convenient for you to keep a watchful eye on and that is away from stairs or elevator.
- Keep the patient's suitcase, street shoes, and street clothes out of sight.
- Assess the patient for pain and treat if needed.
- Plan walks with the patient.
- Use distractions such as a snack or music.
- Take time to talk with the patient.
- Offer a simple, meaningful activity.

Catastrophic Reactions: Patient Feels Overwhelmed and Overreacts to a Situation

Possible Causes

- Fatigue
- Environment is too stimulating
- Patient is asked too many questions at a time
- Too many strangers in a noisy, crowded atmosphere
- Patient is asked to perform a task beyond his abilities
- Fails at a simple task
- Encounters irritable, impatient staff

Possible Strategies

- Remain calm.
- Use a low tone of voice.
- Do not argue with the patient.
- Try the activity or task again later.
- Refrain from forcing or restraining the patient.
- Offer reassurance and try distraction.

- Move the patient to a quieter area.
- Simplify the task for the patient.
- Build in rest periods.
- Simplify communication.
- Be aware of your own body language and what it is saying.

Preventing Catastrophic Reactions

- Maintain a simple, structured, secure environment.
- Follow routines and schedules.
- Limit choices—choose between two items instead of five or six.
- Introduce new treatments slowly.
- Give step-by-step directions.

Disruptive Vocalizations: Calling out or Screaming

Possible Causes

- Fear
- Pain
- Loneliness
- Self-stimulation

Possible Strategies

- Offer the patient reassurance.
- Place the patient where he can see a nurse.
- Spend time with the patient.
- Assess the patient for pain.
- Provide a range of textures in the environment for stimulation.

Chapter 56

Making Decisions about Resuscitation

Introduction

Big issues—and big decisions—confront us when we think about the imminent death of a terminally ill loved one in our care. Among the emotional, legal, and financial considerations are also questions regarding the type of medical assistance your loved one should receive as the end of life approaches. For example, if your loved one suddenly has difficulty breathing, will you allow a paramedic or an emergency room technician to administer CPR (cardiopulmonary resuscitation)? And if CPR revives your loved one, yet he or she still can no longer breathe on his or her own, should you allow a machine—a respirator—to breathe for him or her?

A better understanding of cardiopulmonary resuscitation, or CPR, can be helpful when it comes to making this difficult choice before a crisis occurs. This text specifically addresses the process of CPR and describes the DNR (Do Not Resuscitate) form, the legal document used to indicate to medical professionals your—or your loved one's—wishes. (For a more detailed discussion of the other issues involved in planning for the end of life, see the Family Caregiver Alliance Fact Sheet on End-of-Life Decision Making at http://www.caregiver.org/caregiver/jsp/content_node.jsp?nodeid=401.)

CPR (Cardiopulmonary Resuscitation)

Consider the following scenario: Nancy's husband has had Alzheimer's disease for 8 years, and is now in the final stages of the illness. After a discussion of end-of-life issues with her family, Nancy has decided to "let nature take its course" if anything of an urgent medical nature happens to her husband—in other words, she does not want him to be put on life support. She has told her doctor of this decision, and he has concurred.

One night, Nancy wakes up to find her husband having trouble breathing. Reflexively, without thinking, she calls 911. By the time the paramedics arrive, her husband has stopped breathing completely. The paramedics leap to do their job: they immediately administer CPR and take him to the hospital. By the time Nancy arrives at the hospital, her husband is connected to a ventilator and numerous IVs. Unfortunately, this is exactly what she did not want for him.

Definition

Fully understanding Nancy's scenario requires a deeper understanding of cardiopulmonary resuscitation. Simply put, CPR is the process of restarting the heartbeat and breathing after one or both has stopped. The first step involves creating an artificial heartbeat by pushing on the chest, and attempting to restore breathing by blowing into the person's mouth. A medical professional will then insert a tube through the mouth and down the airway to make the artificial breathing more efficient. Electric shocks may be given to the heart, and various drugs may be given through an intravenous line. If the heartbeat starts again but breathing is still not adequate, a machine called a ventilator may be employed to move air in and out of the person's lungs indefinitely.

On television, CPR is often depicted as the ultimate life-saving technique. However, television does not show this process quite accurately—in real life the process is more brutal. Pushing the center of the chest down about 1 and 1.5 inches, 100 times a minute for several minutes, causes pain, and may even break ribs, damage the liver, or create other significant problems. CPR produces a barely adequate heartbeat, and doing it more gently is not sufficient to circulate enough blood. Electric shocks and a tube in the throat are also harsh treatments, but may be essential to resuscitate someone.

CPR frequently can save a person's life, particularly in the case of some kinds of heart attacks and accidents an otherwise healthy person may experience. CPR is also most successful when the failure of heartbeat and breathing occurs in the hospital, in the Cardiac Care Unit (CCU). Nurses in the unit will instantly recognize the problem and begin sophisticated care.

However, when a person is in failing health from a serious and progressive illness, the heart and breathing will ultimately fail as a result of that illness. In such a circumstance, there is little chance that CPR will succeed at all. Any success will be temporary at best, because the person's weakened condition will soon cause the heartbeat and breathing to fail again.

Another possibility is that CPR may be only partially successful. If the heartbeat is restored but a person is still too weak to breathe on his or her own and remains too weak to do so, he or she may be on a ventilator for days, weeks, months, or longer. Moreover, when breathing or heartbeat fails, the brain is rapidly deprived of oxygen. As a result, within seconds, the brain begins to fail (one loses consciousness), and within a very few minutes permanent damage to the brain occurs. If it takes more than those very few minutes to start effective CPR, the person will not fully recover. The brain damage may mean anything from some mental slowing and loss of memory to complete and permanent unconsciousness and dependency on a ventilator and sophisticated medical life support.

The Role of Emergency Help (Calling 911)

A call to 911 is a request for emergency help; the goal of those who respond to 911 calls is to protect life and property, and the people who respond expect to go to work doing what they are trained to do to accomplish that goal. If your house is on fire, the firefighters don't ask for permission to cut a hole in your roof and spray water all over your living room—they just do what is necessary to stop the fire from destroying your home.

Similarly, when a person's heartbeat and breathing have failed, the 911 responders are not prepared to have a long talk with you about the person's condition and what you think might be best to do. They know that any delay could mean brain damage, so they immediately start CPR and then take the person to the hospital. With one exception, which we will discuss in the next section, their rules require this, and it makes sense if you think about the purpose of the 911 system.

When Nancy called 911 in our scenario, the paramedics simply did what they are trained to do—they revived her husband. However, if Nancy and her doctor had completed a DNR form and kept it in the home, her husband would not have been resuscitated and/or connected to machines when he got to the hospital.

The Do Not Resuscitate (DNR) Form

The "Emergency Medical Systems Prehospital Do Not Resuscitate (DNR) Form" is a legal document that gives the 911 responders permission not to perform CPR. The DNR form is prepared in advance of any situation and kept at home. This prehospital DNR form lists the name of the person to whom it applies, and is signed by that person (or whoever represents that person if he or she is too ill to make medical decisions on his or her own behalf). It is also signed by the person's doctor. Please note this is very important: The form is not valid until the doctor signs it.

The DNR is the only form that affects 911 responders; other documents, such as a Durable Power of Attorney for Health Care or some other Advanced Directives, do not.

If emergency personnel arrive to find a person whose heartbeat and breathing have failed or are failing, they will perform CPR unless they see a correctly completed DNR.

In light of this, the DNR form should be kept near the ill person's bed, perhaps on the wall, so it will be easy to find in case of emergency. When 911 responders see this form, they will still do anything they can to make the sick person comfortable, but they will not perform CPR. In the absence of a DNR form, they must do CPR. The DNR is the only form that gives you control over what they may do. (Note: A DNR may be reversed if you so desire.)

Choices

Why would one choose to prepare a DNR? Because, as we've discussed above, there are times when it may not make sense to perform CPR. When a person is becoming more and more sick, doctors may try various treatments to stop the illness, but eventually it may become clear that treatments are not having the desired effect. Other treatments might provide comfort, and might even partly control the disease, but a point may be reached where nothing will stop the person's decline. At this point, CPR may only prolong dying. Under these circumstances, you might feel there is little reason to attempt CPR. In fact, the original name of the DNR form was "DNAR" for "Do Not Attempt Resuscitation." This name recognized the fact that the form instructed the 911 responders not to undertake something that, despite the best efforts, would not work effectively in the long run. At most, the effort might put the sick person in the hospital, in pain and distress, for the last days of his or her life.

Having a DNR prepared may also relieve the caregiver of making a decision to turn off a machine, which can be an even more difficult decision psychologically.

People might choose to complete a DNR for another reason. As illness progresses, the quality of life declines. Being wheelchair-bound or bed-bound, needing to be fed by others, being in chronic distress of some sort, not being able to manage one's own bowel and urine functions, finding little left in one's life that gives enjoyment or satisfaction, feeling that one's life has become burdensome to others (even if they seem to bear that burden cheerfully)—all these can come to pass with failing health. Advanced age may also mean that most of one's friends and family of one's own generation have died. One may still feel a connection to younger people, but it is not the same. Often, one reaches a point where staying in this world is less attractive than going on to whatever one believes comes next. At this point in life one may realize, in a way younger people do not, that life must come to an end. And one may choose to let it end when it does—peacefully, without a last, frantic attempt at resuscitation.(See the Family Caregiver Alliance Fact Sheet Holding On and Letting Go at http://www.caregiver .org/caregiver/jsp/content_node.jsp?nodeid=400 for more discussions about this issue).

Conclusion

When someone is suffering from a chronic illness, as opposed to an acute illness (the kind that usually requires a hospital visit or stay), the decline is often gradual. As a result, both caregivers and those in their care often forget to talk about the choices the chronically ill person would like to make regarding his or her health care. If you decide that you do not want CPR and are concerned about this decision, it might help to talk with your clergyperson. It is normal, instinctive, to try to save life no matter what, and some people are concerned that not doing everything possible to preserve life is the same as "killing" someone. But it can also simply mean respecting the end stage of a disease as the body shuts down.

There are no right and wrong answers to these questions, and until we face a situation like this, it is difficult to anticipate the kinds of choices we'd make. As we change throughout the course of an illness, our choices might also change. However, the more thoroughly family members have discussed these issues in advance of the need to make a critical decision, the easier it will be on both the person who is ill and those responsible for that person's care. It is never too soon to start the conversation.

Chapter 57

Making Tube Feeding Decisions for People with Advanced Dementia

As their dementia gets worse, nearly all patients will decrease their intake of food and water. This happens for several reasons. First, people with advanced dementia often lose the ability to use the muscles needed to chew and swallow. This change puts them at risk for choking or getting food into their lungs (which is also called "aspirating" their food), where it can block their breathing and cause pneumonia. Second, they often lose the feeling of hunger and the desire to eat. Third, people with advanced dementia can suffer from depression, medication side effects, constipation, and acute illnesses such as infections. These problems also can decrease a person's interest in food.

By the time people with dementia have an eating problem, they often are no longer able to make decisions about their own health care. This means that someone else, usually a family member, must make decisions about medical treatments for the person. One of the therapies the decision maker may need to think about is whether the person with dementia would want a feeding tube. A feeding tube is a tube that goes through the skin and delivers food directly to the stomach. This choice is often difficult for the decision maker because providing and sharing food is such an important caregiving and social activity.

Used with permission from the American Geriatrics Society. "Tube Feeding Decisions for People with Advanced Dementia" http://www.healthinaging.org/public_education/pef/feeding_tube.pdf by Mary Ersek and Laura Hanson from the American Geriatrics Society. For more information visit the AGS online at www.americangeriatrics.org. © 2007.

How is the feeding tube put in?

Most feeding tubes for long-term use are called percutaneous endoscopic gastrostomy tubes, or PEG tubes. Putting in a PEG tube usually takes 15–30 minutes and is done while the patient is sedated using medicine. The doctor uses an x-ray or camera to see where to place the tube. Then, the doctor cuts a small opening through the skin and into the stomach. The PEG tube is inserted through this opening.

What are the risks of the procedure?

Putting in a PEG tube is usually a simple procedure that rarely causes serious or dangerous problems. However, several problems can occur, including bleeding, infection, skin irritation or leakage around the tube, nausea and vomiting, and diarrhea. These problems occur in less than 10% of patients in the first few weeks after the procedure. In studies that followed people for longer periods (for example, several months to a year), more problems, including problems with the tube (e.g., the tube getting blocked or falling out), were reported.

Will the feeding tube help my loved one gain weight and feel better?

When you are thinking about tube feeding, it's important to define the overall goals of care. Some of the goals of tube feeding include improving the person's nutrition, preventing aspiration, and keeping the person comfortable. However, people with advanced dementia generally do not gain weight or have improved physical function when they have a feeding tube. Feeding tubes also do not help wounds heal or prevent pressure sores in people with advanced dementia.

Aspiration pneumonia is a common cause of death in people with late-stage dementia. And while prevention of aspiration is a goal of tube feeding, studies have shown that patients with feeding tubes continue to aspirate at the same rate as they did before the tube was placed. People with feeding tubes are more likely to be hospitalized and have to go through painful procedures. Finally, people who have feeding tubes sometimes have to be tied down to keep them from pulling out the tube.

Will the feeding tube prolong my loved one's life?

This is a hard question to answer based on the available scientific evidence. Several studies have compared dementia patients with and without feeding tubes. All except one of these studies found that a feeding tube did not prolong life for patients with advanced dementia.

Most patients with feeding tubes do not survive very long. Several studies show that 20–30% of patients who get feeding tubes die within a month and 50–60% die within a year.

What are the options for a dementia patient who has difficulty eating or swallowing?

If the patient has decreased appetite from infection, constipation, or depression, then these conditions should be treated to see if the person's appetite gets better. If the loss of appetite is caused by a side effect of a medication, then the medicines may need to be changed.

If the patient can still chew and swallow, caregivers can hand feed the patient. Often, the person is given foods that are easy to eat. Studies show that volunteers and family members can be trained to hand feed people. One important benefit of hand feeding is that it is a time for caregivers and families to interact with the person with dementia. At this time, the person should be fed his or her favorite foods so that eating is a pleasant experience for the person with dementia and his or her family.

Even when people with late-stage dementia can no longer eat because of swallowing problems, they may be able to take small tastes of their favorite foods and beverages. Excellent mouth care is important to maintain the person's hygiene and comfort. Other care includes treating pain and other symptoms, and providing emotional and spiritual support for the person and family. Many people with advanced dementia who cannot eat and drink qualify for hospice care, which can be provided in a home setting or a nursing home.

How can I do what's best for my loved one in this situation?

A decision maker should think about what he or she knows about a loved one's preferences and values. He or she should also learn as much as possible about the person's current medical condition and treatment options.

A decision maker may know what the person with advanced dementia would want based on previous conversations about treatment options. A person's choices about tube feeding or other treatments might also be included in a living will. If these sources of information are not available, the decision should be made based on other factors. First, the decision makers should consider what they know about the person's values. What did the person enjoy in life and what gives his or her life meaning? What is important to him or her? Will inserting a feeding tube improve the person's quality of life based on his or her values and goals?

When the decision maker doesn't know for sure what the person would choose to do, decisions are usually made using the "best interest" standard. The decision maker thinks about the possible risks and benefits of the procedure and decides if the person's quality of life is likely to be better or worse with the feeding tube. In people with advanced dementia, tube feeding is not likely to be helpful and may cause greater discomfort and other problems.

Other factors that affect this decision are family, religious, and community values. Decision makers should discuss the options with their families, clergy, and in some cases, members of their social or ethnic communities if they are uncertain about what to do.

Am I causing my loved one to suffer and starve to death without a feeding tube?

Many family members worry that their loved one will experience hunger and thirst at the end of life without a feeding tube. Although people with advanced dementia cannot tell us if they are hungry or thirsty, we do know from some small studies in terminally ill cancer patients that most patients do not feel hungry or thirsty even if they cannot eat or drink enough. Experts in dementia care say that most of their patients with late-stage dementia do not seem hungry or thirsty.

The doctor suggests putting in a feeding tube for a short time to see if it helps. Is this a good idea?

Sometimes, doctors might suggest using a feeding tube for a short time to see if the patient will get better and be able to eat again. This plan may work for patients who have recently suffered a stroke, because other treatment after the stroke may help them to recover the ability to eat. However, because dementia is not curable or reversible, people with advanced dementia will not regain the urge or ability to eat and drink. People with dementia are less likely to benefit from tube feeding, but are likely to suffer from problems and discomforts related to the feeding tube. In addition, family members and other decision makers often find that stopping the tube feeding and having the tube removed is a more difficult choice to make than deciding to have the feeding tube inserted in the first place.

Where can I get more information?

Here are some resources you can get from the internet or from journals.

- Alzheimer's Association Fact Sheets: "Eating" and "Ethical considerations: Issues in death and dying." Both available at: http://www.alz.org/Resources/FactSheets.asp.

- Hospice and Palliative Nurses Association. Position statement on artificial nutrition and hydration in end-of-life care. Available at: http://www.hpna.org/DisplayPage.aspx?Title=Position Statements.

- Gillick MR, Mitchell SL. Facing eating difficulties in end-stage dementia. *Alzheimer's Care Quarterly*. 2002; 3(3):227–232.

- McCann RM, Judge J. (2005) American Geriatrics Society Clinical Recommendation: Feeding Tube Placement in Elderly Patients with Advanced Dementia.

- Mitchell SL, Tetroe JM, O'Connor AM, Rostom A, Villeneuve C, Hall B. Patient Decision Aid: Making Choices: Long Term Feeding Tube Placement in Elderly Patients. Available at: http://decisionaid.ohri.ca/docs/Tube_Feeding_DA/index.htm.

Chapter 58

Caring for Someone Near the End of Life

As they reach the end of life, people suffering from conditions like Alzheimer disease (AD) or Parkinson disease can present special problems for caregivers. People live with these diseases for years, becoming increasingly disabled. Because they do not die soon after they are diagnosed, it can be hard to think of these as terminal diseases. But they do contribute to death.

Illnesses like Alzheimer disease make it difficult for those who want to provide supportive care at the end of life to know what is needed. Because people with advanced dementia can no longer communicate, they cannot share their concerns. Is Uncle Bert refusing food because he is not hungry or because he's confused? Why does Grandma Ruth seem agitated? Is she in pain and needs medication to relieve it, but can't tell you?

As these conditions progress, they also obstruct efforts to provide emotional or spiritual comfort. How can you let Grandpa know how much his life has meant to you? How do you make peace with your mother if she no longer knows who you are? Someone who has severe memory loss might not take spiritual comfort from sharing family memories or understand when others express what an important part of their life this person has been. Palliative care or hospice can be helpful in many ways to families of people with dementia. Sensory connections—targeting someone's senses, like hearing, touch, or sight—

Excerpted from "End of Life: Helping with Comfort and Care," by the National Institute on Aging (NIA, www.nia.nih.gov), part of the National Institutes of Health, April 2010, pp. 34–37.

can bring comfort to people with Alzheimer disease. Being touched or massaged and listening to music, white noise, or sounds from nature seem to soothe some people and lessen their agitation.

When an illness like Alzheimer disease is first diagnosed, if everyone understands that there is no cure, then plans for the end of life can be made before thinking and speaking abilities fail and people can no longer legally complete documents like advance directives. That didn't happen in Ethel's family. She had been forgetful for years, but even after her family knew that AD was the cause of her forgetfulness, they never talked about what the future would bring. As time passed and the disease eroded Ethel's memory and her ability to think and speak, she became less and less able to share her concerns and desires with those close to her. This made it hard for her daughter Barbara to know what Ethel needed or wanted. Barbara's decisions, therefore, had to be based on what she knew about her mom's values and priorities, rather than on what Ethel actually said she would like.

Quality of life is an important issue when making health care decisions for people with Alzheimer disease. For example, there are medicines available that might slow the progression of this devastating disease for a short time in some patients, generally early in the illness. However, in more advanced AD, some caregivers might not want these drugs prescribed. They may believe that the quality of life is already so diminished and that the medicine is unlikely to make a difference. If the drug has serious side effects, they are even more likely to decide against it.

End-of-life care decisions are more complicated for caregivers if the dying person has not expressed the kind of end-of-life care he or she would prefer. Someone newly diagnosed with Alzheimer disease might not be able to imagine the later stages of the disease. Ethel was like that. She and Barbara never talked about things like feeding tubes, machines that help with breathing, antibiotics for pneumonia, or transfers to the hospital. So when doctors raised some of these questions, Barbara didn't know how to best reflect her mother's wishes. When making care decisions for someone else near the end of life, it is important to consider how a treatment will benefit the person and what the side effects and risks might be. Sometimes you might decide to try the health care team's suggestion for a short time.

Other times you might decide that the best choice is to do nothing. Alzheimer disease and similar conditions often progress slowly and unpredictably. Experts suggest that signs of the final stage of Alzheimer disease include some of the following:

- Being unable to move around on one's own

- Being unable to speak or make oneself understood

- Needing help with most, if not all, daily activities

- Eating problems such as difficulty swallowing or no appetite

Because of their unique experience with what happens at the end of life, hospice and palliative care experts might also be of help identifying when someone in the final stage of Alzheimer disease is beginning to die. Caring for people with Alzheimer disease at home can be demanding and stressful for the family caregiver. Depression is a problem for some family caregivers, as is fatigue, because many feel they are always on call. More than half of one group of family caregivers reported cutting back on work hours or giving up their jobs because of the demands of caregiving.

Most of those family members taking care of dying Alzheimer disease patients at home expressed relief when death happened—for themselves and for the person who died. It is important to realize such feelings are normal. Hospice—whether used at home or in a facility—gives family caregivers needed support near the end of life, as well as help with their grief, both before and after their family member dies.

You will want to understand how the available medical options presented by the health care team fit into your family's particular needs. You might want to ask questions such as how will the approach the doctor is suggesting affect your relative's quality of life? Will it make a difference? If considering hospice for your relative with Alzheimer disease, does the facility have special experience with people with dementia?

Part Seven

Additional Help and Information

Chapter 59

Glossary of Terms Related to AD and Dementia

acetylcholine: A neurotransmitter that plays an important role in many neurological functions, including learning and memory.[1]

Alzheimer disease: The most common cause of dementia in people aged 65 and older. Nearly all brain functions, including memory, movement, language, judgment, behavior, and abstract thinking, are eventually affected.[2]

amygdala: An almond-shaped structure involved in processing and remembering strong emotions such as fear. It is part of the limbic system and located deep inside the brain.[1]

amyloid plaques: Unusual clumps of material found in the tissue between nerve cells. Amyloid plaques, which consist of a protein called beta amyloid along with degenerating bits of neurons and other cells, are a hallmark of Alzheimer disease.[2]

apolipoprotein E: A gene that has been linked to an increased risk of Alzheimer disease. People with a variant form of the gene, called APOE epsilon 4, have about 10 times the risk of developing Alzheimer disease.[2]

ataxia: A loss of muscle control.[2]

Definitions in this chapter were compiled from documents published by two public domain sources. Terms marked 1 are from publications by the National Institute on Aging (NIA, www.nia.nih.gov); terms marked 2 are from publications by the National Institute of Neurological Disorders and Stroke (NINDS, www .ninds.nih.gov).

atherosclerosis: A blood vessel disease characterized by the buildup of plaque, or deposits of fatty substances and other matter in the inner lining of an artery.[2]

axon: The long extension from a neuron that transmits outgoing signals to other cells.[1]

beta amyloid: A protein found in the characteristic clumps of tissue (called plaques) that appear in the brains of Alzheimer patients.[2]

Binswanger disease: A rare form of dementia characterized by damage to small blood vessels in the white matter of the brain. This damage leads to brain lesions, loss of memory, disordered cognition, and mood changes.[2]

brain stem: The portion of the brain that connects to the spinal cord and controls automatic body functions, such as breathing, heart rate, and blood pressure.[1]

capillary: A tiny blood vessel. The brain has billions of capillaries that carry oxygen, glucose (the brain's principal source of energy), nutrients, and hormones to brain cells so they can do their work. Capillaries also carry away carbon dioxide and cell waste products.[1]

cerebellum: The part of the brain responsible for maintaining the body's balance and coordination.[1]

cerebral cortex: The outer layer of nerve cells surrounding the cerebral hemispheres.[1]

cerebral hemispheres: The largest portion of the brain, composed of billions of nerve cells in two structures connected by the corpus callosum. The cerebral hemispheres control conscious thought, language, decision making, emotions, movement, and sensory functions.[1]

cerebrospinal fluid: The fluid found in and around the brain and spinal cord. It protects these organs by acting like a liquid cushion and by providing nutrients.[1]

cholinesterase inhibitors: Drugs that slow the breakdown of the neurotransmitter acetylcholine.[2]

clinical trial: A research study involving humans that rigorously tests safety, side effects, and how well a medication or behavioral treatment works.[1]

cognitive functions: All aspects of conscious thought and mental activity, including learning, perceiving, making decisions, and remembering.[1]

cognitive training: A type of training in which patients practice tasks designed to improve mental performance. Examples include memory aids, such as mnemonics, and computerized recall devices.[2]

computed tomography (CT) scan: A diagnostic procedure that uses special x-ray equipment and computers to create cross-sectional pictures of the body.[1]

cortical atrophy: Degeneration of the brain's cortex (outer layer). Cortical atrophy is common in many forms of dementia and may be visible on a brain scan.[2]

cortical dementia: A type of dementia in which the damage primarily occurs in the brain's cortex, or outer layer.[2]

corticobasal degeneration: A progressive disorder characterized by nerve cell loss and atrophy in multiple areas of the brain.[2]

Creutzfeldt-Jakob disease: A rare, degenerative, fatal brain disorder believed to be linked to an abnormal form of a protein called a prion.[2]

dementia: A term for a collection of symptoms that significantly impair thinking and normal activities and relationships.[2]

dementia pugilistica: A form of dementia caused by head trauma such as that experienced by boxers. It is also called chronic traumatic encephalopathy or Boxer syndrome.[2]

dendrite: A branch-like extension of a neuron that receives messages from other neurons.[1]

early-onset Alzheimer disease: A rare form of AD that usually affects people between ages 30 and 60. It is called familial AD (FAD) if it runs in the family.[1]

electroencephalogram (EEG): A medical procedure that records patterns of electrical activity in the brain.[2]

entorhinal cortex: An area deep within the brain where damage from AD often begins.[1]

enzyme: A protein that causes or speeds up a biochemical reaction.[1]

free radical: A highly reactive molecule (typically oxygen or nitrogen) that combines easily with other molecules because it contains an unpaired electron. The combination with other molecules sometimes damages cells.[1]

frontotemporal dementias: A group of dementias characterized by degeneration of nerve cells, especially those in the frontal and temporal lobes of the brain.[2]

gene: The biologic unit of heredity passed from parent to child. Genes contain instructions that tell a cell how to make specific proteins.[1]

genetic risk factor: A variant in a cell's DNA that does not cause a disease by itself but may increase the chance that a person will develop a disease.[1]

glial cell: A specialized cell that supports, protects, or nourishes nerve cells.[1]

hippocampus: A structure in the brain that plays a major role in learning and memory and is involved in converting short-term to long-term memory.[1]

HIV-associated dementia: A dementia that results from infection with the human immunodeficiency virus (HIV) that causes AIDS (acquired immunodeficiency syndrome). It can cause widespread destruction of the brain's white matter.[2]

Huntington disease: A degenerative hereditary disorder caused by a faulty gene for a protein called huntingtin. The disease causes degeneration in many regions of the brain and spinal cord and patients eventually develop severe dementia.[2]

hypothalamus: A structure in the brain under the thalamus that monitors activities such as body temperature and food intake.[1]

late-onset Alzheimer disease: The most common form of AD. It occurs in people aged 60 and older.[1]

Lewy body dementia: One of the most common types of progressive dementia, characterized by the presence of abnormal structures called Lewy bodies in the brain. In many ways the symptoms of this disease overlap with those of Alzheimer disease.[2]

limbic system: A brain region that links the brain stem with the higher reasoning elements of the cerebral cortex. It controls emotions, instinctive behavior, and the sense of smell.[1]

magnetic resonance imaging (MRI): A diagnostic and research technique that uses magnetic fields to generate a computer image of internal structures in the body. MRIs are very clear and are particularly good for imaging the brain and soft tissues.[1]

metabolism: All of the chemical processes that take place inside the body. In some metabolic reactions, complex molecules are broken down to release energy. In others, the cells use energy to make complex compounds out of simpler ones (like making proteins from amino acids).[1]

microtubule: An internal support structure for a neuron that guides nutrients and molecules from the body of the cell to the end of the axon.[1]

mild cognitive impairment (MCI): A condition in which a person has memory problems greater than those expected for his or her age, but not the personality or cognitive problems that characterize AD.[1]

multi-infarct dementia: A type of vascular dementia caused by numerous small strokes in the brain.[2]

mutation: A permanent change in a cell's DNA that can cause a disease.[1]

myelin: A whitish, fatty layer surrounding an axon that helps the axon rapidly transmit electrical messages from the cell body to the synapse.[1]

nerve growth factor (NGF): A substance that maintains the health of nerve cells. NGF also promotes the growth of axons and dendrites, the parts of the nerve cell that are essential to its ability to communicate with other nerve cells.[1]

neurodegenerative disease: A disease characterized by a progressive decline in the structure, activity, and function of brain tissue. These diseases include AD, Parkinson disease, frontotemporal lobar degeneration, and dementia with Lewy bodies. They are usually more common in older people.[1]

neurofibrillary tangles: Bundles of twisted filaments found within neurons, and a characteristic feature found in the brains of Alzheimer patients. These tangles are largely made up of a protein called tau.[2]

neuron: A nerve cell.[1]

neurotransmitter: A chemical messenger between neurons. These substances are released by the axon on one neuron and excite or inhibit activity in a neighboring neuron.[1]

nucleus: The structure within a cell that contains the chromosomes and controls many of its activities.[1]

oxidative damage: Damage that can occur to cells when they are exposed to too many free radicals.[1]

Parkinson dementia: A secondary dementia that sometimes occurs in people with advanced Parkinson disease, which is primarily a movement disorder. Many Parkinson dementia patients have the characteristic amyloid plaques and neurofibrillary tangles found in Alzheimer disease, but it is not yet clear if the diseases are linked.[2]

Pick disease: A type of frontotemporal dementia where certain nerve cells become abnormal and swollen before they die. The brains of people with Pick disease have abnormal structures, called Pick bodies, inside the neurons. The symptoms are very similar to those of Alzheimer disease.[2]

plaques: Unusual clumps of material found between the tissues of the brain in Alzheimer disease.[2]

positron emission tomography (PET): An imaging technique using radioisotopes that allows researchers to observe and measure activity in different parts of the brain by monitoring blood flow and concentrations of substances such as oxygen and glucose, as well as other specific constituents of brain tissues.[1]

posttraumatic dementia: A dementia brought on by a single traumatic brain injury. It is much like dementia pugilistica, but usually also includes long-term memory problems.[2]

presenilin 1 and 2: Proteins produced by genes that influence susceptibility to early-onset Alzheimer disease.[2]

primary dementia: A dementia, such as Alzheimer disease, that is not the result of another disease.[2]

progressive dementia: A dementia that gets worse over time, gradually interfering with more and more cognitive abilities.[2]

secondary dementia: A dementia that occurs as a consequence of another disease or an injury.[2]

senile dementia: An outdated term that reflects the formerly widespread belief that dementia was a normal part of aging. The word senile is derived from a Latin term that means, roughly, "old age."[2]

single photon emission computed tomography (SPECT): An imaging technique that allows researchers to monitor blood flow to different parts of the brain.[1]

subcortical dementia: Dementia that affects parts of the brain below the outer brain layer, or cortex.[2]

synapse: The tiny gap between nerve cells across which neurotransmitters pass.[1]

tau protein: A protein that helps the functioning of microtubules, which are part of the cell's structural support and help to deliver substances throughout the cell. In Alzheimer disease, tau is changed in a way that causes it to twist into pairs of helical filaments that collect into tangles.[2]

thalamus: A small structure in the front of the cerebral hemispheres that serves as a way station that receives sensory information of all kinds and relays it to the cortex; it also receives information from the cortex.[1]

vascular dementia: A type of dementia caused by brain damage from cerebrovascular or cardiovascular problems—usually strokes. It accounts for up to 20 percent of all dementias.[2]

ventricle: A cavity within the brain that is filled with cerebrospinal fluid.[1]

vesicle: A small container for transporting neurotransmitters and other molecules from one part of the neuron to another.[1]

Chapter 60

Directory of Resources for People with Dementia and Their Caregivers

Government Agencies That Provide Information about Dementia

Administration on Aging (AOA)
One Massachusetts Avenue NW
Washington, DC 20001
Phone: 202-619-0724
Fax: 202-357-3555
Website: www.aoa.gov
E-mail: aoainfo@aoa.hhs.gov

Agency for Healthcare Research and Quality (AHRQ)
Office of Communications and Knowledge Transfer
540 Gaither Road, Suite 2000
Rockville, MD 20850
Phone: 301-427-1104
Website: www.ahrq.gov

Alzheimer's Disease Education and Referral Center (ADEAR)
National Institute on Aging
P.O. Box 8250
Silver Spring, MD 20907-8250
Toll-Free: 800-438-4380
Fax: 301-495-3334
Website: www.alzheimers.nia.nih.gov
E-mail: adear@nia.nih.gov

Resources in this chapter were compiled from several sources deemed reliable; all contact information was verified and updated in March 2011.

Centers for Disease Control and Prevention (CDC)
1600 Clifton Road
Atlanta, GA 30333
Toll-Free: 800-CDC-INFO
(232-4636)
TTY: 888-232-6348
Phone: 404-639-3311
Website: www.cdc.gov
E-mail: cdcinfo@cdc.gov

Eldercare Locator
Toll-Free: 800-677-1116
Website: www.eldercare.gov
E-mail: eldercarelocator@n4a.org

Healthfinder®
National Health Information
Center
P.O. Box 1133
Washington, DC 20013-1133
Toll-Free: 800-336-4797
Phone: 301-565-4167
Fax: 301-984-4256
Website: www.healthfinder.gov
E-mail: healthfinder@nhic.org

National Cancer Institute (NCI)
NCI Office of Communications
and Education
Public Inquiries Office
6116 Executive Boulevard
Suite 300
Bethesda, MD 20892-8322
Toll-Free: 800-4-CANCER
(422-6237)
TTY: 800-332-8615
Website: www.cancer.gov
E-mail:
cancergovstaff@mail.nih.gov

National Center for Complementary and Alternative Medicine (NCCAM)
National Institutes of Health
NCCAM Clearinghouse
P.O. 7923
Gaithersburg, MD 20898-7923
Toll-Free: 888-644-6226
TTY: 866-464-3615
Fax: 866-464-3616
Website: www.nccam.nih.gov
E-mail: info@nccam.nih.gov

National Center for Health Statistics (NCHS)
3311 Toledo Rd
Hyattsville, MD 20782
Toll-Free: 800-232-4636
Website: www.cdc.gov/nchs
E-mail: cdcinfo@cdc.gov

National Institute on Alcohol Abuse and Alcoholism (NIAAA)
5635 Fishers Lane
MSC 9304
Bethesda, MD 20892-9304
Phone: 301-443-3860
Website: www.niaaa.nih.gov
E-mail:
niaaaweb-r@exchange.nih.gov

National Institute on Disability and Rehabilitation Research (NIDRR)

U.S. Department of Education
Office of Special Education and
Rehabilitative Services
400 Maryland Avenue, SW
Washington, DC 20202-7100
Phone: 202-245-7468
TTY: 202-245-7316
Website: www.ed.gov/about/
offices/list/osers/nidrr

National Institute of Mental Health (NIMH)

Science Writing, Press, and
Dissemination Branch
6001 Executive Boulevard
Room 8184
MSC 9663
Bethesda, MD 20892-9663
Toll-Free: 866-615-6464
TTY: 866-415-8051
Phone: 301-443-4513
Fax: 301-443-4279
Website: www.nimh.nih.gov
E-mail: nimhinfo@nih.gov

National Institute of Neurological Disorders and Stroke (NINDS)

NIH Neurological Institute
Brain
P.O. Box 5801
Bethesda, MD 20824
Toll-Free: 800-352-9424
Phone: 301-496-5751
TTY: 301-468-5981
Website: www.ninds.nih.gov
E-mail: braininfo@ninds.nih.gov

National Institutes of Health (NIH)

9000 Rockville Pike
Bethesda, MD 20892
Phone: 301-496-4000
TTY: 301-402-9612
Website: www.nih.gov
E-mail: NIHinfo@od.nih.gov

National Women's Health Information Center (NWHIC)

Office on Women's Health
200 Independence Ave. SW
Washington DC 20201
Toll-Free: 800-994-9662
Toll-Free TTY: 888-220-5446
Website:
www.womenshealth.gov

U.S. Food and Drug Administration (FDA)

10903 New Hampshire Avenue
Silver Spring, MD 20993
Toll-Free: 888-INFO-FDA
(463-6332)
Website: www.fda.gov

U.S. National Library of Medicine (NLM)

8600 Rockville Pike
Bethesda, MD 20894
Toll-Free: 888-FIND-NLM
(346-3656)
TDD: 800-735-2258
Phone: 301-594-5983
Fax: 301-402-1384
Website: www.nlm.nih.gov
E-mail: custserv@nlm.nih.gov

Private Agencies That Provide Information about Dementia

AARP
601 E Street NW
Washington DC 20049
Toll-Free: 888-687-2277
Website: www.aarp.org
E-mail: member@aarp.org

Alzheimer Society of Canada
20 Eglinton Avenue West
Suite 1600
Toronto, ON M4R 1K8
Canada
Toll-Free: 800-616-8816
(Canada only)
Phone: 416-488-8772
Fax: 416-322-6656
Website: www.alzheimer.ca
E-mail: info@alzheimer.ca

Alzheimer's Association
225 North Michigan Avenue, Fl. 17
Chicago, IL 60601-7633
Toll-Free: 800-272-3900
Phone: 312-335-8700
TDD: 312-335-5886
Fax: 866-699-1246
Website: www.alz.org
E-mail: info@alz.org

Alzheimer's Society (UK)
Devon House
58 St. Katherine's Way
London E1W 1JX
United Kingdom
Phone: 44 20 74233500
Fax: 44 20 74233501
Website: alzheimers.org.uk
E-mail:
enquiries@alzheimers.org.uk

Alzheimer's Australia
1 Frewin Place, Scullin
Australia
Phone: 61 02 62544233
Fax: 61 02 62787225
Website:
www.alzheimers.org.au
E-mail:
nat.admin@alzheimers.org.au

Alzheimer's Disease International
64 Great Suffolk Street
London SE1 0BL
United Kingdom
Phone: 44 20 79810880
Fax: 44 20 79282357
Website: www.alz.co.uk
E-mail: info@alz.co.uk

Alzheimer's Drug Discovery Foundation
57 West 57th Street
Suite 904
New York, NY 10019
Phone: 212-901-8000
Website: www.alzdiscovery.org
E-mail: info@alzdiscovery.org

Alzheimer's Foundation of America
322 Eighth Avenue
7th Floor
New York, NY 10001
Toll-Free: 866-232-8484
Fax: 646-638-1546
Website: www.alzfdn.org
E-mail: info@alzfdn.org

American Academy of Neurology
1080 Montreal Avenue
Saint Paul, MN 55116
Toll-Free: 800-879-1960
Phone: 651-695-2717
Fax: 651-695-2791
Website: www.aan.com
E-mail: memberservices@aan.com

American Association for Clinical Chemistry
1850 K Street, NW Suite 625
Washington, DC 20006
Toll-Free: 800-892-1400
Fax: 202-887-5093
Website: www.aacc.org
E-mail: custserv@aacc.org

American Association for Geriatric Psychiatry
7910 Woodmont Avenue
Suite 1050
Bethesda, MD 20814-3004
Phone: 301-654-7850
Fax: 301-654-4137
Website: www.aagpgpa.org
E-mail: main@aagponline.org

American Geriatrics Society Foundation for Health in Aging
The Empire State Building
350 Fifth Avenue, Suite 801
New York, NY 10118
Toll-Free: 800-563-4916
Phone: 212-755-6810
Fax: 212-832-8646
Website: www.healthinaging.org

American Health Assistance Foundation
22512 Gateway Center Drive
Clarksburg, MD 20871
Toll-Free: 800-437-2423
Phone: 301-948-3244
Fax: 301-258-9454
Website: www.ahaf.org/alzheimers
E-mail: info@ahaf.org

American Heart Association
National Center
7272 Greenville Avenue
Dallas, TX 75231
Toll-Free: 800-AHA-USA-1 (242-8721)
Website: www.heart.org

American Medical Association
515 North State Street
Chicago, IL 60654
Toll-Free: 800-621-8335
Website: www.ama-assn.org

American Pain Society
4700 W. Lake Avenue
Glenview, IL 60025
Phone: 847-375-4715
Fax: 866-574-2654
Website: www.ampainsoc.org
E-mail: info@ampainsoc.org

American Psychiatric Association
1000 Wilson Boulevard, Suite 1825
Arlington, VA 22209
Toll-Free: 888-35-PSYCH (357-7924)
Website: www.psych.org
E-mail: apa@psych.org

American Psychological Association
750 First Street NE
Washington, DC 20002-4242
Toll-Free: 800-374-2721
Phone: 202-336-5500
TDD/TTY: 202-336-6123
Website: www.apa.org

American Society on Aging
71 Stevenson Street
Suite 1450
San Francisco, CA 94105-2938
Toll-Free: 800-537-9728
Phone: 415-974-9600
Fax: 415-974-0300
Website: www.asaging.org
E-mail: info@asaging.org

Cleveland Clinic
9500 Euclid Avenue
Cleveland, OH 44195
Toll-Free: 800-223-2273
TTY: 216-444-0261
Website: my.clevelandclinic.org

Dana Alliance for Brain Initiatives
745 Fifth Avenue
Suite 900
New York, NY 10151
Phone: 212-223-4040
Fax: 212-593-7623
Website: www.dana.org
E-mail: dabiinfo@dana.org

Fisher Center for Alzheimer's Research Foundation
One Intrepid Square
West 46th Street & 12th Avenue
New York, NY 10036
Toll-Free: 800-259-4636
Fax: 646-381-5159
Website: www.alzinfo.org
E-mail: info@alzinfo.org

Five Wishes
P.O. Box 1661
Tallahassee FL 32302-1661
Toll-Free: 888-594-7437
Phone: 850-681-2010
Fax: 850-681-2481
Website: www.agingwithdignity
.org/5wishes.html
E-mail: fivewishes@
agingwithdignity.org

Mental Health America
2000 North Beauregard Street
6th Floor
Alexandria, VA 22311
Toll-Free: 800-969-6642
Phone: 703-684-7722
Fax: 703-684-5968
Website: www.nmha.org
E-mail: infoctr@
mentalhealthamerica.net

National Academy of Elder Law Attorneys
1577 Spring Hill Road, Suite 220
Vienna, VA 22182
Toll-Free: 800-677-1116
Phone: 703-942-5711
Fax: 703-563-9504
Website: www.naela.org

National Association of Professional Geriatric Care Managers

3275 West Ina Road, Suite 130
Tucson, AZ 85741-2198
Phone: 520-881-8008
Fax: 520-325-7925
Website:
www.caremanager.org

National Gerontological Nursing Association

3493 Lansdowne Drive
Suite 2
Lexington, KY 40517
Toll-Free: 800-723-0560
Phone: 859-977-7453
Fax: 859-271-0607
Website: www.ngna.org

National Rehabilitation Information Center

8201 Corporate Drive
Suite 600
Landover, MD 20785
Toll-Free: 800-346-2742
Phone: 301-459-5900
Fax: 301-562-2401
Website: www.naric.com
E-mail: naricinfo@
heitechservices.com

National Senior Citizens Law Center

1444 Eye Street NW
Suite 1100
Washington, DC 20005
Phone: 202-289-6976
Fax: 202-289-7224
Website: www.nsclc.org
E-mail: nsclc@nsclc.org

PsychCentral

55 Pleasant Street, Suite 207
Newburyport, MA 01950
Phone: 978-992-0008
Website: www.psychcentral.com
E-mail:
talkback@psychcentral.com

Society of Certified Senior Advisors

1325 South Colorado Boulevard
Suite B-300
Denver, CO 80222
Toll-Free: 800-653-1785
Website: www.society-csa.com

Resources for Information about Other Dementias

American Parkinson Disease Association
135 Parkinson Avenue
Staten Island, NY 10305-1425
Toll-Free: 800-223-2732
Phone: 718-981-8001
Fax: 718-981-4399
Website: www.apdaparkinson.org
E-mail: apda@apdaparkinson.org

Association for Frontotemporal Degeneration
Radnor Station Building #2
Suite 320
290 King of Prussia Road
Radnor, PA 19087
Toll-Free: 866-507-7222
Phone: 267-514-7221
Website: www.FTD-Picks.org
E-mail: info@FTD-Picks.org

Bachmann-Strauss Dystonia and Parkinson Foundation
551 Fifth Avenue
Suite 520
New York, NY 10176
Phone: 212-682-9900
Fax: 212-682-6156
Website:
www.dystonia-parkinsons.org
E-mail: info@bsdpf.org

Brain Injury Association of America, Inc.
1608 Spring Hill Road
Suite 110
Vienna, VA 22182
Toll-Free: 800-444-6443
Phone: 703-761-0750
Fax: 703-761-0755
Website: www.biausa.org
E-mail:
braininjuryinfo@biausa.org

Brain Trauma Foundation
7 World Trade Center
250 Greenwich Street
34th Floor
New York, NY 10017
Phone: 212-772-0608
Fax: 212-772-0357
Website:
www.braintrauma.org
E-mail:
education@braintrauma.org

CJD Aware!
2527 South Carrollton Avenue
New Orleans, LA 70118-3013
Phone: 504-861-4627
Website: www.cjdaware.com
E-mail: info@cjdaware.com

Creutzfeldt-Jakob Disease Foundation Inc.
P.O. Box 5312
Akron, OH 44334
Toll-Free: 800-659-1991
Fax: 330-668-2474
Website: www.cjdfoundation.org
E-mail: help@cjdfoundation.org

CurePSP: Foundation for Progressive Supranuclear Palsy, Corticobasal Degeneration, and Related Brain Diseases
30 E. Padonia Road, Suite 201
Timonium, MD 21093
Toll-Free: 800-457-4777
Phone: 410-785-7004
Fax: 410-785-7009
Website: www.curepsp.org
E-mail: info@curepsp.org

Michael J. Fox Foundation for Parkinson's Research
Church Street Station
P.O. Box 780
New York, NY 10008-0780
Phone: 212-509-0995
Website: www.michaeljfox.org

Huntington's Disease Society of America
505 Eighth Avenue, Suite 902
New York, NY 10018
Toll-Free: 800-345-4372
Phone: 212-242-1968
Fax: 212-239-3430
Website: www.hdsa.org
E-mail: hdsainfo@hdsa.org

Lewy Body Dementia Association
912 Killian Hill Road SW
Lilburn, GA 30047
Toll-Free: 800-539-9767
Phone: 404-935-6444
Fax: 480-422-5434
Website: www.lbda.org
E-mail: lbda@lbda.org

National Down Syndrome Society
666 Broadway, 8th Floor
New York, NY 10012
Toll-Free: 800-221-4602
Fax: 212-979-2873
Website: www.ndss.org
E-mail: info@ndss.org

National Organization for Rare Disorders
55 Kenosia Avenue
P.O. Box 1968
Danbury, CT 06813-1968
Toll-Free: 800-999-6673
Phone: 203-744-0100
Fax: 203-798-2291
Website: www.rarediseases.org
E-mail: orphan@rarediseases.org

National Parkinson Foundation
1501 NW 9th Avenue
Bob Hope Road
Miami, FL 33136-1494
Toll-Free: 800-327-4545
Phone: 305-243-6666
Fax: 305-243-5595
Website: www.parkinson.org
E-mail: contact@parkinson.org

National Stroke Association
9707 East Easter Lane, Suite B
Centennial, CO 80112-3747
Toll-Free: 800-787-6537
Phone: 303-649-9299
Fax: 303-649-1328
Website: www.stroke.org
E-mail: info@stroke.org

601

Parkinson Alliance
P.O. Box 308
Kingston, NJ 08528-0308
Toll-Free: 800-579-8440
Phone: 609-688-0870
Fax: 609-688-0875
Website:
www.parkinsonalliance.org
E-mail: admin@
parkinsonalliance.org

Parkinson's Action Network (PAN)
1025 Vermont Avenue NW
Suite 1120
Washington, DC 20005
Toll-Free: 800-850-4726
Phone: 202-638-4101
Fax: 202-638-7257
Website:
www.parkinsonsaction.org
E-mail: info@parkinsonsaction.org

Parkinson's Disease Foundation
1359 Broadway, Suite 1509
New York, NY 10018
Toll-Free: 800-457-6676
Phone: 212-923-4700
Fax: 212-923-4778
Website: www.pdf.org
E-mail: info@pdf.org

Parkinson's Institute and Clinical Center
675 Almanor Avenue
Sunnyvale, CA 94085
Toll-Free: 800-655-2273
Phone: 408-734-2800
Fax: 408-734-8522
Website: www.thepi.org
E-mail: info@thepi.org

Davis Phinney Foundation
4676 Broadway
Boulder, CO 80304
Toll-Free: 866-358-0285
Phone: 303-733-3340
Fax: 303-733-3350
Website: www.
davisphinneyfoundation.org
E-mail: info@
davisphinneyfoundation.org

WE MOVE (Worldwide Education and Awareness for Movement Disorders)
5731 Mosholu Avenue
Bronx, NY 10024
Phone: 347-843-6132
Fax: 718-601-5112
Website: www.wemove.org
E-mail: wemove@wemove.org

Caregiving, Palliative Care, and Hospice Information

Assisted Living Federation of America
1650 King Street, Suite 602
Alexandria, VA 22314
Phone: 703-894-1805
Website: www.alfa.org

Caring Connections
Toll-Free: 800-658-8898
Website: www.caringinfo.org
E-mail: caringinfo@nhpco.org

Caring.com
Website: www.caring.com

Family Caregiver Alliance
180 Montgomery Street
Suite 900
San Francisco, CA 94104
Toll-Free: 800-445-8106
Phone: 415-434-3388
Website: www.caregiver.org
E-mail: info@caregiver.org

**Hospice Foundation
of America**
1710 Rhode Island Ave NW
Suite 400
Washington, DC 20036
Toll-Free: 800-854-3402
Phone: 202-457-5811
Fax: 202-457-5815
Website:
www.hospicefoundation.org
E-mail: hfaoffice@
hospicefoundation.org

**Meals-on-Wheels
Association of America**
203 S. Union Street
Alexandria, VA 22314
Phone: 703-548-5558
Fax: 703-548-8024
Website: www.mowaa.org
E-mail: mowaa@mowaa.org

**National Adult Day Services
Association**
1421 E. Broad Street
Suite 425
Fuquay Varina, NC 27526
Website: www.nadsa.org
E-mail: NADSAnews@gmail.com

**National Alliance for
Caregiving**
4720 Montgomery Lane
2nd Floor
Bethesda, MD 20814
Website: www.caregiving.org
E-mail: info@caregiving.com

**National Association for
Continence**
P.O. Box 1019
Charleston, SC 29402-1019
Phone: 843-377-0900
Fax: 843-377-0905
Website: www.nafc.org
E-mail:
memberservices@nafc.org

**National Center
on Elder Abuse**
c/o Center for Community
Research and Services
University of Delaware
297 Graham Hall
Newark, DE 19716
Phone: 302-831-3525
Fax: 302-831-4225
Website: www.ncea.aoa.gov
E-mail: ncea-info@aoa.hhs.gov

**National Family Caregivers
Association**
10400 Connecticut Avenue
Suite 500
Kensington, MD 20895-3944
Toll-Free: 800-896-3650
Phone: 301-942-6430
Fax: 301-942-2302
Website: www.nfcacares.org
E-mail:
info@thefamilycaregiver.org

603

National Hospice and Palliative Care Organization/National Hospice Foundation
1731 King Street
Alexandria, VA 22314
Phone: 703-837-1500
Toll-Free: 800-658-8898
Fax: 703-837-1233
Website: www.nhpco.org
E-mail: nhpco_info@nhpco.org

National Palliative Care Research Center
Brookdale Department of
Geriatrics & Adult Development
Box 1070
Mount Sinai School of Medicine
One Gustave L. Levy Place
New York, NY 10029
Phone: 212-241-7447
Fax: 212-241-5977
Website: www.npcrc.org
E-mail: npcrc@mssm.edu

National Respite Network and Resource Center
Website: www.archrespite.org
Respite Locator: www.
archrespite.org/respitelocator

Palliative Care Policy Center
Website: www.medicaring.org
E-mail: info@medicaring.org

Project ACTION
1425 K Street, NW, Suite 200
Washington, DC 20005
Toll-Free: 800-659-6428
Phone: 202-347-3066
Fax: 202-737-7914
TDD: 202-347-7385
Website:
projectaction.easterseals.com

Visiting Nurses Associations of America
900 19th Street NW, Suite 200
Washington, DC 20006
Phone: 202-384-1420
Fax: 202-384-1444
Website: www.vnaa.org
E-mail: vnaa@vnaa.org

Well Spouse Association
63 West Main Street, Suite H
Freehold, NJ 07728
Toll-Free: 800-838-0879
Phone: 732-577-8899
Fax: 732-577-8644
Website: www.wellspouse.org
E-mail: info@wellspouse.org

Chapter 61

Alzheimer Disease Centers (ADCs) Program Directory

What Do the Alzheimer Disease Centers Do?

The National Institute on Aging (NIA) funds Alzheimer's Disease Centers (ADCs) at major medical institutions across the nation. Researchers at these centers are working to translate research advances into improved diagnosis and care for Alzheimer disease (AD) patients while, at the same time, focusing on the program's long-term goal—finding a way to cure and possibly prevent AD.

Areas of investigation range from the basic mechanisms of AD to managing the symptoms and helping families cope with the effects of the disease. Center staff conduct basic, clinical, and behavioral research and train scientists and health care providers who are new to AD research.

Although each center has its own unique area of emphasis, a common goal of the ADCs is to enhance research on AD by providing a network for sharing new ideas as well as research results. Collaborative studies draw upon the expertise of scientists from many different disciplines.

For patients and families affected by AD, the ADCs offer the following:

- Diagnosis and medical management (costs may vary—centers may accept Medicare, Medicaid, and private insurance)

From "AD Research Centers," by the National Institute on Aging (NIA, www .nia.nih.gov), part of the National Institutes of Health, April 22, 2010. Contact information was verified and updated in March 2011.

- Information about the disease, services, and resources

- Opportunities for volunteers to participate in drug trials, support groups, clinical research projects, and other special programs for volunteers and their families

Some ADCs have satellite facilities that offer diagnostic and treatment services and research opportunities in underserved, rural, and minority communities.

National NIA-funded AD resources are listed at the end of the chapter. For more information, contact any of the centers in the directory below.

ADC Directory

Alabama

University of Alabama at
Birmingham
Sparks Research Center
1720 7th Avenue South, Suite 640
Birmingham, AL 35294
Phone: 205-934-3847
Fax: 205-975-7365
Website: www.uab.edu/adc

Arizona

Arizona Alzheimer's Consortium
901 E. Willeta Street
Phoenix, AZ 85006
Phone: 602-239-6500
Fax: 602-239-6253
Website: www.azalz.org

California

Alzheimer's Disease Center
University of California
Davis Medical Center
4860 Y Street, Suite 3900
Sacramento, CA 95817-4540
Phone: 916-734-5496
Fax: 916-703-5290
Website: alzheimer.ucdavis.edu

Alzheimer's Disease Research
Center
University of California, Irvine
UCI Institute for Memory
Impairments and Neurological
Disorders
1100 Gottschalk Medical Plaza
Irvine, CA 92697
Phone: 949-824-2382
Fax: 949-824-2071
Website: www.alz.uci.edu

Alzheimer's Disease Research
Center
University of California, Los
Angeles
10911 Weyburn Avenue
Suite 200
Los Angeles, CA 90095-1769
Phone: 310-794-3665
Fax: 310-794-3148
Website:
www.EastonAD.ucla.edu

Alzheimer's Disease Research
Center
Shiley-Marcos Alzheimer's
Disease Research Center
9500 Gilman Drive
La Jolla, CA 92093-0948
Phone: 858-622-5800
Fax: 858-622-1017
Website: www.adrc.ucsd.edu
E-mail: adrc@ucsd.edu

Alzheimer's Disease Research
Center
University of California, San
Francisco
P.O. Box 1207
350 Parnassus Avenue
Suite 905
San Francisco, CA 94143-1207
Website: www.memory.ucsf.edu
E-mail: adrc@memory.ucsf.edu

Alzheimer's Disease Research
Center
University of Southern
California
Memory and Aging Center
HCCII, Suite 3000
1520 San Pablo Street
Los Angeles, CA 90033
Phone: 323-442-7600
Fax: 323-442-7601
Website: www.adrc.usc.edu
E-mail: gsc@usc.edu

Florida

Florida Alzheimer's Disease
Research Center
Byrd Alzheimer's Institute
4001 East Fletcher Avenue
Tampa, FL 33613
Toll-Free: 866-700-7773
Fax: 813-866-1601
Website: www.floridaadrc.org

Georgia

Alzheimer's Disease Center
Emory University
Wesley Woods Health Center
3rd Floor
1841 Clifton Road NE
Atlanta, GA 30329
Phone: 404-728-6950
Fax: 404-727-3999
Website:
www.med.emory.edu/ADC
E-mail: EmoryADRC@emory.edu

Illinois

Cognitive Neurology and
Alzheimer's Disease Center
Feinberg School of Medicine
Northwestern University
320 E Superior, Searle 11
Chicago, IL 60611
Phone: 312-926-1851
Fax: 312-908-8789
Website: www.brain.
northwestern.edu

Alzheimer's Disease Center
Rush University Medical Center
Armour Academic Center
600 South Paulina Street
Suite 130
Chicago, IL 60612
Phone: 312-942-3333
Fax: 312-563-4605
Website: www.rush.edu/radc

Indiana

Indiana Alzheimer Disease
Center
Department of Pathology and
Lab Medicine
Indiana University School of
Medicine
635 Barnhill Drive, MS-A-138
Indianapolis, IN 46202
Phone: 317-278-5500
Fax: 317-274-4882
Website: www.iadc.iupui.edu
E-mail: iadc@iupui.edu

Kentucky

University of Kentucky
Alzheimer's Disease Center
Sanders-Brown Center on Aging
Room 101
800 South Limestone Street
Lexington, KY 40536-0230
Phone: 859-323-6040
Fax: 859-323-2866
Website: www.mc.uky.edu/coa

Maryland

Alzheimer's Disease Research
Center
Division of Neuropathology
The Johns Hopkins University
Medical Institutions
558 Ross Research Building
720 Rutland Avenue
Baltimore, MD 21205-2196
Phone: 410-502-5164
Fax: 410-955-9777
Website: www.alzresearch.org

Massachusetts

Alzheimer's Disease Center
VA Boston Healthcare System
Neurology Service (127)
150 South Huntington Avenue
Boston, MA 02130
Toll-Free: 888-458-2823
Phone: 857-364-4702
Fax: 857-364-4454
Website: www.bu.edu/
alzresearch
E-mail: bmyoung@bu.edu

Alzheimer's Disease Research
Center
Massachusetts General Hospital
114 16th Street, Room 2009
Charlestown, MA 02129
Phone: 617-726-3987
Fax: 617-724-1480
Website: www.madrc.org

Michigan

Alzheimer's Disease Research
Center
Department of Neurology
2101 Commonwealth, Suite D
Ann Arbor, MI 48105
Phone: 734-936-8281
Fax: 734-763-1752
Website: www.med.umich.edu/
alzheimers
E-mail: ask-madrc@umich.edu

Minnesota

Alzheimer's Disease Research
Center
Mayo Clinic
200 First Street SW
Rochester, MN 55905
Phone: 507-284-2511
Website: mayoresearch.mayo
.edu/alzheimers_center
E-mail: mayoADC@mayo.edu

Missouri

Alzheimer's Disease Research
Center
Washington University School of
Medicine
Department of Neurology
4488 Forest Park Avenue
St. Louis, MO 63108
Phone: 314-286-2881
Fax: 314-286-2763
Website:
www.alzheimer.wustl.edu

New York

Columbia University Alzheimer's
Disease Center
630 West 168th Street
P&S Box 16
New York, NY 10032
Phone: 212-305-1818
Fax: 212-342-2849
Website:
www.alzheimercenter.org

Alzheimer's Disease Research
Center
Department of Psychiatry
Mount Sinai School of Medicine
One Gustave Levy Place
Box 1230
New York, NY 10029-6574
Phone: 212-241-6500
Fax: 718-562-9120
Website: www.mssm.edu/
research/centers/alzheimers
-disease-research-center

NYU Langone Medical Center
Center of Excellence on Brain
Aging
145 E 32nd Street, 2nd Floor
New York, NY 10016
Phone: 212-263-8088
Fax: 212-263-6991
Website: www.med.nyu.edu/adc

North Carolina

Joseph and Kathleen Bryan
Alzheimer's Disease Research
Center
Duke University
2200 West Main Street
Suite A-200
Durham, NC 27705
Toll-Free: 866-444-2372
Fax: 919-668-0828
Website: adrc.mc.duke.edu

Oregon

Aging and Alzheimer's Disease
Center CR 131
Oregon Health and Science
University
3181 SW Sam Jackson Park
Road
Portland, OR 97239-3098
Phone: 503-494-8311
Fax: 503-494-7499
Website: www.ohsu.edu/research/
alzheimers

Pennsylvania

Alzheimer's Disease Center
Department of Pathology and
Laboratory Medicine
University of Pennsylvania
School of Medicine
Ralston House
3615 Chestnut Street
Philadelphia, PA 19104
Phone: 215-662-6830
Fax: 215-349-5909
Website: www.uphs.upenn.edu/
ADC

Alzheimer's Disease Research
Center
Fourth Floor Montefiore
Suite 421W
200 Lothrop Street
Pittsburgh, PA 15213-2582
Phone: 412-692-2700
Fax: 412-692-2710
Website: www.adrc.pitt.edu

Texas

Alzheimer's Disease Research
Center
Department of Neurology
University of Texas SW Medical
Center
5323 Harry Hines Boulevard
Dallas, TX 75390-9129
Phone: 214-648-3111
Fax: 214-648-6824
Website: www.utsouthwestern
.edu/alzheimers/research

Washington

Alzheimer's Disease Center
VA Puget Sound Health Care
System
S-116 6 East
1660 S. Columbian Way
Seattle, WA 98108
Toll-Free: 800-317-5382
Fax: 206-768-5456
Website: www.uwadrc.org
E-mail:
adrcweb@u.washington.edu

Wisconsin

University of Wisconsin
Alzheimer's Disease Center
UW Hospital
600 Highland Avenue, J5/1
Mezzanine, Mail Code: 2420
Madison, WI 53792
Toll-Free: 866-636-7764
Phone: 608-263-2582
Fax: 608-265-3091
Website: www.wcmp.wisc.edu

National NIA-Funded Alzheimer Disease Resources

Alzheimer's Disease Cooperative Study (ADCS)

University of California,
San Diego
9500 Gilman Drive–0949
La Jolla, CA 92093-0949
Website: www.adcs.org
E-mail: brainlink@ucsd.edu

Alzheimer's Disease Education and Referral Center

PO Box 8250
Silver Spring, MD 20907-8250
Toll-Free: 800-438-4380
Fax: 301-495-3334
Website: www.nia.nih.gov/
Alzheimers
E-mail: adear@nia.nih.gov

National Alzheimer's Coordinating Center

4311 11th Avenue NE, #300
Seattle, WA 98105
Phone: 206-543-8637
Fax: 206-616-5927
Website:
www.alz.washington.edu
E-mail:
naccmail@u.washington.edu

National Cell Repository for Alzheimer's Disease

Indiana University Medical
Center
Department of Medical and
Molecular Genetics
975 West Walnut Street
Room IB-130
Indianapolis, IN 46202-5251
Toll-Free: 800-526-2839
Fax: 317-274-2387
Website: www.ncrad.org
E-mail: alzstudy@iupui.edu

611

Index

Index

Page numbers followed by 'n' indicate a footnote. Page numbers in *italics* indicate a table or illustration.

615

National Institute of Neurological
 Disorders and Stroke (NINDS)
 contact information 595
 publications
  Binswanger disease 202n
  CADASIL 204n
  corticobasal degeneration 160n
  Creutzfeldt-Jakob disease 208n
  dementia overview 21n
  dementia risk factors 35n
  heredity 315n
  Huntington disease 172n
  hydrocephalus 225n
  medications 279n
  multi-infarct dementia 205n
  Parkinson disease 176n
  traumatic brain injury 121n
National Institute on Aging (NIA),
 publications
 AD diagnosis 250n, 254n
 AD overview 65n
 AD prevention 295n
 AD research centers 605n
 AD symptoms 83n
 amyloid deposits 308n
 biomarker testing 271n
 brain, AD 73n
 brain, aging 11n
 brain overview 3n
 caregiver guide 445n
 clinical trials 287n
 end-of-life care 579n
 forgetfulness 231n
 future planning 416n
 genetics 104n
 home safety 494n
 hospitalizations 555n
 long-distance caregiving 457n
 memory loss 15n
 physician communication 237n
 planning documents 424n
 sleep changes 366n
 treatment options 275n
National Institute on Alcohol Abuse
 and Alcoholism (NIAAA), contact
 information 594
National Institute on Disability and
 Rehabilitation Research (NIDRR),
 contact information 595

National Institutes of Health (NIH)
 contact information 595
 genes publication 108n
National Library of Medicine (NLM)
 APOE gene publication 110n
 contact information 595
National Organization for Rare
 Disorders, contact information 601
National Palliative Care Research
 Center, contact information 604
National Parkinson Foundation,
 contact information 601
National Rehabilitation
 Information Center,
 contact information 599
National Respite Network and
 Resource Center, contact
 information 604
National Senior Citizens Law
 Center, contact information 599
National Stroke Association
 contact information 601
National Stroke Association,
 vascular dementia publication 200n
National Women's Health Information
 Center (NWHIC), contact
 information 595
Nauert, Rick 143n
Navane (thiothixene),
 AIDS dementia complex 218
NCCAM *see* National Center for
 Complementary and Alternative
 Medicine
NCEA *see* National Center on
 Elder Abuse
NCHS *see* National Center for
 Health Statistics
NCI *see* National Cancer Institute
NDMA antagonists *see* N-methyl
 D-aspartate antagonists
Negri, Mario 315
neprilysin, research 50
nerve cells *see* neurons
nerve growth factor (NGF),
 defined 589
"Neurocognitive Testing"
 (A.D.A.M., Inc.) 260n
neurodegenerative disease,
 defined 589

635

Health Reference Series

Adolescent Health Sourcebook, 3rd Edition

Adult Health Concerns Sourcebook

AIDS Sourcebook, 5th Edition

Alcoholism Sourcebook, 3rd Edition

Allergies Sourcebook, 4th Edition

Alzheimer Disease Sourcebook, 5th Edition

Arthritis Sourcebook, 3rd Edition

Asthma Sourcebook, 3rd Edition

Attention Deficit Disorder Sourcebook

Autism & Pervasive Developmental Disorders
Sourcebook, 2nd Edition

Back & Neck Sourcebook, 2nd Edition

Blood & Circulatory Disorders Sourcebook,
3rd Edition

Brain Disorders Sourcebook, 3rd Edition

Breast Cancer Sourcebook, 3rd Edition

Breastfeeding Sourcebook

Burns Sourcebook

Cancer Sourcebook for Women, 4th Edition

Cancer Sourcebook, 6th Edition

Cancer Survivorship Sourcebook

Cardiovascular Disorders Sourcebook,
4th Edition

Caregiving Sourcebook

Child Abuse Sourcebook, 2nd Edition

Childhood Diseases & Disorders Sourcebook,
2nd Edition

Colds, Flu & Other Common Ailments
Sourcebook

Communication Disorders Sourcebook

Complementary & Alternative Medicine
Sourcebook, 4th Edition

Congenital Disorders Sourcebook, 2nd Edition

Contagious Diseases Sourcebook, 2nd Edition

Cosmetic & Reconstructive Surgery Sourcebook,
2nd Edition

Death & Dying Sourcebook, 2nd Edition

Dental Care & Oral Health Sourcebook,
3rd Edition

Depression Sourcebook, 2nd Edition

Dermatological Disorders Sourcebook,
2nd Edition

Diabetes Sourcebook, 5th Edition

Diet & Nutrition Sourcebook, 4th Edition

Digestive Diseases & Disorder Sourcebook

Disabilities Sourcebook, 2nd Edition

Disease Management Sourcebook

Domestic Violence Sourcebook, 3rd Edition

Drug Abuse Sourcebook, 3rd Edition

Ear, Nose & Throat Disorders Sourcebook,
2nd Edition

Eating Disorders Sourcebook, 3rd Edition

Emergency Medical Services Sourcebook

Endocrine & Metabolic Disorders Sourcebook,
2nd Edition

Environmental Health Sourcebook, 3rd Edition

Ethnic Diseases Sourcebook

Eye Care Sourcebook, 4th Edition

Family Planning Sourcebook

Fitness & Exercise Sourcebook, 4th Edition

Food Safety Sourcebook

Forensic Medicine Sourcebook

Gastrointestinal Diseases & Disorders
Sourcebook, 2nd Edition

Genetic Disorders Sourcebook, 4th Edition

Head Trauma Sourcebook

Headache Sourcebook

Health Insurance Sourcebook

Healthy Aging Sourcebook

Healthy Children Sourcebook

Healthy Heart Sourcebook for Women

Hepatitis Sourcebook

Household Safety Sourcebook

Hypertension Sourcebook

Immune System Disorders Sourcebook,
2nd Edition

Infant & Toddler Health Sourcebook

Infectious Diseases Sourcebook